D0838133

Guide to
Healthy Restaurant Eating
2nd Edition

Hope S. Warshaw,
MMSc, RD, CDE

American Diabetes Association.
Cure • Care • Commitment℠

Book Acquisitions, Sherrye Landrum; *Editor*, Mary Beth Oelkers-Keegan; *Production Manager*, Peggy M. Rote; *Desktop Publishing & Text Design*, Circle Graphics, Inc.; *Cover Design*, VC Graphics; *Printer*, Transcontinental Printing.

©2002 by Hope S. Warshaw. All Rights Reserved. No part of this publication may be reproduced or transmitted in any form or by any means, electronic or mechanical, including duplication, recording, or any information storage and retrieval system, without the prior written permission of the American Diabetes Association.

Trademarks and brand names are property of the contributing restaurants.

Printed in Canada
1 3 5 7 9 10 8 6 4 2

The suggestions and information contained in this publication are generally consistent with the *Clinical Practice Recommendations* and other policies of the American Diabetes Association, but they do not represent the policy or position of the Association or any of its boards or committees. Reasonable steps have been taken to ensure the accuracy of the information presented. However, the American Diabetes Association cannot ensure the safety or efficacy of any product or service described in this publication. Individuals are advised to consult a physician or other appropriate health care professional before undertaking any diet or exercise program or taking any medication referred to in this publication. Professionals must use and apply their own professional judgment, experience, and training and should not rely solely on the information contained in this publication before prescribing any diet, exercise, or medication. The American Diabetes Association—its officers, directors, employees, volunteers, and members—assumes no responsibility or liability for personal or other injury, loss, or damage that may result from the suggestions or information in this publication.

ADA titles may be purchased for business or promotional use or for special sales. For information, please write to: Lee Romano Sequeira, Special Sales & Promotions, at the address below.

Published by American Diabetes Association, Inc., 1701 N. Beauregard Street, Alexandria, Virginia 22311.

Library of Congress Cataloging-in-Publication Data

Warshaw, Hope S., 1954–
    The American Diabetes Association guide to healthy restaurant eating / Hope S. Warshaw.–2nd ed.
        p.   cm.
    ISBN 1-58040-152-X (pbk. : alk. paper)
    1. Diabetes–Diet therapy. 2. Food exchange lists. 3. Restaurants.
I. Title: Guide to healthy restaurant eating. II. American Diabetes Association. III. Title.
RC662 .W3155 2002
616.4'620654–dc21

2002018475

*To people with diabetes who, on a daily basis,
strive to control blood glucose to stay healthy
and prevent diabetes complications.
May the knowledge and information
you gain from this book help you
stay healthy and complication free.*

— HSW

Contents

Alphabetical Index of Restaurants

Preface

Four years have elapsed since the first edition of *Guide to Healthy Restaurant Eating* was published. Have things changed? The answer is YES and NO.

More nutrition information is available from what I call "walk up and order" national chain restaurants. Much of that information is now available on the Internet sites of these restaurants. That's commendable! However, little additional information is available from those "sit down and order" national chain restaurants. They don't seem to want you or I to know. That's not commendable! In addition, virtually no information is available from independent chains, single unit restaurants, or most ethnic restaurants (beyond the fast food Mexican and Italian).

I hope the tips in *Put Your Best Guess Forward* (page 29), help you get better at estimating the nutrient content of foods when you don't have information from the restaurant. With so many people tightly managing their blood glucose levels and adjusting medications (usually insulin) based on carbohydrate intake, the skills of being a good guestimater have become even more important.

Restaurant serving sizes are still out of control. You are pushed to overeat with meal deals, buffet style restaurants, and ever-growing serving sizes. If you want to control portions—and you need to if you want to eat healthfully and control weight—try the strategies in the pages ahead. Added fats and salt continue to be a big problem in restaurant food preparation, so we also provide ways to lighten up on added fat and salt.

Restaurant meals, whether eaten in or taken out, continue to be a way of life in our fast-paced world. This means you need all the advice and nutrition information you can get. I hope the content of this second edition of the *Guide to Healthy Restaurant Eating* helps with your quest to eat healthy, control your blood glucose, and stay healthy for many years to come. I encourage you to continue to ask for the nutrition information from restaurants for which it is not yet available. Perhaps if enough of us keep asking, they will come forward with the facts.

Acknowledgments

This book would have been impossible to create without the cooperation and assistance from many people at the corporate headquarters of many restaurant chains and the willingness of many other chains to provide their nutrition information on their web sites. On behalf of people with diabetes who will use and benefit from the information in the pages ahead, I am indebted to these restaurant chains. These restaurants set an example of public responsibility to the rest of the chain restaurant industry.

No book is completed by just the author alone. In this case, many manuscript pages and a large nutrient database became a book with many people's ideas and countless hours. Thanks to all those at ADA who supported this effort: Sherrye Landrum, Acquisitions Editor; John Fedor, Director of Publishing; and Len Boswell, Vice President, Publications.

Thanks also to Tina Katserikas, a dietetic intern who assisted with the development of the nutrient database.

A last thanks goes to my professional colleagues who consistently lent their ears and ideas to make this book the best it could be. They continue to be a source of inspiration and encouragement.

Today's Diabetes Eating Goals

During the 1990s the diabetes eating goals underwent a minor revolution. In fact, the phrase "a diabetic diet" is now a misnomer. No such diet exists. No longer must you ax sugary foods and sweets from your list of acceptable foods. Now you can savor the taste of a few slices of pizza at your local pizza parlor or cruise to the drive-thru for a hamburger and french fries when time is not on your side. The bottom line is, the current diabetes eating goals encourage you to eat healthfully and to do what it takes to keep your blood glucose in the normal range as much as possible. Your diabetes plan needs to be worked around your needs and lifestyle. The end goal, of course, is to prevent or slow down long-term diabetes complications, such as eye, heart, and kidney problems. These occur, to a great degree, because of high blood glucose levels day after day.

Diabetes Eating Goals in a Nutshell

In 1994 the American Diabetes Association (ADA) put forth six nutrition goals. These were again reinforced in the 2002 nutrition goals:

1. Hold blood glucose (blood sugar) as near to normal as possible. Balance what you eat with insulin or diabetes pills (if you need diabetes medicine to control your blood glucose) and physical activity.

2. Keep or get your blood lipid (blood fat) levels as close to levels recommended by ADA as possible. Blood lipids include cholesterol, low-density lipoproteins (LDL, or "bad" cholesterol), high-density lipoproteins (HDL, or "good" cholesterol), and triglycerides (the form in which your body stores fat in fat cells for ready energy).

3. Eat enough calories to stay at or get to a healthy weight for you. If you are a child or teenager or if you are pregnant or breastfeeding, eat enough calories to grow and develop normally.

4. Prevent or treat problems caused by high or low blood glucose. For instance, eat on time to prevent low blood glucose (hypoglycemia).

5. Prevent, slow down, or treat long-term diabetes problems. For example, eat less saturated fat to prevent heart problems, or eat a moderate amount of protein to slow kidney problems if you have them.

6. Improve your overall health by choosing foods and eating the way all Americans are encouraged to eat. This means eating what you know is healthy for your whole family.

Those are the nutrition goals. But what foods should you eat to reach these goals? Here are general pointers to focus on:

- Eat more (6 or more servings) grains, beans, and starchy vegetables each day.
- Eat more fruits and vegetables. Strive for at least 5 servings a day from a combination of fruits and vegetables. More is better!
- Include at least 2 servings of fat-free or low-fat dairy foods—milk, yogurt, and cheese—within your calorie allotment. They provide calcium and other nutrients.

- Eat a moderate amount of meat and other protein foods. Two 3-oz servings each day is enough for most people. Not only does eating less meat help you eat less protein, it also makes it easier for you to eat less total fat, saturated fat, and cholesterol.
- Go light on fats and oils (especially those high in saturated fat, such as coconut and palm oils).
- Limit foods high in cholesterol (such as whole-milk dairy foods, egg yolks, and organ meats).
- Eat small amounts of sugary foods and sweets only once in a while. If you have some pounds to shed or your blood sugar or blood fats are not in a good range, you'll need to eat sweets even more sparingly. If you're on the slim side, you can splurge on sweets a bit more often if you want to.
- Drink no more than one alcoholic drink a day if you are a woman and two drinks a day if you are a man. One drink is defined as 1½ oz of hard liquor (a shot), 12 oz of beer, or 6 oz of wine.

Everybody Sings the Same Song

Take note: ADA recommendations for healthy eating echo the way all Americans are encouraged to eat—even Americans at risk for heart disease or some cancers. Whether it's the American Heart Association, the American Cancer Society, or the U.S. government, every organization sings the same nutrition song.

This means that as a person with diabetes, you don't need to stick out like a sore thumb because you strive to eat healthfully. That's not to make healthy eating sound simple or not to acknowledge that at times you feel like a fish swimming upstream because so many Americans chow down on downright unhealthy foods and large portions of them. Remember, it's not easy to eat healthfully. And that is particularly true with restaurant foods.

How Much Should You Eat?

Base what you eat each day on what you like to eat, as long as you eat these foods in reasonable amounts. The quantities of food you eat and when you eat must match your lifestyle and schedule. Another critical element is to determine what foods and times for meals and snacks work best to help you keep your blood glucose, blood lipids, and blood pressure in control. Lastly, what's best for your diabetes is what allows you to feel good day to day and what helps prevent or slow down the development of diabetes problems.

No set number of calories is right for everyone with diabetes. The number of calories you need depends on many factors. A few of them are your height, your age, your current weight and whether you want to lose weight or are at a healthy weight, your daily activity level, the type of exercise you do, and more. Always have a meal plan and method of meal planning that fits you and your lifestyle. To develop a meal plan and/or healthy eating goals that you are comfortable with and one that factors in your individual needs, work with a registered dietitian (RD) with diabetes expertise (preferably a certified diabetes educator, or CDE). A dietitian can help you learn how to work almost any food into your meal plan or to solve meal planning dilemmas (for instance, maybe you travel several days a week and eat all your meals in restaurants). (To find diabetes education programs, see "Help Is Nearby" on page 6.) Several books on the topic of food, nutrition, and meal planning published by the ADA give more in-depth information about how much and what you should eat.

Myriad Approaches to Meal Planning

Once you know what and how much you should eat, you and your dietitian can zero in on a meal planning approach that fits your needs. If you want a simple approach, for example, then the diabetes food pyramid may be best for you. Or if you are willing to check your blood glucose several times a day and do some math, then you might opt for carbohydrate counting.

You may be familiar with the diabetes exchange system as the way some people with diabetes learn to plan meals. The ADA and the American Dietetic Association's *Exchange Lists for Meal Planning* date back to 1950. The exchange system has been revised a number of times. The last revision was in 1995. Today, the exchange system is no longer the only way to do diabetes meal planning. You can use the diabetes food pyramid, carbohydrate gram counting, fat gram counting, or the point system, to name a few options. The right meal planning approach for you is the one that you can learn and put to work. One approach might be right for you when you first develop diabetes, then down the road another approach may work best.

Any Meal Planning Approach Works in Restaurants

No matter which meal planning approach you use, you can take advantage of the information in this book. If you opt for the exchange system or the diabetes food pyramid, use the food servings or exchanges noted in the charts. If you do carbohydrate counting, then the grams of carbohydrate and grams of dietary fiber are where you want to focus. Zero in on the calories and fat if fat gram counting is part of your meal planning method.

Help Is Nearby

Whether you have just found out you have diabetes or you have been doing the diabetes balancing act for years, you can always learn more. Get to know a diabetes educator. Your diabetes educator will help you tailor your diabetes management plan and offer tips for dealing with diabetes. The following resources are a good start to link you up with quality diabetes care:

- To find a Recognized Diabetes Education Program (a teaching program approved by the American Diabetes Association) near you, call 1-800-DIABETES (1-800-342-2383), look at ADA's Internet home page http://www.diabetes.org, or go straight to http://www.diabetes.org/education/eduprogram.asp.
- To find diabetes educators (who may be dietitians, nurses, pharmacists, counselors, or other health professionals) near you, call the American Association of Diabetes Educators (AADE) toll-free at 1-800-TEAMUP4 (1-800-832-6874) or go to AADE's internet site at www.aadenet.org and go to "Find an Educator."

Here's more good news: It may now be easier for you to take advantage of the services of a diabetes educator or diabetes education program as well as a dietitian. Medicare now covers diabetes education and nutrition counseling for diabetes in many new settings for those with Medicare part B or managed care. Also, in nearly all states across the country, those private insurers and managed care organizations that are regulated by the state must pay for diabetes education. If you have questions about whether or not your diabetes education will be covered, contact your health care company, your state insurance commissioner's office, the local Medicare office, or the American Diabetes Association.

Restaurant Pitfalls and Strategies for Self-Defense

To eat out healthfully is no small task. You need will-power and perseverance. It's tough enough to eat healthfully in your own house. But even more challenges confront you when you pick and choose from a menu and are not able to sneak a peek in the kitchen. You can't march into the kitchen and hold the cook's hand when he or she ladles more butter or shakes more salt onto your once healthy vegetables. Healthy restaurant eating is, no doubt, a challenge. That's because there are lots of pitfalls—from sky-high portions to fat, fat everywhere. The good news is that you can choose to eat healthfully in 99 percent of restaurants. *Choose* is the critical word here. It's important to learn the pitfalls of restaurant eating and tuck the strategies to eat more healthfully in restaurants into your brain.

Pitfalls of Restaurant Eating

- **You think of restaurant ventures as special occasions.** Yes, once upon a time, people only ate in restaurants to celebrate a birthday, Mother's Day, or an anniversary. Not today. The average American eats four meals away from home each week. And personally you may top that number. When you eat that many meals away from home each week, your waistline quickly spreads if you eat as if each meal is a special occasion or even eat the portion served in most restaurants. Today, restaurant meals for most people are just part of our fast-paced life. They're hardly special occasions.

- **You're not the cook.** The cook is in the kitchen and you can't peek. Your methods of control are to ask questions about the food on the menu, to make special requests to get an item delivered the way you want it, and to practice portion control when you order and eat.

- **Fats are here, there, and everywhere.** Remember, fat makes food taste good and stay moist. Restaurants, therefore, love it. Extra fat is in high-fat ingredients, such as butter, sour cream, or cream; in high-fat foods, such as cheese, bacon, or potato chips; and in high-fat cooking methods, such as deep-fat frying, breading and frying, and sautéing. And it's at the table in fried Chinese noodles, tortilla chips, or butter. You need to master the craft of being a fat sleuth.

- **Sodium can skyrocket.** Along with fat, salt makes food taste good. So, many restaurants pour it aplenty. If you're watching your sodium intake, you'll need to shy away from certain items and make some special requests.

- **Portions are oversized.** Restaurants simply serve too much food. The portions are often enough for two. You need to develop and use strategies that help you not overeat. Restaurants, and many Americans, believe more is better.

- **Meat (protein) is front and center.** A primary focus of the American diner is summed up in the catchphrase "Where's the beef?" Whether it is fish, chicken, or beef, the protein often takes center stage in restaurant meals. And most plates contain too much of it. A steak is often 8 oz or more cooked. A chicken breast is often a whole chicken breast. Your goal is to put the meat on the side of your plate and fill the rest of your plate with sides.

Americans Eat Out: How Much and How Often?

An average American today spends almost half of every food dollar on food eaten away from home. In 1950, according to the National Restaurant Association, the average American spent only a quarter of his or her food dollar eating away from home. The average American today eats four meals out of the house each week. Lunch is the meal eaten out most often, with dinner a close second. Breakfast is eaten out least often. And men eat out more than women. Fast-food restaurants—from hamburger joints to pizza and sub shops—represent about a quarter of all restaurants. As for ethnic food, Americans' favorites are Mexican, Chinese, and Italian.

Let's face it, restaurant meals—eaten in or out—are just part of dealing with our fast-paced world. You might ask, "Is that a problem if I have diabetes?" The answer is no, as long as you learn to eat healthy restaurant meals most of the time. And remember, whether you eat in the restaurant or take food out to the soccer field, your office, or the kitchen table, you face the same kinds of decisions. In fact, you have to make similar choices in today's supermarkets, because they have begun to look a bit like restaurants, with ready-to-eat meal components, complete meals, sandwiches, and salad bars. Of course, one advantage in the supermarket is that frequently the nutrition facts stare you in the face. Not so in restaurants.

Ten Strategies for Eating Out Healthfully

1. **Develop a can-do attitude.** Too many of us think in negative equations: Eating out equals pigging out; a restaurant meal must be a special occasion; eating out means blowing your diet. These attitudes defeat your efforts to eat healthfully. It's time to develop a can-do attitude about restaurant meals. Build confidence to believe that you can enjoy a healthy meal when you eat out. Slowly begin to change how you order and the types of restaurants in which you choose to eat.

2. **Decide when to eat out—or not.** Take a look at how often you eat out. If the count verges on the excessive, then ask yourself why you eat out so frequently and how you can reduce your restaurant meals. Also, if you eat out more frequently, you need to keep splurges to a minimum. If you eat out only once a month, you might take a few more liberties—perhaps with an alcoholic drink or a dessert.

3. **Zero in on the site.** Seek out restaurants that offer at least a smattering of healthier options. Remember, there is an advantage to eating in chain restaurants. You can master the menu and plan ahead, no matter which one of the chain's locations you pop into.

4. **Set your game plan.** On your way to the restaurant—whether it's a quick fast-food lunch or a leisurely weekend dinner—envision a healthy and

enjoyable outcome. Plan your strategy, or at least what you might have if you aren't familiar with the restaurant, before you cross the threshold. Don't become a victim of hasty choices.

5. **Become a fat sleuth.** Learn to focus on fats. Fat is the densest form of calories, and it often gets lost in the sauce, so to speak—or on the salad, on the bread, or in the chips. Watch out for high-fat ingredients—butter, cream, sour cream. Be alert for high-fat foods—cheese, avocado, sausage. Steer clear of high-fat preparation methods—frying of any kind. Look out for high-fat dishes—Mexican chimichangas, broccoli with cheese sauce, or stuffed potato skins, for starters.

6. **Let your food plan be your guide.** Keep a miniaturized version of your food plan with you. Choose foods with your meal plan in mind. Try to fulfill each food group with menu items or substitute foods to make your meal complete. For instance, replace a serving of milk or a fruit serving, which are often hard to get in restaurants, with another starch serving so that you will keep your carbohydrate intake consistent—an important goal.

7. **Practice portion control from the start.** The best way not to eat too much is to order less. Order with your stomach in mind, not your eyes. You need to outsmart the menu to get the right amount of food for you.

8. **Be creative with the menu.** You outsmart the menu by being creative. You also control portions by being creative. Remember, no sign at the entrance says, "All who enter must order an entree." Your options are to take advantage of appetizers, soups, and salads; to split menu items,

including the entree, with your dining partner; to order one or two fewer dishes than the number of people at the table and eat family style; or to mix and match two entrees to achieve nutritional balance. For example, in a steak house, one person orders the steak, baked potato, and salad bar and the other orders just the potato and salad bar, then they split the steak. In an Italian restaurant, one person orders pasta with a tomato-based sauce and the other orders a chicken or veal dish with a vegetable.

9. **Get foods made to order.** Don't be afraid to ask for what you want, even in a fast-food restaurant. Restaurants today need your business and want you back. Make sure your requests are practical—leave an item such as potato chips off the plate; substitute mustard for mayonnaise on a sandwich; make a sandwich on whole-wheat bread rather than on a croissant; or serve the salad dressing on the side. Restaurants can abide these requests. However, don't expect to have your special requests greeted with a smile at noon in a fast-food restaurant or when you try to remake a menu item. Be reasonable and pleasant.

10. **Know when enough is enough.** Many of us grew up being members of the clean-plate club. Now you need to reserve a membership in the "leave-a-few-bites-on-your-plate club." To keep from overeating, don't order too much, order creatively, and push your plate away when you meet your calorie needs. Remember, take-home containers are at-the-ready in most restaurants.

Diabetes Dining Dilemmas

Many people who eat restaurant meals have concerns about their health and have the need to ask questions. So, as a person with diabetes, your questions and special requests are nothing out of the ordinary. However, as someone with diabetes, you deal with dining dilemmas beyond just the food, due to your schedule for medications and your blood glucose control. This section provides you with guidance to face these additional challenges.

Delayed Meals

A big challenge, if you take a diabetes medication that can cause your blood glucose to get too low (see list below), may be how to manage delayed meals. For example, if you are used to eating lunch between noon and 12:30 pm, how can you safely delay your meal until 1:00 pm when your friends or business associates want to meet. Or what should you do if you want to dine at 7:30 pm on a Saturday night, when your usual dinner time during the week is 6:00 pm.

A big and positive change in the management of diabetes today is that there are new oral diabetes medications and new types of insulin that better mesh with the realities of life in the 21st century. Several of these medications help your health care providers, diabetes educators, and you work out a medication schedule that best controls your blood glucose while allowing you the flexibility you need to live your life in the manner that best suits your needs. What's important in developing a medication plan is that you communicate your lifestyle and schedule to your health care providers and diabetes educators. If they don't know your habits, then they are less able to develop a medication plan to suit you.

The biggest concern in delaying meals is if you have taken a diabetes medication that can cause your blood glucose to go too low if you don't eat on time. Prior to the availability of new oral medications and newer insulins, this was more of a concern than it is today. But it is certainly still a concern for you if you are taking a medication that can cause low blood glucose. On page 17 is a list of the diabetes medications that can cause blood glucose to go too low (cause hypoglycemia) and those that cannot. If you take one or more of the medications then you need to pay special attention to your meal times.

Do keep in mind, though, that several of the newer diabetes medications that can cause hypoglycemia are very quick acting, such as the insulins lispro (Humalog) and aspart (Novolog) and the oral pills Prandin and Starlix. Their job is to quickly lower your blood glucose after you eat. If you take one of these medications along with other medications that are not likely to cause low blood glucose, then you should take these quick acting medications when you start to eat your meal rather than at your usual meal time.

If you take a pre-mixed combination of insulin, such as 70/30 or 75/25, or just take insulin twice a day, such as a mixture of NPH or Lente and regular, it becomes more important for you to eat on time.

TABLE 1 Diabetes Medications and Hypoglycemia

Diabetes medications that can cause hypoglycemia	Diabetes medications that do not cause hypoglycemia
Sulfonylureas: Amaryl, Glucotrol, Glucotrol XL, Glyburide, Glipizide, DiaBeta, Glynase, Micronase, Orinase, Tolinase, Diabinese, Dymelor	Metformin: Glucophage, Glucophage XR
	Alpha-glucosidase inhibitors: Precose and Glyset
Combination pill: Glucovance (combination of metformin and glyburide, the glyburide portion can cause hypoglycemia)	Glitazones: Avandia and Actos
Meglitinides: repaglinide (Prandin)	
d-phenylalanine: nateglinide (Starlix)	
Insulin: all types	

These insulin regimens do not allow much flexibility in meal times. If you regularly need more flexibility in your schedule, then talk to your health care providers and diabetes educators about your needs. Today there are much more flexible insulin regimens including the use of an insulin pump or the use of the insulin glargine (Lantus) with quick acting lispro (Humalog) or aspart (Novolog).

Steps to Take If Low Blood Sugar Is Possible

If you will delay a meal and you take a longer acting pill or insulin that can cause your blood glucose to get too low, you need to take precautions to prevent this. Follow these steps.

Check your blood glucose at the usual time of your meal.

- If it is high (> 150 mg/dl), wait awhile before eating. But do check again if you feel your blood glucose is getting too low prior to your meal.
- If your blood glucose level is around your pre-meal goal (90–130 mg/dl*) and you feel it will fall too low before you get to eat, eat some carbohydrate (start with 15 grams) to make sure it doesn't go too low prior to your meal.
- If you will be delaying your meal more than one hour and your blood glucose is around your pre-meal goal, you may need to eat more than 15 grams of carbohydrate to keep it from going too low prior to your meal.

It is always a smart idea to keep quick and easy carbohydrate foods at the ready in places such as your desk, briefcase, purse, locker, or glove compartment. Also, it is ideal to carry one of these foods with you into restaurants. That's especially true for sit down restaurants. After all, you never know what will happen in restaurants. The restaurant might not have your reservation, they might not be able to seat you quickly, your meal-mate might be late, the kitchen might be slow, or there may be a mix up with your order. And the list goes on. As the saying goes, "It's better to be safe than sorry."

---

*The numbers used for blood glucose values are based on plasma glucose goals, not whole blood. Today, most blood glucose meters read results as plasma, not whole blood.

Suggested foods that contain carbohydrate are: dried fruit, cans of juice, pretzels, milk, yogurt, gum drops, gummy bears, or snack crackers. Check the nutrition facts on the food to determine the amount equivalent to 15 grams of carbohydrate.

If your blood glucose is lower than 80 mg/dl and/or you feel the symptoms of low blood glucose, then you should use 15 grams of glucose tablets or gel to treat your hypoglycemia and should eat your meal as soon as your blood glucose returns to normal.

These suggestions offer you general rules of thumb. Check with your health care providers or diabetes educator to learn what are the best alternatives for you based on your diabetes medication plan. But if your diabetes medication plan is not fitting with your lifestyle, recognize that there are alternatives.

Alcohol

Clearly there are numerous reasons not to drink alcohol. Alcohol is high in calories (unhealthy calories). It can raise blood lipid levels, especially triglycerides. It can cause low blood glucose if you take sulfonylureas, Prandin/Starlix, or insulin. And it can cause problems if you take metformin (Glucophage, Glucophage XR, Glucovance). It can lead to health problems with overuse, can slow your responses, and can be dangerous if you drink and drive. However, if your blood glucose and blood lipids are in good control and you drink sensibly, there is no reason you cannot enjoy some alcohol. And a common time to drink alcohol is when you eat in a restaurant. Here's how to drink smartly with diabetes.

Tips to Sip By

- Don't drink when your blood glucose is too low.
- Remember that alcohol can cause low blood glucose soon after you drink it (if your medicine is working hardest and/or you need to eat). It can continue to cause low blood glucose 8–12 hours after you drink it, especially if you drink in excess and take too much medicine or don't eat enough.
- Don't drink on an empty stomach. Either munch on a carbohydrate source (popcorn or pretzels) as you drink or wait to drink until you get your meal.
- Alcohol can also make blood glucose too high. This is true for anyone with diabetes, no matter how they control it. High blood glucose can be caused by the calories from carbohydrate in the alcoholic beverage, such as wine or beer, or in a mixer, such as orange juice.
- Avoid mixers that add lots of carbohydrates and calories—tonic water, regular soda, syrups, juices, and liqueurs.
- Check your blood glucose to help you decide whether you should drink and when you need to eat something.
- Wear or carry identification that states you have diabetes.
- Sip a drink to make it last.
- At a meal have a noncaloric, nonalcoholic beverage by your side to quench your thirst.
- If you do not take a diabetes medicine that can cause low blood glucose and you have some pounds to shed, you can substitute an alcoholic drink for fats in your meal plan.
- If you do not have to lose weight, then just have an occasional drink and don't worry about the extra calories.

- Do not drive for several hours after you drink alcohol. Never drink and drive.

Sugars and Sweets

It is common to want a sweet dessert to end a restaurant meal. As you know by now, you can fit sweets into your diabetes food plan as long as you substitute them for other foods or compensate for their extra carbohydrates, fat, and calories with your diabetes medicines to keep your blood glucose close to normal. To set healthy goals with sweets, you also need to consider your weight and blood fats. Work with a dietitian to figure out how to fit sweets into your meal plan. In the meantime, here are a few pointers.

Hints for Sweet Tooths

- Prioritize your personal diabetes goals. Which is most important for you: blood glucose control, weight loss, or lower blood fats? Your priorities dictate how you strike a balance with sugars and sweets.
- Choose a few favorite desserts. Decide how often to eat them and how to fit them into your meal plan.
- Perhaps it is best for you to limit desserts just to when you eat in restaurants. That way you keep sweets out of your home.
- Split a dessert in a restaurant or take half home. Portions are generally too big.
- Take advantage of smaller portions available in restaurants or ice cream spots—kiddie, small, or regular are the words to look for.
- Use the nutrition information you find in this book and information you find in restaurants to learn about the calorie, carbohydrate, fat, saturated fat, and cholesterol content of desserts.

- When you eat a sweet, check your blood glucose about two hours later to see how it has been affected. You might find, for instance, that because of the fat content, the same quantity of ice cream raises your blood glucose more slowly than does frozen yogurt, which contains less fat and more carbohydrate.
- Keep an eye on your glycated hemoglobin (your longer-range blood glucose measure, also known as hemoglobin A1C or glycosylated hemoglobin) and your blood fat (lipid) levels to see whether eating more sweets leads to an unwanted rise in these numbers.

These are basic guidelines and suggestions to deal with diabetes dining dilemmas. Each person with diabetes is different. So talk with your health care provider or diabetes educator to get specific information pertinent to the way you manage your diabetes.

Restaurants Help or Hinder Your Healthy Eating Efforts

The pendulum swings back and forth. During the 1980s and early 1990s, when the voices of people concerned about what they ate and about their health were loud, restaurants gave in. Lower-calorie and lower-fat menu items were introduced. Restaurateurs willingly made lower-fat milk and reduced calorie salad dressings available. Some restaurants even marked their menus with little hearts or other notations to indicate which menu items met specific health criteria.

Now the pendulum in restaurants has swung back toward a lax attitude about healthy eating. McDonald's no longer carries the McLean hamburger or meal-sized salads. Belly busting portions are commonplace. Taco Bell's Border Lights line bombed because it was introduced toward the end of the health craze. We've entered the era of new giant burgers, super-sized meals, and more all-you-can-eat buffets. But don't blame it on the restaurants. They cannot stock menu items that customers don't order. Unfortunately, a majority of Americans cast all health and nutrition cares to the wind when they set foot in a restaurant. And you can see where that is leading us. Today over 50 percent of Americans are overweight and type 2 diabetes is growing exponentially.

The "no cares" nutrition attitude makes it harder for those who are still health conscious. But don't feel pessimistic. Lower-fat milk, reduced calorie salad dressings, and lower-fat frozen desserts are still available, and there's a greater ease in making special requests. With skills and a bit of fortitude, you can eat healthfully at most restaurants. Granted, you still have to pick and choose among the menu offerings.

Your voice still matters and can make a difference. If you and thousands of other people with concerns about their health continue to make special requests, eventually your voices will be heard loud and clear. Maybe then the pendulum will once again swing toward an abundant supply of healthy menu items offered in reasonable portions.

Chains That Give the Nutrition Lowdown

For this book, menu and nutrition information was sought from about 80 large family and chain restaurants—from large hamburger chains to smaller Italian table-service chains. (See "How This Book Can Work for You" to find more information about the restaurant selection process we used.)

Since writing the first edition of this book in 1997, we've seen information available via the internet explode. And nutrition information for restaurant foods is no exception. It is now relatively easy to access nutrition information for the fast-food hamburger chains—from the large McDonald's and Burger King to the smaller Carl's Jr. and Sonic, America's Drive-In. Among the categories of restaurants and chains that make nutrition information available on their web sites are those selling pizza, chicken, Mexican food, desserts and ice cream, subs and sandwiches, and donuts and bagels.

The types of restaurants that, for the most part, either do not have or do not give out nutrition information are sit-down restaurants (such as Applebee's, Chili's, Friday's and Outback). Several of these restaurants are willing to provide information to you about a couple of items or their healthier ones. However, they either don't have the information or are unwilling to disclose it for everything.

Why don't some restaurants provide nutrition information? There are a few reasons. First, it's expensive to obtain nutritional analyses on all menu items. Second, restaurants that do not provide information tend to change their menus frequently. As soon as they would print nutrition information, it would need to be revised. Third, they want you to stay blindfolded to the nutrition lowdown on their foods. An important point here is that you—a person with diabetes concerned about your health—need to keep asking for nutrition information at restaurants that don't give it.

How to Get the Latest Nutrition Lowdown

If you do not find a particular restaurant chain in this book or there is a new menu item introduced for a restaurant that is included, here are a few hints on how to get the nutrition information.

■ If you have access to the internet, use it. We have added the internet addresses for all the restaurants and have indicated which ones have nutrition information on their web site.

- If you don't have internet access, ask for nutrition information at the location you frequent. You might get lucky and have a nutrition pamphlet put right into your hands. Sometimes they have run out or just don't keep them in stock. Make sure you check the date on the nutrition pamphlet to be sure it is current.
- If the restaurant does not have the information, ask where you can call or write for it. You might need to call or write the corporate headquarters and have them send you a pamphlet.
- If you have a question about the nutrition content or ingredients used in a few items, contact the company either through the internet or via the phone.

A Bit of Help from Your Government

The nutrition facts panel on most canned and packaged foods in the supermarket hardly seems new. But you only started to see it in 1994. How come the same type of nutrition labeling is not required for restaurants? There are a number of reasons. The most important reason is that the content of menu items varies too much and that menu items change often. However, as part of the Nutrition Labeling and Education Act (NLEA), which is the federal legislation that changed the nutrition label and increased the number of foods with information, restaurants must comply with several aspects of this law.

In January 1993, NLEA regulations required restaurants to provide nutrition information to customers when nutrition and health claims were made on signs and placards. Menu claims were exempt at that point. Since May 1997, if any restaurant makes a health claim about a food, that it is "low-fat," for instance, the nutrition information has to comply with the meaning of the term according to the NLEA. This helps you know that when you see the word "healthy" to describe a can of beans or a fast-food sandwich, it has the same meaning. Restaurants from small one-unit sandwich shops to McDonald's will have to abide by the regulations. Table 2 (see page 28) gives terms you might see on restaurant menu items and their definitions.

The new law permits restaurants to make

- specific claims about a menu item's nutritional content.
- one of the approved health claims about the relationship between a nutrient or food and a disease or health condition. The criteria to make the health claim must be met.

If the restaurant makes a nutrition or health claim, it must provide you with the nutrition information to back it up. The claim can be substantiated by a nutrition database, nutrition information in the cookbook from which the recipe was made, or another source that provides nutrition information. Further, restaurants do not have to give you the information in the nutrition label format you are familiar with from the supermarket. They can provide it in any format they choose.

TABLE 2 Meaning of Nutrition Claims* on Restaurant Menus, Signs, and Placards

Nutrition Claim	Meaning
Cholesterol-Free	Less than 2 mg of cholesterol per serving and 2 g or less of saturated fat per serving
Low-Cholesterol	20 mg or less of cholesterol per serving and 2 g or less of saturated fat per serving
Fat-Free	Less than 0.5 g of fat per serving
Low-Fat	3 g or less of fat per serving
Light or Lite	Cannot be used by restaurants as a nutrient content claim, but can be used to describe a menu item, such as "lighter fare" or "light size"
Sodium-Free	Less than 5 mg of sodium per serving
Low-Sodium	140 mg or less of sodium per serving
Sugar-Free	Less than 0.5 g of sugar per serving
Low-Sugar	May not be used as a nutrient claim
Healthy	The food item is low in fat, low in saturated fat, has limited amounts of cholesterol and sodium, and provides significant amounts of one or more key nutrients—vitamins A and C, iron, calcium, protein, or fiber.
Heart Healthy (These claims will indicate that a diet low in saturated fat and cholesterol may reduce the risk of heart disease.)	The item is low in fat, saturated fat, and cholesterol, and provides without fortification (added nutrients) significant amounts of one or more key nutrients—vitamins A and C, iron, calcium, protein, or fiber. OR The item is low in fat, saturated fat, and cholesterol, and provides without fortification (added nutrients) significant amounts of one or more key nutrients—vitamins A and C, iron, calcium, protein—and is a significant source of soluble fiber.

*The definitions of these claims are the same as those used for food labels in the supermarket.

Put Your Best Guess Forward

When you've got the nutrition information in hand, it makes knowing what you are eating a snap. And the listings in this book help a great deal when you choose to eat in one of the nearly 60 restaurants whose information is provided in the pages ahead.

The reality is, however, that nutrition information is simply not available from some of the restaurants in which you may choose to eat. They might be sit-down chain restaurants unwilling to provide information or smaller local chains that weren't large enough to include in this book. Or they might be independent single-location restaurants who are unlikely to have any nutrition information. Assessing the nutrient content of what you are eating in these restaurants is more of a challenge. These tips should help you learn to put your best guess forward.

Another reality, this time on the plus side, is that most people regularly eat just 25 to 50 foods, including restaurant foods. People tend to frequent the same restaurants, usually because they like certain dishes. For this reason, it does make sense to spend some time estimating the nutrient content of your favorite restaurant items for which nutrition information is not available. Once you have this figured out, put it in a notebook or develop a computer file that you print out and keep with you.

Keep in mind that most restaurants serve portions that are larger than most average-sized people need to eat. So, even if you choose healthy foods that combine to make a healthy meal, you will likely also need to limit the amount you eat. Portion control is clearly not an easy task. Learn some techniques by reading the "Strategies for Self-Defense" on pages 13–14.

A word to the wise: avoid all-you-can-eat restaurants and other settings that simply promote overeating, such as hotel breakfast buffets or salad or food bars. This is best if you don't have much willpower or it bothers you to think that the restaurant is making money on you because you will not walk out feeling like a stuffed turkey. However, if you feel these settings work well because they help you control portions, use them to your advantage.

Tips to Put Your Best Guess Forward

■ Have measuring equipment at home and use it. Have a set of measuring spoons and measuring cups as well as an inexpensive food scale. Weigh and measure foods at home. Do this on a regular basis as you start to familiarize yourself with the portions you should eat. Then on occasion, say once a month, weigh and measure foods, especially the starches, fruits, and meats. Weighing and measuring foods at home familiarizes you with portion sizes and helps you closely estimate them in restaurants. Estimating portions correctly helps you estimate the nutrient content.

- Use these "handy" hand guides to estimate portions:
  - Tip of the thumb (to first knuckle)—1 teaspoon
  - Whole thumb—1 tablespoon
  - Palm of your hand—3 ounces (this is the portion size of cooked meat that most people need at a meal). Others: the size of a deck of regular size playing cards or the size of a household bar of soap.
  - Tight fist—1/2 cup
  - Loose fist or open handful—1 cup
    Note: These guidelines hold true for most women's hand, but some men's hands are much larger. Check the size of your hands out for yourself with real weighing and measuring equipment.
- Use the scales in the produce aisle of the supermarket to educate yourself about the servings of food you may be served in a restaurant, such as baked white or sweet potatoes, an ear of corn, or a banana. Weigh individual pieces of these foods. Check out how many ounces a usual potato or an ear of corn is that you may be served in a restaurant. Note that you are weighing these foods raw, but their weight doesn't change that much when cooked.
- If there are no data for a particular restaurant you frequent, use the information available from other similar restaurants in the pages of this book. If you want to get a feel for the nutrient content of a food like french fries, baked potato, stuffing, pizza, or bagels, look at the serving size and nutrition information for those foods in restaurants that are included. You might want to take a few examples and then do an average. For example: if you regularly

eat at a local pizza shop rather than a national chain and they have no nutrition information, take the nutrition information from this book for two slices of medium-sized regular crust cheese pizza from three restaurants. Then do an average. You will come pretty close to the nutrition content of the two slices of cheese pizza you eat.

- You can also use the nutrition information from the nutrition facts of foods in the supermarket to estimate what you might be eating in a restaurant. You might find some similar foods in the frozen or packaged convenience foods area. Again, take a couple of examples and then average.

- If you regularly eat particular ethnic foods for which you find no nutrition information, you might want to get a few cookbooks out of the library (or use your own) that contain recipes for the foods you enjoy. Then use a nutrient database or book with nutrition information (see page 33) to determine the estimated nutrient content for each ingredient. Do this for a couple of similar recipes. Then get an average to help you estimate the nutrient content of what you are eating in the restaurant. This might work well for ethnic foods such as Indian, Mexican, or Chinese.

If you frequently eat particular items in large chain restaurants for which nutrition information is not available in this book, contact the restaurants. Several restaurants noted that while they were unwilling to provide the nutrition information for all their items for this book, if a customer contacted them, they would provide information for several items.

Resources to determine nutrient content:

B O O K S :

1. *The Diabetes Carbohydrate and Fat Gram Guide,* by Lea Ann Holzmeister, RD, CDE. American Diabetes Association, 2nd edition, 2000. This book provides the carbohydrate count and other nutrition information for thousands of basic and brand name convenience foods.
2. *Calories and Carbohydrates,* by Barbara Kraus, Mass Market Paperback, 14th edition, 2001. This book provides the carbohydrate and calorie count for more than 8,000 basic and brand name convenience foods.
3. The Corinne T. Netzer *Carbohydrate Counter,* by Corinne T. Netzer, Dell Publishing, 2nd edition, 1998. This book provides the carbohydrate count for thousands of basic and brand name convenience foods.
4. *Bowes and Church Food Values of Portions Commonly Used,* by Janet Pennington. 17th ed, J.P. Lippincott Company, 1998, Cost $36. To order, call 1-800-777-2295.

I N T E R N E T :

www.nal.usda.gov gets you to the Federal Government Nutrient Databases. You can download this information for free.

How This Book Can Work for You

You might open this book and be thrilled to see many of the restaurants you frequent. Then again, you might wonder why a certain restaurant that you've never laid eyes on is included, or why your favorite hamburger or pizza stop is nowhere to be found.

Each July, a restaurant trade association magazine, *Restaurants and Institutions*, publishes a list of the top 400 restaurant chains. The 60 largest chains were culled from a recent list. The restaurants were selected based on the number of locations they operate and whether the business was growing or in the red.

If one of your favorite restaurants is not included, it is for one of the following reasons:

- The restaurant might not have been willing or able to provide sufficient menu and/or nutrition information to warrant their inclusion.

- The restaurant chain may not be large enough across the country, although it appears to you that in your area there's an outlet on every corner.

Where to Find the Restaurant

Clearly, you know to look in "Burgers and More" to find McDonald's or Wendy's, or in "Pizza, Pasta, and All Else Italian" to find Domino's or Pizza Hut. But because Boston Market's menu today includes more than just chicken, you might not guess that it is in the section "Sit-Down Family Fare." Let's just say we used the "best-fit" approach. Nine times out of 10 you'll guess correctly. But if you don't find a restaurant in the chapter where you think it should be, then check the alphabetical listing of restaurants on page ix in the beginning of the book.

Close but Not Exact

You should be aware that the nutrition information from restaurants is close but not exact. Many restaurants state that their nutrition information is based on the specified ingredients and preparation. However, the same restaurant has locations all over the country, and different regions purchase their ingredients and foods from different food wholesalers. For example, a Wendy's in California might purchase lettuce, tomatoes, and hamburger buns from one food supplier, whereas a Wendy's in Connecticut will buy foods from another company. The nutrition analysis of these items is close, but not identical. However, it is close enough to help you to make food decisions and manage your blood glucose.

Restaurant foods are also prepared by different people. Even in the same restaurant, on different days you might get more or less cheese on your pizza, more pickles or ketchup on your hamburger, or a slightly smaller or larger steak even though you order the 6-oz filet. Wherever humans are involved, portions can't be exact. Consider these differences if one day you notice that your blood glucose goes up more or less than you expect from a restaurant meal you've eaten again and again.

Restaurants are concerned that you know their nutrition information is close but not exact. That's because they have been called on the carpet by some public interest groups who evaluate their food for its nutrients and find that the foods they choose to sample do not exactly match the nutrition information published by the restaurant.

What's In, What's Out

Nutrition information that was made available by the restaurants is included in the pages ahead. Some restaurants provided nutrition information for only their "core menu items," the items that every one of their outlets must serve. An outlet you visit might serve a few foods that are not part of the core menu. So you might find foods that are not included in this book.

Also, there are two categories of items that are not listed separately in the information provided for each restaurant. The first is beverages. Regularly sweetened drinks, such as carbonated beverages (soda, or pop), lemonade, noncarbonated fruit drinks, and the like, are not listed individually because from a nutrition standpoint, they are loaded with sugar and provide almost no nutritional value. Most restaurants also serve a similar variety of noncaloric beverages as well as milk and orange juice. To avoid repeating information on the same products, we've put the nutrition information for the most commonly served regular and diet beverages in Table 3 on page 38.

The second category of items not listed for individual restaurants is common condiments, such as ketchup, mustard, mayonnaise, and honey. Don't despair, we've put the nutrition information for these condiments in Table 4 on page 41.

TABLE 3 Nutrition Information for Beverages

Beverage	Amount	Cal.	Fat (g)	Sat. Fat (g)	Chol. (mg)	Sod. (mg)	Carb. (g)	Pro. (g)	Servings/Exchanges
Beer (regular)	12 oz	140	0	0	0	11	13	1	1 carb, 2 fat*
Beer (light)	12 oz	99	0	0	0	18	5	1	2 fat*
Coffee, black (regular and decaffeinated)	8 oz	5	0	0	0	4	1	0	free
Coke (regular)	12 oz	144	0	0	0	6	43	0	3 carb
Coke (diet)	12 oz	1	0	0	0	6	0	0	free
Iced Tea (unsweetened)	12 oz	4	0	0	0	6	1	0	free
Liquor (any type)	1 1/2 oz	96	0	0	0	0	0	0	2 fat*
Lemonade (regular)	12 oz	160	0	0	0	0	42	0	3 carb
Milk (whole)	8 oz	150	8	5	33	120	12	8	1 whole milk
✔Milk (reduced-fat/2%)	8 oz	120	5	3	18	122	12	8	1 low-fat milk

✔Milk (fat-free)	8 oz	86	0	0	4	126	12	8	1 fat-free milk
✔Orange juice	8 oz	112	0	0	0	2	27	2	2 fruit
Pepsi (regular)	12 oz	144	0	0	0	6	43	0	3 carb
Pepsi (diet)	12 oz	1	0	0	0	6	0	0	free
Sprite (regular)	12 oz	148	0	0	0	3	37	0	2 1/2 carb
Sprite (diet)	12 oz	1	0	0	0	6	0	0	free
Tea (hot, nothing added)	8 oz	2	0	0	0	7	1	0	free
Wine, white	6 oz	120	0	0	0	9	1	0	2 fat*
Wine, red	6 oz	120	0	0	0	114	3	1	2 fat*

*Talk to your diabetes educator or health care provider about whether you can work alcoholic beverages into your meal plan and how to do so.

✔Healthiest Bets.

The Nutrition Numbers Ahead

All the nutrition information you need to know to fit foods into your meal plan is in the pages ahead, unless the information was not available from the restaurant. Whether you use the diabetes exchange system or the diabetes food pyramid, do carbohydrate counting or fat gram counting for meal planning, the numbers are here. This is the nutrition information you'll find, in this order:

- Calories
- Fat (in grams) and
  - Percentage of calories from fat. Look at this in relation to grams of fat. Keep in mind that the percentage of calories from fat might be high, but the grams of fat might be low, or vice versa.
  - Saturated fat (in grams). Saturated fat is the type of fat that raises blood cholesterol levels. You should keep your saturated fat intake to 10 percent or less of your total calories.

- Cholesterol (in milligrams)
- Sodium (in milligrams)
- Carbohydrate (in grams)
  - Dietary fiber (in grams). Dietary fiber is a component of carbohydrate. Generally, Americans don't eat enough dietary fiber. Try to eat 20–35 grams of dietary fiber each day. If you count carbohydrates, you might have been taught to subtract grams of dietary fiber from your carbohydrate count if a serving of the food or the meal has more than 5 grams of dietary fiber.

- Protein (in grams)

TABLE 4 Nutrition Information for Condiments

Condiment	Amount	Cal.	Fat (g)	Sat. Fat (g)	Chol. (mg)	Sod. (mg)	Carb. (g)	Pro. (g)	Servings/Exchanges
Bacon, thinly sliced	1 slice	36	3	1	5	101	0	2	1 fat
Butter	1 t	30	4	2	10	39	0	0	1 fat
Cheese, American	1-oz slice	106	9	6	27	405	1	6	1 high-fat meat
Cheese, Swiss	1-oz slice	107	8	5	26	74	1	8	1 high-fat meat
Cheese, mozzarella, whole-milk	1/4 cup shredded/1 oz	80	6	4	22	106	1	6	1 medium-fat meat
Cream Cheese (regular)	1 T	50	5	3	15	45	1	1	1 fat
Cream Cheese (light)	1 T	30	3	2	5	80	1	2	1/2 fat
Half & Half	1/2 oz/1 T	20	2	1	6	6	1	0	free
Honey	1 t	22	0	0	0	0	6	0	1/2 carb
Honey Mustard	1 t	15	1	n/a	n/a	75	2	0	free

(Continued)

TABLE 4 **Nutrition Information for Condiments** *(Continued)*

Condiment	Amount	Cal.	Fat (g)	Sat. Fat (g)	Chol. (mg)	Sod. (mg)	Carb. (g)	Pro. (g)	Servings/Exchanges
Ketchup	1 T	16	0	0	0	137	4	0	free
Margarine (regular stick)	1 t	34	4	1	0	44	0	0	1 fat
Margarine (regular tub)	1 t	34	4	1	0	51	0	0	1 fat
Margarine (light)	1 t	17	2	0	0	17	0	0	free
Mayonnaise (regular)	1 T	100	11	2	8	78	0	0	2 fat
Mayonnaise (light)	1 T	40	4	0	5	15	1	0	1 fat
Mustard	1 t	5	0	0	0	65	0	0	free
Non-Dairy Creamer	1/2 oz/1 T	16	1	0	0	5	2	0	free
Olive Oil	1 t	40	5	2	0	0	0	0	1 fat
Pancake Syrup (regular)	1 T	50	0	0	0	13	13	0	1 carb
Pancake Syrup (light)	1 T	25	0	0	0	56	7	0	1/2 carb

Pancake Syrup (low-calorie)	1 T	23	0	0	0	57	6	0	1/2 carb
Relish, pickle-type	1 T	19	0	0	0	164	5	0	free
Salsa, tomato-based	1 T	3	3	0	0	112	1	0	free
Sour Cream (regular)	1 T	31	3	2	6	8	1	0	1/2 fat
Sour Cream (light)	1 T	18	1	0	5	10	1	1	free
Soy Sauce	1 t	3	0	0	0	343	1	0	free
Vinegar (all types)	1 t	2	0	0	0	0	1	0	free

n/a, not available

■ Food servings/exchanges. Servings and exchanges are virtually the same. They have been calculated using the *1995 Exchange Lists for Meal Planning*, published by the ADA and the American Dietetic Association, and the book *Diabetes Meal Planning Made Easy*, 2nd edition, published by ADA in 2000.

A "best-fit" approach was used to calculate servings or exchanges. There is no one right way to fit restaurant foods into your meal plan. Figuring out what food group the grams of carbohydrate come from is the biggest challenge to figuring servings or exchanges. This is how we approached it: When it appears that the grams of carbohydrate come from a starch—be it potato, bread, or starchy vegetable—we've called the servings or exchanges starches. If the carbohydrate comes from vegetable, fruit, or milk, we've designated the servings or exchanges as such.

A new food group in the *1995 Exchange Lists for Meal Planning* is the "other carbohydrate" group. This group contains foods such as sweets, frozen desserts, spaghetti sauce, jam, and maple syrup, to name a few. The calories and carbohydrates in many of these foods come from simple sugars. Therefore, in calculating the servings or exchanges for this book, we've called foods that fit into the "other carbohydrate" group "carb." Exchanges for fast-food shakes and frozen and regular desserts, for example, are calculated as carbs.

When it comes to meat dishes, we've tried to calculate the servings or exchanges based on the group that the meat itself fits into regardless of how it's prepared. For example, fish fillet sandwiches and chicken fingers are considered to fall into the lean meat group even though they have a lot of fat by the time they are served. On the other hand, sausage in any form is classified as a high-fat meat because that's the food group sausage fits into.

It is worth noting that some restaurants that provide nutrition information also provide exchanges. These were not used in this book. The author calculated exchanges/servings based on ADA methodology. The author has often found inconsistencies between the restaurant's exchange calculations and the ones she obtains using ADA guidelines.

Putting It All Together

Perhaps one of the hardest parts of meal planning is figuring out how to put together healthy, well-balanced meals. This is a particular challenge in restaurants. To show you how to design healthier restaurant meals, we've put together two sample meals for most of the restaurants. We applied the following criteria to put together the meals. (Please note that the criteria might be less strict than what you would consider for a healthy meal at home. That's because restaurant meals tend to be higher in calories, fat, etc.) We have not designed meals for several of the restaurants, including all those in the "Sweets and Frozen Treats" chapter, because of their limited menus.

The Light 'n Lean Choice

- 400–700 calories (based on about 1,200–1,600 calories per day)
- 30–40 percent of calories from fat
- 100–200 milligrams of cholesterol (total per day should be 300 milligrams or less)

- 1,000–2,000 milligrams of sodium (total per day should be 2,400–3,000 milligrams)

The Healthy 'n Hearty Choice

- 600–1,000 calories (based on about 1,800–2,400 calories per day)
- 30–40 percent of calories from fat
- 100–200 milligrams of cholesterol (total per day should be 300 milligrams or less)
- 1,000–2,000 milligrams of sodium (total per day should be 2,400–3,000 milligrams)

Healthiest Bets

With nutrition information in hand, we've also made it easy for you to zero in on healthier restaurant offerings. We've marked these "Healthiest Bets" with a ✔. Remember, foods that are not marked as Healthiest Bets are not necessarily foods you should never eat. Healthiest Bets just steer you toward healthier choices.

When you're putting together healthy meals, don't look at only the Healthiest Bets. You can feel free to mix and match healthier and less healthy foods to make up overall healthy meals. Also keep in mind that if you split or share some less healthy bets, such as shakes, desserts, or fried items, they then fit into Healthiest Bets. That's why you'll see some Healthiest Bets and some less healthy items mixed and matched in the sample meals for each restaurant. What's most important is that you eat a healthy balance over the course of the day and from week to week. So if you want a juicy hamburger and french fries for lunch one day a month, go ahead and enjoy.

The Healthiest Bets were chosen on the basis of the following criteria:

- Breakfast entrees: Less than 400 calories per serving, with less than 15 grams of fat (3 fat exchanges [about 30 percent fat]) and 1,000 milligrams of sodium.
- Lunch or dinner entrees, including entree salads: Less than 600–750 calories, with less than 20 grams of fat (4 fat exchanges [about 30 percent fat]) and 1,000 milligrams of sodium.
- Pizza, sandwiches (including breakfast sandwiches), hamburgers, etc.: Less than 500 calories per reasonable serving (for example, 2 slices of pizza), 20 grams of fat (4 fat exchanges [about 30% fat]), and 1,000 milligrams of sodium.
- Side items: For items such as fruit, vegetables (raw and cooked), grains, legumes, starches, and meats, no more than 5 grams of fat (1 fat exchange). For fried items, such as french fries, hash browns, chicken pieces, fried chicken, onion rings, and potato chips, less than 10 grams of fat (2 fat exchanges); less than 500 milligrams of sodium per serving.
- Soups: Less than 10 grams of fat (2 fat exchanges) and 1,000 milligrams of sodium per serving.
- Salad dressings, cream cheeses, spreads, and condiments: Less than 50 calories, 5 grams of fat (1 fat exchange), and 250 milligrams of sodium per tablespoon.
- Breads (such as rolls, biscuits, bagels, bread, croissants, scones, donuts, muffins, pretzels, and scones): Less than 400 calories, 10 grams of fat (2 fat exchanges), and 800 milligrams of sodium per serving.
- Desserts: Less than 300 calories, 10 grams of fat (2 fat exchanges), and 30 grams of carbohydrate per serving.

- Beverages (such as milk, juice, milk shakes, and special coffees): Less than 300 calories, 30 grams of carbohydrate, and 5 grams of fat (1 fat exchange). Less than 400 milligrams of sodium. (Coffee and diet beverages, though minimal in calories, were not checked as Healthiest Bets.)

Bon Appetit!

Breakfast Eats, Donuts, Coffees, Snacks, and More

RESTAURANTS

Auntie Anne's Hand-Rolled Soft Pretzels

Bruegger's Bagels

Dunkin' Donuts

Einstein Bros Bagels

Krispy Kreme Doughnuts

Manhattan Bagel Company

Starbucks

Tim Hortons

Note: Restaurants in this chapter devote their menu to bagels, donuts, coffees, pretzels, and more. They are the usual American breakfast spots. Look in "Burgers, Fries, and More" for fast-food breakfasts. Look in "Sit-Down Family Fare" for restaurants that serve breakfast and brunch as well as lunch and dinner. Look in "Soups, Sandwiches, and Subs" for Au Bon Pain and Panera Bread, which also serve breakfast items.

The healthy meal choices for the restaurants in this section will have slightly fewer calories and other nutrients than the criteria noted on page 46. That's because meals you eat in these restaurants are most likely breakfasts, light meals, or snacks.

NUTRITION PROS

- Bagels are the rage. That's great because they are low in fat—as long as you apply spreads thinly and wisely.

Healthy Tips

★ Stick with coffee without a lot of added cream, whole milk, or sugar. They add fat and empty calories. Use a sugar substitute. They are always available.

★ Try a soft-baked pretzel as an accompaniment to a sandwich or salad.

★ Opt for one of the light bagel spreads, but keep in mind that they are hardly calorie or fat free. Spread them thinly.

★ Cake donuts have slightly less fat than yeast donuts.

★ Do eat breakfast. Skipping breakfast just keeps your engine in low gear and helps you rationalize overeating at meals during the rest of the day. Plus, if you take diabetes medications to lower your blood sugar, skipping breakfast is not a smart move.

★ Steer clear of tuna, chicken, or seafood salads. They're chock full of fat. Stick with unadulterated meats and cheese.

★ Read the fine print when you see the words "low-fat," "fat-free," or "sugar-free." They don't mean there are no calories or no carbohydrate. In fact, some of these foods can contain more carbohydrate and/or more calories than the regular food.

★ If jam or jelly is an option, take it. Jams and jellies have no fat. Spread them thinly all the same.

- Light cream cheese spreads are available in most bagel shops.
- Soft-baked pretzels unadulterated with lots of fat or sugar are a healthy snack or side item. But you might not want to eat the whole thing.
- Pretzels and bagels are a source of dietary fiber.
- No longer is it donuts-only at Dunkin' Donuts and other donut shops. They serve bagels, low-fat muffins, and various coffees too.
- Muffin mania has died down, but you'll still find them at many breakfast spots. Often low-fat muffins are up for grabs. Even regular muffins are a better choice than some donuts or loaded bagels. But do watch the size. They can be huge.
- English muffins and yeast rolls are healthy choices as long as you use only a light amount of butter or margarine.

NUTRITION CONS

- Bagels can quickly become high fat and high calorie if they are topped with a quarter inch of high-fat cream cheese or spread.
- Bagels in most bagels shops average at least 3–4 oz and 250–340 calories. They're often equal to at least three or four slices of bread, not two.
- Pretzels sound healthy, but their calories and fat rise when they are rolled in lots of glaze or butter, or dipped in cheese sauce, cream cheese, or caramel.
- Croissants are high fat by nature—that's how they become flaky. You add insult to injury when you stuff a croissant with items such as bacon, sausage, cheese, tuna salad, or chicken salad.

- Donuts are high in fat (but surprisingly, not as bad as you might think). Save them for a once-in-a-while splurge.
- Biscuits are loaded with fat. When sausage, bacon, egg, and/or cheese is sandwiched between them, they give you your fat for one day in one fell swoop.
- The newfangled coffees—mocha or Starbucks' Frappuccino—are not just coffee. The sugar is blended through and through.
- One of the quickest and healthiest breakfast foods—dry or cooked cereal with fat-free (skim) milk—is rarely served. When it's an option, grab it.

Get It Your Way

- ★ Order bagel spreads on the side so that you can control how much is spread.
- ★ Order butter or margarine on the side.
- ★ Opt for fat-free milk in specialty coffees.
- ★ Order a sandwich on a bagel or roll, not on a high-fat croissant.

Auntie Anne's Hand-Rolled Soft Pretzels

❖Auntie Anne's Hand-Rolled Soft Pretzels provides nutrition information for all of its menu items on their website at www.auntieannes.com.

Light 'n Lean Choice

Jalapeno Pretzel, without butter

Calories......................270	Sodium (mg) 780
Fat (g) 1	Carbohydrate (g).........58
% calories from fat ...3	Fiber (g) 2
Saturated fat (g)........0	Protein (g) 8
Cholesterol (mg) 0	

Exchanges: 4 starch

Healthy 'n Hearty Choice

Sour Cream & Onion Pretzel, without butter

Calories......................310	Sodium (mg) 920
Fat (g) 1	Carbohydrate (g).........66
% calories from fat ...3	Fiber (g) 2
Saturated fat (g)........0	Protein (g) 9
Cholesterol (mg) 0	

Exchanges: 4 1/2 starch

(*Continued*)

Auntie Anne's Hand-Rolled Soft Pretzels

	Amount	Cal.	Fat (g)	% Cal. Fat	Sat. Fat (g)	Chol. (mg)	Sod. (mg)	Carb. (g)	Fiber (g)	Pro. (g)	Servings/Exchanges
DIPS											
Caramel Dip	1.5 oz	135	3	20	1.5	5	110	27	0	1	2 carb
Cheese Sauce	1.25 oz	100	8	72	4	10	510	4	0	3	2 fat
Chocolate Flavored Dip	1.25 oz	130	4	28	1.5	2	65	24	1	1	1 1/2 carb
Hot Salsa Cheese	1.25 oz	100	8	72	4	10	550	4	0	2	2 fat
Light Cream Cheese	1.25 oz	70	6	77	4	25	140	1	0	3	1 fat
✔Marinara Sauce	1.25 oz	10	0	0	0	0	180	4	0	0	free
Strawberry Cream Cheese	1.25 oz	110	10	82	6	35	105	4	0	2	2 fat
✔Sweet Mustard	1.25 oz	60	1.5	23	1	40	120	8	0	1	1/2 carb

DUTCH ICE

Auntie Anne's Lemonade	22 oz	180	0	0	0	0	0	43	0	0	3 carb
Blue Raspberry Dutch Ice (large)	20 oz	230	0	0	0	0	30	55	0	0	3 1/2 carb
Blue Raspberry Dutch Ice (regular)	14 oz	165	0	0	0	0	20	38	0	0	2 1/2 carb
Kiwi-Banana Dutch Ice (large)	20 oz	270	0	0	0	0	40	63	0	0	4 carb
Kiwi-Banana Dutch Ice (regular)	14 oz	190	0	0	0	0	30	44	0	0	3 carb
Lemonade Dutch Ice (large)	20 oz	450	0	0	0	0	0	110	0	0	7 carb
Lemonade Dutch Ice (regular)	14 oz	315	0	0	0	0	0	77	0	0	5 carb

✔ = Healthiest Bets; n/a = not available

(Continued)

DUTCH ICE (*Continued*)	Amount	Cal.	Fat (g)	% Cal. Fat	Sat. Fat (g)	Chol. (mg)	Sod. (mg)	Carb. (g)	Fiber (g)	Pro. (g)	Servings/Exchanges
Mocha Dutch Ice (large)	20 oz	570	15	24	12.5	0	150	105	0	0	7 carb, 2 fat
Mocha Dutch Ice (regular)	14 oz	400	10	23	9	0	100	74	0	0	5 carb, 2 fat
Orange Creme Dutch Ice (large)	20 oz	400	0	0	0	0	50	92	0	0	6 carb
Orange Creme Dutch Ice (regular)	14 oz	280	0	0	0	0	35	64	0	0	4 carb
Pina Colada Dutch Ice	14 oz	220	0	0	0	0	15	53	0	0	3 1/2 carb
Pina Colada Dutch Ice	20 oz	535	0	0	0	0	50	125	0	0	8 carb
Strawberry Dutch Ice (large)	20 oz	315	0	0	0	0	60	72	0	0	5 carb
Strawberry Dutch Ice (regular)	14 oz	220	0	0	0	0	40	50	0	0	3 carb

	Amount	Cal.	Fat (g)	% Fat Cal.	Sat. Fat (g)	Chol. (mg)	Sod. (mg)	Carb. (g)	Fiber (g)	Prot. (g)	Exchanges/Choices
Wild Cherry Dutch Ice	20 oz	300	0	0	0	0	35	69	0	0	4 1/2 carb
Wild Cherry Dutch Ice	14 oz	210	0	0	0	0	25	48	0	0	3 carb
PRETZELS WITH BUTTER											
✔Almond	1	400	8	18	5	20	400	72	2	9	5 starch, 1 fat
Cinnamon Sugar	1	450	9	18	5	25	430	83	3	8	4 1/2 starch, 1 carb, 2 fat
Garlic	1	350	5	13	2.5	10	850	68	2	9	4 1/2 starch, 1 fat
Glazin' Raisin	1	510	4	7	2	10	480	107	4	11	5 starch, 2 carb, 1 fat
Jalapeno	1	310	5	15	2.5	10	940	59	2	8	4 starch, 1 fat
✔Kidstix	4 sticks	247	3	11	1	7	620	48	2	7	3 starch, 1/2 fat
Original	1	370	4	10	2	10	930	72	3	10	5 starch, 1 fat
Parmesan Herb	1	440	13	27	7	30	660	72	9	10	3 1/2 starch, 2 fat

✔ = Healthiest Bets; n/a = not available

PRETZELS WITH BUTTER (*Continued*)	Amount	Cal.	Fat (g)	% Cal. Fat	Sat. Fat (g)	Chol. (mg)	Sod. (mg)	Carb. (g)	Fiber (g)	Pro. (g)	Servings/Exchanges
Sesame	1	410	12	26	4	15	860	64	7	12	4 starch, 2 fat
Sour Cream & Onion	1	340	5	13	3	10	930	66	2	9	4 1/2 starch, 1 fat
Whole Wheat	1	370	5	12	1.5	10	1120	72	7	11	5 starch, 1 fat
PRETZELS WITHOUT BUTTER											
✔ Almond	1	350	2	5	0.5	0	390	72	2	9	4 starch, 1 carb
✔ Cinnamon Sugar	1	350	2	5	0	0	410	74	2	9	4 starch, 1 carb
✔ Garlic	1	320	1	3	0	0	830	66	2	9	4 1/2 starch
Glazin' Raisin	1	470	1	2	0	0	460	104	3	11	5 starch, 2 carb
✔ Jalapeno	1	270	1	3	0	0	780	58	2	8	4 starch
Kidstix	4 sticks	227	1	4	0	0	600	48	2	7	3 starch
Original	1	340	1	3	0	0	900	72	3	10	5 starch

✔Parmesan Herb	1	390	5	12	2.5	10	780	74	4	11	5 starch, 1 fat
Sesame	1	350	6	15	1	0	840	63	3	11	4 starch, 1 fat
Sour Cream & Onion	1	310	1	3	0	0	920	66	2	9	4 1/2 starch
Whole Wheat	1	350	2	5	0	0	1100	72	7	11	5 starch

✔ = Healthiest Bets; n/a = not available

Bruegger's Bagels

❖Bruegger's Bagels provides nutrition information for all of its menu items on its website at www.brueggersbagels.com.

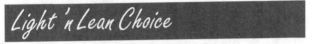

Light 'n Lean Choice

**Sundried Tomato Bagel
Light Herb Garlic Cream Cheese**
(order cream cheese on the side, use 2 T)

Calories......................380	Sodium (mg)..............715
Fat (g) 7	Carbohydrate (g).........67
% calories from fat..17	Fiber (g) 3
Saturated fat (g).....2.5	Protein (g) 16
Cholesterol (mg) 15	

Exchanges: 4 1/2 starch, 1 fat

Healthy 'n Hearty Choice

Chicken Fajita Bagel Sandwich

Calories......................500	Sodium (mg)..............970
Fat (g) 12	Carbohydrate (g).........74
% calories from fat..22	Fiber (g) 5
Saturated fat (g).....4.5	Protein (g) 28
Cholesterol (mg) 85	

Exchanges: 5 starch, 2 lean meat, 1 fat

Bruegger's Bagels

	Amount	Cal.	Fat (g)	% Cal. Fat	Sat. Fat (g)	Chol. (mg)	Sod. (mg)	Carb. (g)	Fiber (g)	Pro. (g)	Servings/Exchanges
BAGELS											
✔Blueberry	1	330	2	5	0	0	530	68	4	11	4 1/2 starch
✔Chocolate Chip	1	310	5	15	1.5	0	500	69	4	11	4 1/2 starch
✔Cinnamon Raisin	1	320	2	6	0	0	510	68	4	11	4 1/2 starch
✔Cranberry Orange	1	330	2	5	0	0	510	68	4	11	4 1/2 starch
✔Everything	1	310	2	6	0	0	710	62	4	12	4 starch
✔Garlic	1	310	2	6	0	0	540	62	4	12	4 starch
✔Honey Grain Bagel	1	330	3	8	0	0	500	64	5	13	4 starch
✔Jalapeno	1	310	2	6	0	0	550	63	4	12	4 starch
✔Onion	1	310	2	6	0	0	540	62	4	12	4 starch

✔ = Healthiest Bets; n/a = not available

(Continued)

	Amount	Cal.	Fat (g)	% Cal. Fat	Sat. Fat (g)	Chol. (mg)	Sod. (mg)	Carb. (g)	Fiber (g)	Pro. (g)	Servings/Exchanges
✔ Plain	1	300	2	6	0	0	540	61	4	12	4 starch
✔ Poppy Seed	1	310	3	9	0	0	540	61	4	12	4 starch
✔ Pumpernickel	1	320	3	8	0	0	600	64	5	12	4 starch
✔ Rosemary Olive Oil	1	350	6	15	1	0	530	62	4	11	4 starch, 1 fat
Salt	1	300	2	6	0	0	1540	61	4	12	4 starch
✔ Sesame	1	320	2	6	0	0	540	61	4	12	4 starch
✔ Sun Dried Tomato	1	310	2	6	0	0	630	64	4	12	4 starch
BREAKFAST SANDWICHES											
Egg and Cheese	1	480	15	28	6	190	840	66	4	22	4 starch, 2 medium-fat meat
Egg, Cheese, Bacon	1	560	22	35	9	200	1070	66	4	26	4 starch, 2 medium-fat meat, 2 fat

Egg, Cheese, Ham	1	520	17	29	7	205	1350	66	4	28	4 starch, 2 medium-fat meat, 2 fat
Egg, Cheese, Sausage	1	680	33	44	12	235	1570	66	4	33	4 starch, 3 medium-fat meat, 3 fat

CREAM CHEESES

✔ Bacon Scallion	2 T	100	8	72	5	30	105	4	0	2	1 1/2 fat
✔ Chive	2 T	100	9	81	5	30	90	2	0	2	2 fat
✔ Garden Veggie	2 T	90	8	80	4.5	25	95	3	0	2	1 1/2 fat
Honey Walnut	2 T	110	8	65	4.5	25	85	5	0	2	1 1/2 fat
✔ Jalapeno	2 T	100	9	81	5	30	100	3	0	2	2 fat
✔ Light Garden Veggie	2 T	60	4	60	2.5	15	75	2	0	4	1 fat
✔ Light Herb Garlic	2 T	70	5	64	2.5	15	85	3	0	4	1 fat

✔ = Healthiest Bets; n/a = not available

(Continued)

	Amount	Cal.	Fat (g)	% Cal. Fat	Sat. Fat (g)	Chol. (mg)	Sod. (mg)	Carb. (g)	Fiber (g)	Pro. (g)	Servings/Exchanges
CREAM CHEESES (*Continued*)											
✔Light Plain	2 T	70	5	64	2	15	90	3	0	2	1 fat
✔Light Strawberry	2 T	70	4	51	2.5	15	85	4	0	4	1 fat
✔Olive Pimento	2 T	100	9	81	4	30	90	2	0	2	2 fat
✔Plain	2 T	90	8	80	5	25	85	4	0	2	1 1/2 fat
✔Smoked Salmon	2 T	100	9	81	4.5	25	105	2	0	2	2 fat
✔Wildberry	2 T	100	9	81	5	25	85	4	0	2	2 fat
DESSERTS											
Blondies	1	370	23	56	6	25	220	42	2	5	3 carb, 3 fat
Bruegger Bar	1	420	24	51	11	15	240	47	3	6	3 carb, 4 fat
Cappuccino Bar	1	420	25	54	9	60	125	45	1	5	3 carb, 4 fat
Chocolate Chunk Brownie	1	330	19	52	7	55	150	39	2	4	2 1/2 carb, 3 fat

✔ = Healthiest Bets; n/a = not available

Luscious Lemon Bars	1	350	20	51	7	85	260	39	0	4	2 1/2 carb, 3 fat
Mint Brownie	1	300	17	51	7	40	95	34	0	3	2 carb, 3 fat
Oatmeal Cranberry Mountains	1	430	24	50	13	60	320	49	3	7	3 carb, 4 fat
Pecan Chocolate Chunk	1	350	24	62	9	80	160	32	1	4	2 carb, 4 fat
Raspberry Sammies	1	270	13	43	8	35	130	36	1	3	2 1/2 carb, 2 fat
MEAT / FISH											
✔Atlantic Smoked Salmon	1	90	3	30	1	30	840	1	0	15	2 lean meat
SANDWICHES											
✔Atlantic Smoked Sandwich	1	470	12	23	6	55	590	66	4	26	4 starch, 2 lean meat, 1 fat
Chicken Breast	1	440	6	12	1.5	60	1230	62	4	37	4 starch, 3 lean meat
✔Chicken Fajita	1	500	12	22	4.5	85	970	74	5	28	5 starch, 2 lean meat, 1 fat
✔Chicken Salad with Mayo	1	460	12	23	1.5	55	820	67	4	24	4 starch, 2 lean meat, 1 fat

(Continued)

✔ = Healthiest Bets; n/a = not available

SANDWICHES (*Continued*)	Amount	Cal.	Fat (g)	% Cal. Fat	Sat. Fat (g)	Chol. (mg)	Sod. (mg)	Carb. (g)	Fiber (g)	Pro. (g)	Servings/Exchanges
Deli-Style Ham with Honey Mustard	1	440	5	10	1	30	1440	77	4	24	4 starch, 2 lean meat
✓Garden Veggie	1	390	6	14	2.5	15	580	70	5	17	4 starch, 1 vegetable, 1 lean meat
✓Herby Turkey	1	530	14	24	7	55	1180	73	4	28	5 starch, 2 lean meat, 1 fat
✓Leonardo da Veggie	1	460	11	22	6	40	740	69	4	19	4 1/2 starch, 1 medium-fat meat, 1 fat
Santa Fe Turkey	1	480	10	19	4	55	1630	71	4	29	4 1/2 starch, 2 lean meat, 1/2 fat
Turkey with Mayo	1	480	14	26	1.5	35	1220	65	4	25	4 starch, 2 lean meat, 1 fat
SOUPS											
✓Aztec Chicken	8 oz	90	3	30	.5	15	500	10	2	7	1/2 starch, 1/2 fat

✔Bean and Bacon	8 oz	160	4	23	0	10	920	23	13	11	1 1/2 starch, 1 fat
Big Chili (Beef Chili with Beans)	8 oz	240	9	34	3.5	50	1130	20	7	23	1 starch, 2 medium-fat meat
Chicken Noodle	8 oz	110	7	57	2	25	1150	6	1	7	1/2 starch, 1 lean meat, 1 fat
Chicken Wild Rice	8 oz	260	19	66	11	75	1170	16	1	9	1 starch, 1 lean meat, 3 fat
Clam Chowder	8 oz	170	7	37	2	10	1230	18	1	8	1 starch, 1 very lean meat, 1 fat
Garden Split Pea	8 oz	150	6	36	3	10	1050	19	3	4	1 starch, 1 1/2 fat
✔Gazpacho	8 oz	80	4	45	0	0	480	13	2	2	2 vegetable, 1 fat
✔Marcello Minestrone	8 oz	90	1	10	0	0	890	18	2	4	1 starch
Ratatouille Stew	8 oz	140	9	58	1.5	0	1100	12	3	2	2 vegetable, 2 fat
✔Spinach Tortellini	8 oz	240	9	34	4.5	25	890	31	3	9	2 starch, 2 fat
✔Sweet Corn Chowder	8 oz	180	9	45	5	60	740	29	3	4	2 starch, 1 1/2 fat

✔ = Healthiest Bets; n/a = not available

(Continued)

SOUPS (*Continued*)	Amount	Cal.	Fat (g)	% Cal. Fat	Sat. Fat (g)	Chol. (mg)	Sod. (mg)	Carb. (g)	Fiber (g)	Pro. (g)	Servings/Exchanges
✔Tuscan Minestrone	8 oz	200	3	14	.5	0	700	34	19	11	2 starch, 1 1/2 fat
✔Velvet Veggie Cheese	8 oz	140	8	51	5	25	750	14	2	4	1 starch, 1 1/2 fat
SPREADS											
✔Bruegger's Hummus	2 T	60	4	60	.5	0	85	4	2	2	1 fat
Orval Kent Tuna Salad	5 T	180	14	70	2	20	440	6	0	8	1/2 carb, 3 fat

✔ = Healthiest Bets; n/a = not available

Dunkin' Donuts

❖Dunkin' Donuts provides nutrition information for all of its menu items on their website at www.dunkindonuts.com.

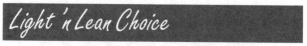

1 English Muffin with Ham/Egg/Cheese
4 oz Orange Juice

Calories	380	Sodium (mg)	1,340
Fat (g)	12	Carbohydrate (g)	46
% calories from fat	28	Fiber (g)	2
Saturated fat (g)	6	Protein (g)	22
Cholesterol (mg)	195		

Exchanges: 2 starch, 1 fruit, 2 medium-fat meat

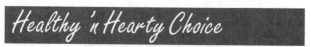

2 Glazed Yeast Donuts

Calories	360	Sodium (mg)	500
Fat (g)	16	Carbohydrate (g)	50
% calories from fat	40	Fiber (g)	2
Saturated fat (g)	3	Protein (g)	6
Cholesterol (mg)	0		

Exchanges: 3 carb, 3 fat

(Continued)

Dunkin' Donuts

	Amount	Cal.	Fat (g)	% Cal. Fat	Sat. Fat (g)	Chol. (mg)	Sod. (mg)	Carb. (g)	Fiber (g)	Pro. (g)	Servings/Exchanges
BAGELS											
✔Berry Berry	1	340	3	8	.5	0	540	69	4	11	4 1/2 starch
✔Blueberry	1	340	3	8	.5	0	630	69	2	11	4 1/2 starch
✔Cinnamon Raisin	1	340	4	11	.5	0	600	69	3	11	4 1/2 starch
✔Everything	1	360	3	8	.5	0	710	67	2	12	4 1/2 starch
✔Garlic	1	360	3	8	.5	0	720	68	2	12	4 1/2 starch
✔Onion	1	350	4	10	.5	0	660	66	3	12	4 1/2 starch, 1 fat
✔Plain	1	340	3	8	.5	0	680	67	2	12	4 1/2 starch
✔Poppy	1	360	4	10	.5	0	710	68	2	12	4 1/2 starch, 1 fat
Salt	1	340	3	8	.5	0	3030	67	2	12	4 1/2 starch

	Amount	Cal	Fat (g)	% Cal from Fat	Sat Fat (g)	Chol (mg)	Sodium (mg)	Carb (g)	Fiber (g)	Pro (g)	Exchanges
✔ Sesame	1	380	5	12	.5	0	720	74	3	12	5 starch
✔ Sundried Tomato	1	330	3	8	.5	0	700	66	3	13	4 1/2 starch
✔ Wheat	1	350	5	13	1	0	640	67	4	13	4 1/2 starch
BEVERAGES											
Coffee Coolatta (18% Fat Cream)	16 oz	410	22	48	14	75	65	51	0	3	3 1/2 carb, 4 fat
Coffee Coolatta (2% Low-fat Milk)	16 oz	240	2	8	1.5	10	80	52	0	4	3 1/2 carb
Coffee Coolatta (Skim Milk)	16 oz	230	0	0	0	5	80	52	0	4	3 1/2 carb
Coffee Coolatta (Whole Milk)	16 oz	260	4	14	2.5	15	75	52	0	4	3 1/2 carb, 1 fat
Coffee Coolatta with Cream	16 oz	460	24	47	14	75	120	58	0	4	4 carb, 3 fat
& Chocolate Mint Cookie Coolatta Whirl-Ins											

✔ = Healthiest Bets; n/a = not available

(Continued)

BEVERAGES *(Continued)*	Amount	Cal.	Fat (g)	% Cal. Fat	Sat. Fat (g)	Chol. (mg)	Sod. (mg)	Carb. (g)	Fiber (g)	Pro. (g)	Servings/Exchanges
Coffee Coolatta with Cream & Coolatta Whirl-Ins made with Oreo Cookie	16 oz	460	24	47	14	75	150	58	0	4	4 carb, 3 fat
Coffee Coolatta with Milk & Chocolate Mint Cookie Coolatta Whirl-Ins	16 oz	310	6	17	3	15	130	59	0	4	4 carb, 1 fat
Coffee Coolatta with Milk & Coolatta Whirl-Ins made with Oreo Cookie	16 oz	300	5	15	3	15	160	60	0	4	4 carb, 1 fat
Coffee Coolatta with Skim Milk & Chocolate Mint Cookie Coolatta Whirl-Ins	16 oz	280	3	10	0	5	135	59	0	4	4 carb, 1 fat
Coffee Coolatta with Skim Milk & Coolatta Whirl-Ins made with Oreo Cookie	16 oz	270	2	7	0	5	160	60	0	5	4 carb, 1 fat
Dunkaccino	10 oz	250	11	40	3.5	10	240	34	0	2	2 carb, 2 fat
Hot Chocolate	10 oz	230	8	31	2	0	310	38	2	2	2 1/2 carb, 1 fat

Orange Mango Fruit Coolatta	16 oz	290	0	0	0	0	30	71	0	0	4 1/2 carb
Pina Coolatta	16 oz	270	4	13	3	0	65	57	0	1	3 1/2 carb, 1 fat
Strawberry Fruit Coolatta	16 oz	280	0	0	0	0	30	70	1	0	4 1/2 carb
Vanilla Bean Coolatta & Coolatta Whirl-Ins made with Oreo Cookie	16 oz	500	18	32	15	0	170	83	0	2	5 1/2 carb, 3 fat
Vanilla Bean Coolatta (Skim Milk)	16 oz	450	7	14	4	0	170	94	0	1	6 carb, 1 fat
Vanilla Bean Coolatta with Chocolate Mint Cookie Coolatta Whirl-Ins	16 oz	500	19	34	15	0	150	82	0	2	5 1/2 carb, 3 fat

BREAKFAST CROISSANT SANDWICHES

Bagel, Bacon Cheddar Omwich	1	600	21	32	8	295	1630	79	0	26	5 starch, 1 medium-fat meat, 3 fat
Bagel, Pizza Omwich	1	560	19	31	6	255	1305	74	2	25	5 starch, 1 medium-fat meat, 2 fat

✔ = Healthiest Bets; n/a = not available

(Continued)

BREAKFAST CROISSANT SANDWICHES (*Continued*)	Amount	Cal.	Fat (g)	% Cal. Fat	Sat. Fat (g)	Chol. (mg)	Sod. (mg)	Carb. (g)	Fiber (g)	Pro. (g)	Servings/Exchanges
Biscuit, Egg & Cheese	1	380	22	52	8	180	1250	30	0	17	2 starch, 2 medium-fat meat, 2 fat
Biscuit, Bacon & Cheddar Omwich	1	500	32	58	11	300	1660	33	1	21	2 starch, 2 medium-fat meat, 4 fat
Biscuit, Egg, Sausage & Cheese	1	590	42	64	15	220	1620	31	0	25	2 starch, 3 medium-fat meat, 5 fat
Biscuit, Pizza Omwich	1	500	30	54	9	255	1475	39	0	19	2 1/2 starch, 2 medium-fat meat, 3 fat
Biscuit, Spanish Omwich	1	470	29	56	9	285	1400	34	1	19	2 starch, 2 medium-fat meat, 2 fat
Croissant, Bacon & Cheddar Omwich	1	560	38	61	13	295	1190	33	1	21	2 starch, 2 medium-fat meat, 6 fat

Croissant, Spanish & Cheese Omwich	1	530	36	61	11	285	930	33	1	19	2 starch, 2 medium-fat meat, 5 fat
English Muffin, Bacon & Cheddar Omwich	1	400	21	47	8	295	1440	33	2	21	2 starch, 2 medium-fat meat, 2 fat
English Muffin, Egg, Ham & Cheese	1	320	12	34	6	195	1340	31	2	22	2 starch, 2 medium-fat meat
English Muffin, Pizza Omwich	1	350	17	44	6	255	1145	33	1	17	2 starch, 2 medium-fat meat, 1 fat
English Muffin, Spanish Omwich	1	370	18	44	6	280	1180	34	2	18	2 starch, 2 medium-fat meat, 1 fat

CAKE DONUTS

Blueberry	1	290	16	50	3.5	10	400	35	1	3	2 carb, 2 fat
✓ Blueberry Crumb	1	240	10	38	3	0	260	36	1	3	2 1/2 carb, 1 fat

(Continued)

✓ = Healthiest Bets; n/a = not available

CAKE DONUTS (Continued)	Amount	Cal.	Fat (g)	% Cal. Fat	Sat. Fat (g)	Chol. (mg)	Sod. (mg)	Carb. (g)	Fiber (g)	Pro. (g)	Servings/Exchanges
Butternut	1	300	16	48	4.5	0	360	36	1	3	2 1/2 carb, 2 fat
Chocolate Coconut	1	300	19	57	6	0	370	31	1	4	2 carb, 3 fat
Chocolate Glazed	1	290	16	50	3.5	0	370	33	1	3	2 carb, 3 fat
Cinnamon	1	270	15	50	3	0	360	31	1	3	2 carb, 3 fat
Coconut	1	290	17	53	5	0	360	33	1	3	2 carb, 3 fat
Double Chocolate	1	310	17	49	3.5	0	370	37	2	3	2 1/2 carb, 2 1/2 fat
Old Fashioned	1	250	15	54	3	0	360	26	1	3	1 1/2 carb, 3 fat
Powdered	1	270	15	50	3	0	350	32	1	3	2 carb, 2 1/2 fat
Sugared	1	250	15	54	3	0	350	27	1	3	2 carb, 2 1/2 fat
Toasted Coconut	1	300	17	51	5	0	370	35	1	3	2 carb, 3 fat
Whole Wheat Glazed	1	310	19	55	4	0	380	32	2	4	2 carb, 2 1/2 fat

CAKE MUNCHKINS

Butternut	3	200	11	50	3	0	240	25	1	2	1 1/2 carb, 2 fat
✔ Chocolate Glazed	3	200	10	45	2	0	250	26	1	2	1 1/2 carb, 2 fat
Cinnamon	4	250	14	50	3	0	330	30	1	3	2 carb, 2 1/2 fat
Coconut	3	200	12	54	3.5	0	240	23	1	2	1 1/2 carb, 2 fat
✔ Glazed Cake	3	200	10	45	2	0	250	22	1	2	2 carb, 2 fat
Plain	4	220	14	57	3	0	310	22	1	2	1 1/2 carb, 2 1/2 fat
Powdered Sugar	4	250	14	50	3	0	310	29	1	2	2 carb, 2 1/2 fat
Sugared	4	240	14	53	3	0	310	28	1	2	2 carb, 2 1/2 fat
Toasted Coconut	3	200	11	50	3	0	250	24	1	2	1 1/2 carb, 2 fat

COOKIES

Chocolate Chocolate Chunk	1	210	11	47	7	35	110	26	2	3	1 1/2 carb, 2 fat
Chocolate Chunk	1	220	11	45	7	35	105	28	1	3	2 carb, 2 fat

✔ = Healthiest Bets; n/a = not available

(Continued)

COOKIES *(Continued)*	Amount	Cal.	Fat (g)	% Cal. Fat	Sat. Fat (g)	Chol. (mg)	Sod. (mg)	Carb. (g)	Fiber (g)	Pro. (g)	Servings/Exchanges
Chocolate Chunk w/ Nuts	1	230	12	47	6	35	110	27	1	3	2 carb, 2 fat
Chocolate White Chocolate Chunk	1	230	12	47	7	35	120	28	1	3	2 carb, 2 fat
✔Oatmeal Raisin Pecan	1	220	10	41	5	30	110	29	1	3	2 carb, 2 fat
Peanut Butter Chocolate Chunk w/ Nuts	1	240	14	53	6	25	125	24	2	4	1 1/2 carb, 2 fat
Peanut Butter w/ Nuts	1	240	14	53	6	30	150	24	1	5	1 1/2 carb, 2 fat
CREAM CHEESES											
✔Classic Lite	1 Packet	130	11	76	7	30	250	3	0	5	2 fat
Classic Plain	1 Packet	200	19	86	13	60	230	3	0	4	4 fat
Garden Veggie	1 Packet	180	17	85	11	45	310	3	1	3	4 fat
Savory Chive	1 Packet	190	19	90	13	55	220	3	1	3	4 fat

Smoked Salmon	1 Packet	180	17	85	11	50	150	2	0	5	4 fat
Strawberry	1 Packet	180	16	80	9	0	0	9	0	2	4 fat

CROISSANTS

Plain	1	290	18	56	6	5	270	26	1	5	1 1/2 starch, 3 fat

CRULLERS/STICKS

Glazed Chocolate Cruller	1	280	15	48	3	0	360	35	1	3	2 carb, 3 fat
Glazed Cruller	1	290	15	47	3	0	350	37	2	3	2 1/2 carb, 3 fat
Jelly Stick	1	290	12	37	2.5	0	390	44	1	3	3 carb, 2 fat
Plain Cruller	1	240	15	56	3	0	350	32	1	3	2 carb, 3 fat
Powdered Cruller	1	270	15	50	3	0	340	30	1	3	2 carb, 3 fat
Sugar Cruller	1	250	15	54	3	0	340	27	1	3	2 carb, 3 fat

FANCIES

Apple Fritter	1	300	14	42	3	0	360	41	1	4	2 1/2 carb, 2 1/2 fat

(Continued)

✓ = Healthiest Bets; n/a = not available

FANCIES (*Continued*)	Amount	Cal.	Fat (g)	% Cal. Fat	Sat. Fat (g)	Chol. (mg)	Sod. (mg)	Carb. (g)	Fiber (g)	Pro. (g)	Servings/Exchanges
Bismark, Chocolate Iced	1	340	15	40	3.5	0	290	50	1	3	3 carb, 3 fat
Bow Tie	1	300	17	51	3.5	0	340	34	1	4	2 carb, 3 fat
Chocolate Frosted Coffee Roll	1	290	15	47	3	0	340	36	1	4	2 1/2 carb, 3 fat
Cinnamon Bun	1	510	15	26	4	0	420	85	0	8	5 1/2 carb, 3 fat
Coffee Roll	1	270	14	47	3	0	340	33	1	4	2 carb, 2 1/2 fat
Eclair	1	270	11	37	2.5	0	290	39	1	3	2 1/2 carb, 2 fat
Glazed Fritter	1	260	14	48	3	0	330	31	1	4	3 carb, 2 1/2 fat
Maple Frosted Coffee Roll	1	290	14	43	3	0	340	36	1	4	2 1/2 carb, 2 fat
✓Vanilla Frosted Coffee Roll	1	290	9	28	2	0	260	30	1	3	2 carb, 2 fat
LOW-FAT MUFFINS											
Blueberry	1	450	12	24	9	65	590	77	2	8	5 starch, 2 fat

MUFFINS

Apple Cinnamon Pecan	1	510	21	37	6	70	590	74	1	8	5 starch, 3 fat
Banana Nut	1	530	23	39	6	75	540	72	2	11	5 starch, 3 fat
Blueberry	1	490	17	31	6	75	610	76	2	8	5 starch, 3 fat
Chocolate Chip	1	590	24	37	10	75	560	88	3	9	6 starch, 3 fat
Corn	1	500	16	29	4.5	80	920	78	1	10	5 starch, 3 fat
Cranberry Orange	1	470	15	29	5	75	600	76	2	8	5 starch, 3 fat
Honey Raisin Bran	1	490	16	29	3.5	30	880	84	5	7	5 1/2 starch, 3 fat
Lemon Poppy Seed	1	580	19	29	6	85	620	94	2	10	6 starch, 3 fat

YEAST DONUTS

✔ Apple Crumb	1	230	10	39	3	0	270	34	1	3	2 carb, 1 1/2 fat
✔ Apple n' Spice	1	200	8	36	1.5	0	270	29	1	3	2 carb, 1 fat
✔ Bavarian Kreme	1	210	9	39	2	0	270	30	1	3	2 carb, 2 fat

✔ = Healthiest Bets; n/a = not available

(Continued)

YEAST DONUTS (*Continued*)	Amount	Cal.	Fat (g)	% Cal. Fat	Sat. Fat (g)	Chol. (mg)	Sod. (mg)	Carb. (g)	Fiber (g)	Pro. (g)	Servings/Exchanges
✔Black Raspberry	1	210	8	34	1.5	0	280	32	1	3	2 carb, 2 fat
✔Boston Kreme	1	240	9	34	2	0	280	36	1	3	2 1/2 carb, 2 fat
Caramel Apple Krunch	1	300	14	42	3	0	310	41	1	4	2 1/2 carb, 3 fat
✔Chocolate Frosted	1	200	9	41	2	0	260	29	1	3	2 carb, 1 1/2 fat
Chocolate Kreme Filled	1	270	13	43	3	0	260	35	0	3	2 carb, 2 1/2 fat
✔Glazed	1	180	8	40	1.5	0	250	25	1	3	1 1/2 carb, 1 1/2 fat
✔Jelly Filled	1	210	8	34	1.5	0	280	32	1	3	2 carb, 1 1/2 fat
✔Lemon	1	200	9	41	2	0	270	28	1	3	2 carb, 1 1/2 fat
✔Maple Frosted	1	210	9	39	2	0	260	30	1	3	2 carb, 1 1/2 fat
✔Marble Frosted	1	200	9	41	2	0	260	29	1	3	2 carb, 1 1/2 fat
✔Strawberry	1	210	8	34	1.5	0	260	32	1	3	2 carb, 1 1/2 fat
✔Strawberry Frosted	1	210	9	39	2	0	260	30	1	3	2 carb, 1 1/2 fat

✔ Sugar Raised	1	170	8	42	1.5	0	250	22	1	3	1 1/2 carb, 1 1/2 fat
✔ Vanilla Frosted	1	210	9	39	2	0	260	30	1	3	2 carb, 1 1/2 fat
Vanilla Kreme Filled Donut	1	270	13	43	3	0	250	36	1	3	2 1/2 carb, 2 fat

YEAST MUNCHKINS

✔ Glazed Raised	5	200	9	41	2	0	220	27	1	3	2 carb, 1 1/2 fat
✔ Jelly	5	210	9	39	2	0	240	30	1	3	2 carb, 1 1/2 fat
✔ Lemon	4	170	8	42	1.5	0	190	23	1	2	1 1/2 carb, 1 1/2 fat
✔ Sugar Raised	6	220	12	49	2.5	0	290	26	1	4	1 1/2 carb, 2 fat

✔ = Healthiest Bets; n/a = not available

Einstein Bros Bagels

❖Einstein Bros Bagels provided nutrition
information for their menu items for this book;
the information is not on their website at
www.einsteinbros.com.

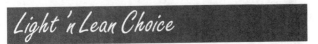

Light 'n Lean Choice

Red Beans & Rice Soup *(bowl)*
1/2 Tuna Sandwich on 12 Grain Bread

Calories 415	Sodium (mg) 1,530
Fat (g) 5	Carbohydrate (g).........67
% calories from fat..11	Fiber (g) 12
Saturated fat (g)........1	Protein (g) 22
Cholesterol (mg) 15	

Exchanges: 4 starch, 2 lean meat

Healthy 'n Hearty Choice

Dark Pumpernickel Bagel with
2 T Sun-Dried Tomato & Basil Cream Cheese
Cappuccino, regular nonfat

Calories......................440	Sodium (mg) 875
Fat (g) 6	Carbohydrate (g).........79
% calories from fat..12	Fiber (g) 3
Saturated fat (g).....3.5	Protein (g) 18
Cholesterol (mg) 20	

Exchanges: 4 starch, 1 fat-free milk, 1 fat

Einstein Bros Bagels

12 GRAIN BREAD SANDWICHES

	Amount	Cal.	Fat (g)	% Cal. Fat	Sat. Fat (g)	Chol. (mg)	Sod. (mg)	Carb. (g)	Fiber (g)	Pro. (g)	Servings/Exchanges
Chicken Salad	1	470	15	29	2	50	1230	59	6	26	4 starch, 2 lean meat, 1 fat
Egg Salad	1	490	21	39	4	315	800	57	5	18	4 starch, 1 medium-fat meat, 2 fat
Ham	1	560	25	40	7	75	1680	55	5	29	3 1/2 starch, 3 lean meat, 2 fat
Roast Beef	1	560	24	39	7	80	1170	56	5	34	3 1/2 starch, 3 lean meat, 3 fat
Smoked Turkey	1	530	21	36	6	70	1700	56	5	31	3 1/2 starch, 3 lean meat, 2 fat

(Continued)

✓ = Healthiest Bets; n/a = not available

12 GRAIN BREAD SANDWICHES (*Continued*)	Amount	Cal.	Fat (g)	% Cal. Fat	Sat. Fat (g)	Chol. (mg)	Sod. (mg)	Carb. (g)	Fiber (g)	Pro. (g)	Servings/Exchanges
✓Tuna Salad	1	430	10	21	1.5	30	990	54	5	30	3 1/2 starch, 3 lean meat
Turkey Pastrami	1	540	21	35	6	70	1900	55	5	34	3 1/2 starch, 3 lean meat, 2 fat
Ultimate Toasted Cheese w/ Tomato	1	770	49	57	24	110	1130	53	4	32	3 1/2 starch, 3 high-fat meat, 4 fat
BAGEL SANDWICHES											
Chicago Bagel Dog, Asiago	1	740	34	41	15	80	1360	78	2	29	5 starch, 2 high-fat meat, 3 fat
Chicago Bagel Dog, everything	1	730	34	42	12	70	1850	80	3	26	5 starch, 2 high-fat meat, 3 fat
Chicago Bagel Dog, onion, no cheese	1	680	30	40	12	70	1220	78	2	25	5 starch, 2 high-fat meat, 2 fat

										Exchanges/Choices
Chicago Chili Cheese Bagel Dog	1	810	38	42	17	105	1550	83	4	33	5 1/2 starch, 2 high-fat meat, 3 fat
Egg (original)	1	480	10	19	4	270	680	74	2	23	5 starch, 1 medium-fat meat
Egg and Ham	1	530	13	22	5	295	1120	74	2	31	5 starch, 2 medium-fat meat
Egg and Sausage	1	550	14	23	5	295	1000	74	2	33	5 starch, 2 medium-fat meat
Egg Salad	1	560	18	29	4.5	315	860	79	3	20	5 starch, 1 medium-fat meat, 2 fat
Egg Santa Fe	1	650	24	33	8	300	1210	78	2	30	5 starch, 2 medium-fat meat, 2 fat
Egg with Bacon	1	580	19	29	7	285	970	74	2	29	5 starch, 2 medium-fat meat, 1 fat
Egg, Salmon Shmear	1	650	22	30	12	310	1040	82	3	31	5 1/2 starch, 2 medium-fat meat, 1 fat

(Continued)

✔ = Healthiest Bets; n/a = not available

BAGEL SANDWICHES (*Continued*)	Amount	Cal.	Fat (g)	% Cal. Fat	Sat. Fat (g)	Chol. (mg)	Sod. (mg)	Carb. (g)	Fiber (g)	Pro. (g)	Servings/Exchanges
Ham	1	450	6	12	1.5	45	1390	74	3	26	5 starch, 2 lean meat
Harvest Chicken Salad	1	540	12	20	2.5	50	1360	81	4	28	5 starch, 2 lean meat
Holey Cow	1	900	50	50	13	105	1450	77	3	36	5 starch, 3 medium-fat meats, 6 fat
Hummus & Feta	1	540	13	22	4	15	880	89	5	18	6 starch, 2 fat
New York Lox & Bagels	1	660	27	37	19	85	1150	79	3	26	5 starch, 2 medium-fat meat, 3 fat
Roast Beef	1	460	4	8	1.5	45	880	76	3	31	5 starch, 2 lean meat
Smoked Turkey	1	420	2	4	0	30	1270	75	3	25	5 starch, 2 very lean meat
Tasty Turkey	1	600	21	32	12	100	1510	78	3	27	5 starch, 2 lean meat, 2 fat
The Veg Out	1	490	13	24	7	30	850	77	3	17	5 starch, 2 fat
Tuna Salad	1	500	7	13	1.5	30	1060	77	3	32	5 starch, 2 lean meat, 2 fat

Turkey Pastrami Deli	1	440	2	4	0	40	1610	76	3	31	5 starch, 2 lean meat
Turkey Pastrami Reuben Deli	1	660	19	26	6	65	2590	83	4	39	5 1/2 starch, 3 medium-fat meat

BAGEL SHTICKS

Asiago	1	450	9	18	5	15	770	72	2	20	5 starch, 1 fat
Cinnamon Sugar	1	570	24	38	4	0	800	79	2	11	5 starch, 4 fat
Everything	1	380	5	12	0	0	1130	73	3	12	5 starch, 1 fat
✔Potato	1	350	5	13	1	0	590	69	2	10	4 starch, 1 fat
✔Sesame	1	420	8	17	1	0	510	75	5	13	5 starch, 1 fat

BAGEL SHTICKS MINI

✔Corn Meal	1/2	170	0	0	0	0	260	38	1	6	2 1/2 starch
✔Sesame	1/2	180	2	10	0	0	260	36	2	6	2 1/2 starch

(Continued)

✔ = Healthiest Bets; n/a = not available

	Amount	Cal.	Fat (g)	% Cal. Fat	Sat. Fat (g)	Chol. (mg)	Sod. (mg)	Carb. (g)	Fiber (g)	Pro. (g)	Servings/Exchanges
BAGELS											
✓Asiago Cheese	1	360	3	8	1.5	5	570	71	2	13	4 1/2 starch, 1/2 fat
✓Chocolate Chip	1	370	3	7	2	0	500	76	3	11	5 starch, 1/2 fat
✓Chopped Garlic	1	380	3	7	1	0	680	79	4	13	5 starch
✓Chopped Onion	1	330	1	3	0	0	500	71	2	11	4 1/2 starch
✓Cinnamon Raisin Swirl	1	350	1	3	0	0	490	78	2	11	5 starch
✓Cinnamon Sugar	1	330	1	3	0	0	490	74	2	10	5 starch
✓Cranberry	1	350	1	3	0	0	490	78	3	10	5 starch
✓Dark Pumpernickel	1	320	1	3	0	0	730	68	3	11	4 1/2 starch
✓Egg	1	340	3	8	1	35	510	69	2	11	4 1/2 starch, 1 fat
✓Everything	1	340	2	5	0	0	820	75	2	13	5 starch
✓Honey Whole Wheat	1	320	1	3	0	0	470	71	3	10	4 1/2 starch

✔Jalapeno	1	330	1	3	0	0	510	71	2	11	4 1/2 starch
✔Lucky Green	1	320	1	3	0	0	520	71	2	11	4 1/2 starch
✔Mango	1	360	1	3	0	0	490	80	2	10	5 starch
✔Marble Rye	1	340	2	5	0	0	690	73	3	11	5 starch
✔Nutty Banana	1	360	3	8	1	0	510	74	2	11	5 starch, 1/2 fat
✔Plain	1	320	1	3	0	0	520	71	2	11	4 1/2 starch
✔Poppy Dip'd Bagel	1	350	2	5	0	0	680	74	2	12	5 starch
✔Potato Bagel	1	350	5	13	1	0	590	69	2	10	4 1/2 starch, 1 fat
Power	1	410	5	11	0.5	0	310	81	4	13	5 1/2 starch, 1 fat
Power with Peanut Butter	1	750	34	41	6	0	780	92	7	27	5 1/2 starch, 2 high-fat meat, 2 fat
✔Pumpkin	1	330	2	5	0	0	470	72	3	10	5 starch
Salt	1	330	1	3	0	0	1790	73	2	11	5 starch

✔ = Healthiest Bets; n/a = not available

(Continued)

BAGELS (Continued)	Amount	Cal.	Fat (g)	% Cal. Fat	Sat. Fat (g)	Chol. (mg)	Sod. (mg)	Carb. (g)	Fiber (g)	Pro. (g)	Servings/Exchanges
✔Sesame Dip'd	1	280	5	16	1	0	680	75	3	11	5 starch, 1 fat
✔Sun Dried Tomato	1	320	1	3	0	0	520	69	3	11	4 1/2 starch
✔Wild Blueberry	1	350	1	3	0	0	510	77	3	11	5 starch
BEVERAGES											
✔Café Latte	12 oz	140	5	32	3.5	20	140	13	0	9	1 fat-free milk, 1 fat
Café Latte	16 oz	200	8	36	5	30	210	20	0	13	1 1/2 fat-free milk, 1 fat
Café Latte	20 oz	250	9	32	6	35	250	24	0	16	2 fat-free milk, 1 1/2 fat
✔Caffé Latte, nonfat	12 oz	100	0	0	0	5	140	14	0	9	1 fat-free milk
✔Caffé Latte, nonfat	16 oz	140	1	6	0.5	5	210	20	0	14	1 1/2 fat-free milk
✔Caffé Latte, nonfat	20 oz	180	1	5	0.5	10	260	25	0	16	2 fat-free milk
✔Cappuccino	12 oz	90	4	40	2	15	95	9	0	6	1 fat-free milk
Cappuccino	16 oz	190	7	33	4.5	30	190	19	0	12	1 1/2 fat-free milk, 1 fat

Cappuccino	20 oz	230	9	35	5	35	240	23	0	15	2 fat-free milk, 1 1/2 fat
✔Cappuccino, low fat	16 oz	130	1	7	0	5	200	19	0	13	1 1/2 fat-free milk
Cappuccino, low fat	20 oz	150	6	36	3.5	20	150	15	0	10	1 fat-free milk, 1 fat
✔Cappuccino, nonfat	12 oz	60	0	0	0	5	95	9	0	6	1 fat-free milk
✔Espresso	1.5 oz	1	0	0	0	0	0	0	0	0	free
Hot Cocoa	12 oz	290	11	34	8	20	160	39	0	9	1 fat-free milk, 1 carb, 2 fat
✔Hot Cocoa, low fat	12 oz	260	7	24	6	5	160	39	0	9	1 fat-free milk, 1 carb, 1 fat
✔Iced Latte	16 oz	120	5	38	3	20	125	12	0	8	1 fat-free milk, 1 fat
✔Iced Latte, nonfat	16 oz	90	0	0	0	5	130	12	0	8	1 fat-free milk
Iced Mocha	16 oz	210	6	26	4	15	120	33	0	7	1 fat-free milk, 1 carb, 1 fat
✔Iced Mocha, lowfat	16 oz	25	3	108	2	5	115	32	0	7	1 fat-free milk, 1 carb
Mocha	12 oz	230	6	23	4.5	15	135	34	0	8	1 fat-free milk, 1 carb, 1 fat
Mocha	16 oz	390	20	46	12	75	170	42	1	10	1 fat-free milk, 2 carb, 3 fat

(Continued)

✔ = Healthiest Bets; n/a = not available

BEVERAGES *(Continued)*	Amount	Cal.	Fat (g)	% Cal. Fat	Sat. Fat (g)	Chol. (mg)	Sod. (mg)	Carb. (g)	Fiber (g)	Pro. (g)	Servings/Exchanges
Mocha	20 oz	470	22	42	13	85	230	56	1	13	2 fat-free milk, 2 carb, 3 fat
Mocha Smoothie	16 oz	470	5	10	3	20	170	98	0	9	2 fat-free milk, 4 carb
✔ Mocha, low fat	12 oz	190	3	14	2	5	130	34	0	8	1 fat-free milk, 1 carb
Mocha, low fat	16 oz	350	15	39	9	60	180	42	1	10	1 fat-free milk, 2 carb, 2 fat
Mocha, low fat	20 oz	420	16	34	9	65	240	56	1	15	2 fat-free milk, 2 carb, 2 fat
✔ Odwalla Fresh Squeezed Orange Juice	10 oz	143	0	0	0	0	71	34	2	1	1 1/2 fruit
CHALLAH SANDWICHES											
✔ BBQ Chicken	1	380	8	19	2	80	1000	52	2	27	3 1/2 starch, 2 lean meat
Chicken Salad	1	410	14	31	3	80	1040	47	3	26	3 starch, 2 lean meat, 1 fat
Club Mex	1	750	45	54	14	135	2290	47	2	39	3 starch, 4 medium-fat meat, 5 fat

Cobbie	1	630	33	47	12	110	1920	45	4	37	3 starch, 4 medium-fat meat, 2 fat
✔ Egg Salad	1	430	20	42	5	345	540	45	2	18	3 starch, 1 medium-fat meat, 3 fat
Pastrami	1	480	21	39	7	100	1650	43	2	34	3 starch, 4 lean meat
Roast Beef	1	500	23	41	8	110	920	44	2	34	3 starch, 4 lean meat, 1 fat
Roasted Chicken & Smoked Gouda	1	440	13	27	6	110	1010	47	2	36	3 starch, 4 lean meat
Smoked Turkey	1	470	21	40	7	100	1450	44	2	31	3 starch, 3 lean meat, 1 1/2 fat
✔ Tuna Salad	1	370	10	24	2.5	60	740	42	2	30	3 starch, 3 lean meat
Turkey Ham	1	500	25	45	8	105	1430	43	2	29	3 starch, 3 lean meat, 2 fat

(Continued)

✔ = Healthiest Bets; n/a = not available

	Amount	Cal.	Fat (g)	% Cal. Fat	Sat. Fat (g)	Chol. (mg)	Sod. (mg)	Carb. (g)	Fiber (g)	Pro. (g)	Servings/Exchanges
COFFEE EXTRAS											
Almond Syrup	2 T	90	0	0	0	0	0	23	0	0	1 1/2 carb
✔Caramel, sugar free	2 T	0	0	0	0	0	0	0	0	0	free
Hazelnut Syrup	2 T	80	0	0	0	0	0	20	0	0	1 carb
Light Whipped Cream	2 T	30	2	60	1.5	10	0	2	0	0	1/2 fat
✔On Top Reduced Fat Topping	2 T	20	2	90	1	0	5	2	0	0	free
Raspberry Syrup	2 T	80	0	0	0	0	0	20	0	0	1 carb
Vanilla Syrup	2 T	80	0	0	0	0	0	19	0	0	1 carb
✔Vanilla, sugar free	2 T	0	0	0	0	0	0	0	0	0	free
CONDIMENTS											
✔Ancho Lime Mayo	1 T	50	5	90	1	5	160	1	0	0	1 fat
✔Ancho Lime Salsa	1/4 cup/4 T	20	1	45	0	0	670	3	0	0	free

	Amount										Exchanges
✔Honey Mustard	1 t	15	0	0	0	0	45	2	0	0	free
✔Marinated Red Onions	4 oz	150	12	72	2	0	160	9	2	1	2 vegetable, 2 fat
✔Raspberry Mustard	2 T	50	2	36	0	2	190	7	0	1	1/2 carb
✔Whole Kosher Pickle	1	5	0	0	0	0	650	1	1	0	free
COOKIES											
Chocolate Chunk	1	600	28	42	10	45	480	78	3	8	5 carb, 4 fat
Ginger White Chocolate	1	510	17	30	8	25	350	81	1	7	5 carb, 2 fat
Oatmeal Raisin	1	550	21	34	5	40	320	82	4	8	5 1/2 carb, 2 fat
Peanut Butter	1	620	35	51	10	55	620	66	2	10	4 1/2 carb, 6 fat
Sugar	1	610	32	47	8	55	490	73	1	7	5 carb, 5 fat
COUNTRY WHITE SANDWICHES											
Chicken Salad	1	570	17	27	4	50	1770	79	4	30	5 starch, 2 lean meat, 1 fat

(Continued)

✔ = Healthiest Bets; n/a = not available

COUNTRY WHITE SANDWICHES *(Continued)*	Amount	Cal.	Fat (g)	% Cal. Fat	Sat. Fat (g)	Chol. (mg)	Sod. (mg)	Carb. (g)	Fiber (g)	Pro. (g)	Servings/Exchanges
Egg Salad	1	590	23	35	6	315	1280	77	3	22	5 starch, 1 medium-fat meat, 3 fat
Ham	1	660	27	37	9	15	2160	75	3	33	5 starch, 3 lean meat, 2 fat
Roast Beef	1	660	26	35	9	80	1650	76	3	38	5 starch, 3 lean meat, 2 fat
Smoked Turkey	1	630	23	33	8	70	2180	76	3	35	5 starch, 3 lean meat, 1 1/2 fat
Tuna Salad	1	530	12	20	3.5	30	1470	74	3	34	5 starch, 3 lean meat
Turkey Pastrami	1	640	23	32	8	70	2380	75	3	38	5 starch, 3 lean meat, 2 fat
Ultimate Toasted Cheese w/ Tomato	1	870	51	53	26	110	1610	73	2	36	5 starch, 3 high-fat meat, 4 fat
CREAM CHEESES											
✔Blueberry	2 T	70	4	51	3	1	45	6	0	1	1/2 carb, 1 fat

✔Cappuccino	2 T	70	5	64	3.5	15	50	4	0	2	1 fat
✔Garden Vegetable	2 T	60	5	75	3.5	15	105	2	0	1	1 fat
✔Honey Almond Reduced Fat	2 T	70	5	64	3	15	40	5	0	1	1 fat
✔Jalapeno Salsa	2 T	60	5	75	3	15	95	3	0	1	1 fat
✔Maple Raisin Walnut	2 T	60	5	75	3.5	15	45	4	0	1	1 fat
✔Onion and Chive	2 T	70	6	77	4	20	70	2	0	1	1 fat
✔Plain	2 T	70	7	90	4.5	20	65	1	0	1	1 fat
✔Plain Reduced Fat	2 T	60	5	75	3.5	15	85	2	0	1	1 fat
✔Smoked Salmon	2 T	60	5	75	3.5	15	115	3	0	1	1 fat
✔Strawberry	2 T	70	5	64	3.5	15	50	5	0	1	1 fat
✔Sun-Dried Tomato & Basil	2 T	60	5	75	3.5	15	50	2	0	1	1 fat
DESSERTS											
Brownie	1	500	21	38	4	30	280	76	2	4	5 carb, 3 fat

✔ = Healthiest Bets; n/a = not available

(Continued)

DESSERTS (*Continued*)	Amount	Cal.	Fat (g)	% Cal. Fat	Sat. Fat (g)	Chol. (mg)	Sod. (mg)	Carb. (g)	Fiber (g)	Pro. (g)	Servings/Exchanges
✔Cinnamon Bun w/ Icing	1	380	10	24	2	0	310	64	2	8	4 carb, 1 fat
✔Fresh Fruit Cup	8 oz	110	1	8	0	0	10	25	2	1	1 1/2 fruit
Pound Cake, Lemon Iced	1 slice	540	24	40	13	155	420	74	0	7	5 carb, 3 fat
Pound Cake, Marble	1 slice	460	24	47	12	150	430	57	1	7	4 carb, 3 fat
Rice Krispy Bar	1	420	8	17	1.5	0	610	83	1	5	5 1/2 carb
Sticky Bun	1	470	13	25	1.5	0	280	77	3	9	5 carb, 2 fat
FLAT BREADS											
Peanut Sesame	1	650	15	21	2	0	1520	111	5	18	7 1/2 starch, 2 fat
Rosemary & Asiago	1	520	9	16	3.5	5	1010	92	3	18	6 starch, 2 fat
FOCACCIA											
Cheese Pizza	1	500	11	20	7	35	1010	75	3	25	5 starch, 1 high-fat meat
Margherita	1	400	17	38	1.5	5	580	76	3	14	5 starch, 2 fats

	Amount										
Pepperoni Pizza	1	590	19	29	10	55	1380	76	3	29	5 starch, 2 high-fat meat
MUFFINS											
Banana Nut	1	520	29	50	5	95	430	59	3	9	4 starch, 4 fat
Blueberry	1	460	24	47	2.5	90	410	57	2	6	4 starch, 3 fat
Chocolate Chip	1	240	13	49	3	40	180	67	0	3	4 1/2 starch, 2 fat
Morning Harvest	1	460	19	37	3.5	70	370	69	4	7	4 1/2 starch, 2 fat
✔ Poppy Seed, low fat	1	370	7	17	1	0	560	69	1	8	4 1/2 starch
Pumpkin Pecan	1	480	30	56	5	80	360	50	3	6	3 starch, 5 fat
ROLL-UPS											
Albuquerque Turkey	1	790	39	44	15	85	2040	81	5	31	5 1/2 carb, 2 lean meat, 5 fat
Thai Vegetable	1	630	21	30	2	0	1310	97	5	24	6 starch, 2 vegetable, 2 fat
Thai Vegetable w/ Chicken	1	670	18	24	1	40	1850	99	4	27	6 starch, 2 vegetable, 1 lean meat, 3 fat

(Continued)

✔ = Healthiest Bets; n/a = not available

	Amount	Cal.	Fat (g)	% Cal. Fat	Sat. Fat (g)	Chol. (mg)	Sod. (mg)	Carb. (g)	Fiber (g)	Pro. (g)	Servings/Exchanges
ROLLS											
✔Challah	1	200	4	18	1	30	190	36	1	8	2 1/2 starch
SALAD DRESSINGS											
Asian Sesame	2 T	80	2	23	0	0	600	16	0	1	1 carb
Caesar	2 T	150	16	96	2.5	10	360	1	0	1	3 fat
✔Chicken & Tuna	2 T	52	5	87	1	10	250	2	0	0	1 fat
✔Chipotle BBQ	2 T	110	11	90	1.5	0	220	4	0	0	2 fat
✔Harvest Chicken Salad	2 T	90	8	80	1.5	15	410	3	0	1	1 1/2 fat
✔Honey Chipotle	2 T	140	10	64	1.5	0	210	12	0	0	1/2 carb, 2 fat
Horseradish Sauce	2 T	170	18	95	3	20	190	1	0	0	4 fat
Raspberry Vinaigrette	2 T	160	14	79	2	0	80	8	0	0	1 carb, 3 fat
✔Thousand Island	2 T	110	9	74	20	10	210	5	0	0	2 fat

	Amount	Cal.	Fat (g)	% Cal. Fat	Sat. Fat (g)	Chol. (mg)	Sod. (mg)	Carb. (g)	Fiber (g)	Pro. (g)	Exchanges/Choices
✓Wasabi Oriental	2 T	80	8	90	0	0	320	5	0	1	1 1/2 fat
SALAD EXTRAS											
✓Bagel Croutons	2 T	25	1	36	0	0	75	4	0	1	free
Sweet Roasted Walnuts	2 T	180	15	75	1.5	0	85	7	1	5	1/2 carb, 3 fat
SALADS											
Asian Chicken w/ Peanut Sesame Flat Bread	1	480	5	9	1	55	1520	84	4	24	5 starch, 2 vegetable, 1 very lean meat
Bros Bistro w/ Rosemary Asiago Flat Bread	1	1050	52	45	14	30	1640	117	5	28	7 starch, 2 vegetables, 3 medium-fat meat, 5 fat
Caesar—small side	1	220	17	70	3	10	520	12	1	4	2 vegetable, 2 fat
Chicken Chipotle Spinach Salad w/ Mini Shticks	1	640	44	62	10	80	1420	33	5	32	2 vegetable, 1 1/2 starch, 3 lean meat, 7 fat
Egg	1/2 cup/4 oz	200	17	77	4	310	340	5	0	9	1 medium-fat meat, 3 fat

(Continued)

✓ = Healthiest Bets; n/a = not available

SALADS (*Continued*)	Amount	Cal.	Fat (g)	% Cal. Fat	Sat. Fat (g)	Chol. (mg)	Sod. (mg)	Carb. (g)	Fiber (g)	Pro. (g)	Servings/Exchanges
Harvest Chicken w/ Rosemary & Asiago Flat Bread	1	730	20	25	5	55	1880	103	5	36	6 starch, 2 vegetable, 3 lean meat, 1 fat
Mind-Bageling Side	1	220	18	74	3	0	380	13	1	2	1 starch, 3 fat
Potato	1/2 cup/4 oz	290	21	65	3	15	600	21	2	3	1 1/2 starch, 4 fat
Roasted Chicken Caesar w/ Rosemary & Asiago Flat Bread	1	890	42	42	9	85	2-50	86	4	40	5 starch, 2 vegetable, 3 lean meat, 7 fat
✓Roasted Corn	1	90	3	30	0	0	150	13	4	2	1 starch
✓Tuna	1/4 cup/2 oz	150	6	36	1	30	540	3	0	21	3 lean meat
Wasabi Salmon Spinach Salad w/ Mini Shticks	1	430	3	6	2.5	105	1750	28	3	20	1 starch, 2 vegetables, 2 lean meat, 1 fat
SCONES											
Blueberry w/ Icing	1	450	18	36	8	55	460	64	2	7	4 starch, 3 fat

Item	Serving	Cal	Fat (g)	% Fat	Sat Fat (g)	Chol (mg)	Sodium (mg)	Carb (g)	Fiber (g)	Prot (g)	Exchanges/Choices
✔ Raspberry, low fat	1	350	3	8	0.5	25	330	74	2	7	5 starch
SIDE ITEMS											
✔ Fruit & Yogurt Parfait	10 oz	190	1	5	0	5	115	38	4	7	1 fat-free milk, 1 carb
✔ Potato Chips, Kettle Classic Natural	1 oz	100	10	90	2	0	130	11	1	1	1/2 starch, 2 fat
SOUPS											
Chicken & Wild Rice	bowl	320	16	45	3	40	1710	30	3	20	2 starch, 2 lean meat, 1 fat
✔ Chicken & Wild Rice	cup	190	10	47	2	25	990	18	2	10	1 starch, 1 lean meat, 1 fat
✔ Chicken Noodle	bowl	210	7	30	0	5	1070	30	4	7	2 starch, 1 fat
✔ Chicken Noodle	cup	140	5	32	0	35	680	19	2	10	1 starch, 1 lean meat
Cream of Potato	bowl	280	13	42	4	5	1280	35	5	7	2 starch, 3 fat
✔ Cream of Potato	cup	180	8	40	2.5	5	830	23	3	10	1 1/2 starch, 1 1/2 fat
✔ Red Beans & Rice	bowl	200	0	0	0	0	1040	40	9	7	2 1/2 starch

✔ = Healthiest Bets; n/a = not available

(Continued)

SOUPS *(Continued)*	Amount	Cal.	Fat (g)	% Cal. Fat	Sat. Fat (g)	Chol. (mg)	Sod. (mg)	Carb. (g)	Fiber (g)	Pro. (g)	Servings/Exchanges
✔Red Beans & Rice	cup	130	0	0	0	0	680	26	6	6	1 1/2 starch
Turkey Chili w/ Beans	bowl	340	17	45	3.5	50	1630	28	3	10	2 starch, 1 lean meat, 3 fat
Turkey Chili w/ Beans	cup	240	12	45	2.5	35	1160	20	2	12	1 starch, 1 lean meat, 2 fat
✔Vegetarian Black Bean	bowl	240	6	23	1.5	0	1030	34	10	14	2 starch, 1 lean meat, 1 fat
✔Vegetarian Black Bean	cup	160	4	23	1	0	690	23	7	9	1 starch, 1 lean meat
Zesty Lentil	bowl	220	5	20	0.5	0	1140	34	11	10	2 starch, 1 lean meat
✔Zesty Lentil	cup	130	3	21	0	0	680	20	7	6	1 starch, 1 lean meat

✔ = Healthiest Bets; n/a = not available

Krispy Kreme Doughnuts

❖Krispy Kreme Doughnuts provides nutrition
information for all their menu items on their
website at www.krispykreme.com.

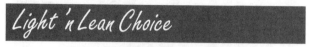

1 Traditional Cake Doughnut
8 oz Fat-Free Milk

Calories......................286	Sodium (mg).............406
Fat (g) 11	Carbohydrate (g).........34
% calories from fat..35	Fiber (g) 0
Saturated fat (g)........3	Protein (g) 11
Cholesterol (mg).........15	

Exchanges: 1 1/2 carb, 1 fat-free milk, 2 fat

Healthy 'n Hearty Choice

1 Original Glazed Doughnut
8 oz Orange Juice

Calories......................322	Sodium (mg)...............67
Fat (g) 12	Carbohydrate (g).........49
% calories from fat..34	Fiber (g) 0
Saturated fat (g)........4	Protein (g) 4
Cholesterol (mg)...........5	

Exchanges: 1 1/2 carb, 2 fruit, 2 fat

(Continued)

Krispy Kreme Doughnuts

	Amount	Cal.	Fat (g)	% Cal. Fat	Sat. Fat (g)	Chol. (mg)	Sod. (mg)	Carb. (g)	Fiber (g)	Pro. (g)	Servings/Exchanges
CAKE DOUGHNUTS											
Fudge Iced Cake	1	230	12	47	3	15	280	28	1	3	2 carb, 1 1/2 fat
Traditional Cake	1	200	11	50	3	15	280	22	1	3	1 1/2 carb, 2 fat
CRULLERS											
Glazed	1	250	16	58	4	5	190	24	0	2	1 1/2 carb, 3 fat
Fudge Iced Cruller	1	240	12	45	3	10	160	31	1	2	2 carb, 2 fat
DOUGHNUTS											
Cinnamon Bun	1	220	11	45	3	0	160	23	4	5	1 1/2 carb, 2 fat
Cinnamon Twist	1	220	11	45	3	5	150	27	1	4	2 carb, 1 1/2 fat
Fudge Iced Glazed	1	280	14	45	4	5	75	26	1	3	1 1/2 carb, 3 fat

✔Fudge Iced Sprinkles	1	220	10	41	2.5	5	95	31	1	2	2 carb, 1 1/2 fat
Glazed Blueberry	1	300	15	45	3	5	200	37	1	2	2 1/2 carb, 2 fat
Glazed Devil's Food	1	390	24	55	5	5	250	41	5	2	2 1/2 carb, 4 fat
✔Maple Iced Glazed	1	200	9	41	2.5	0	100	28	2	3	2 carb, 1 fat
Original Glazed	1	210	12	51	4		65	22	0	2	1 1/2 carb, 2 fat
FILLED DOUGHNUTS											
Cinnamon Apple Filled	1	280	13	42	3	5	180	35	3	5	2 carb, 3 fat
Fudge Iced Crème Filled	1	340	18	48	5	5	160	39	4	5	2 1/2 carb, 3 fat
Fudge Iced Custard Filled	1	310	16	46	4	5	170	39	5	4	2 1/2 carb, 2 1/2 fat
Glazed Crème Filled	1	350	20	51	5	5	135	39	1	4	2 1/2 carb, 3 fat
Glazed Raspberry Filled	1	270	12	40	3	5	170	37	2	4	2 1/2 carb, 2 fat
Powdered Blueberry Filled	1	270	13	43	4	5	170	33	1	5	2 carb, 2 fat
Glazed Lemon Filled	1	280	14	45	4	5	160	33	1	5	2 carb, 2 fat

✔ = Healthiest Bets; n/a = not available

Manhattan Bagel Company

❖Manhattan Bagel Company provided nutrition information for its bagels and cream cheeses for this book.

Light 'n Lean Choice

Jalapeno Cheddar Bagel
Light Plain Cream Cheese (*2 T*)

Calories......................330	Sodium (mg)..............385
Fat (g) 8	Carbohydrate (g).........53
% calories from fat..22	Fiber (g) 3
Saturated fat (g)........4	Protein (g) 13
Cholesterol (mg).........20	

Exchanges: 3 1/2 starch, 1 1/2 fat

Healthy 'n Hearty Choice

Oat Goodness Bagel with
Light Raisin Walnut Cream Cheese (*2 T*)

Calories......................360	Sodium (mg)..............465
Fat (g) 8	Carbohydrate (g).........61
% calories from fat..20	Fiber (g) 3
Saturated fat (g)........3	Protein (g) 12
Cholesterol (mg).........15	

Exchanges: 4 starch, 1 fat

Manhattan Bagel Company

	Amount	Cal.	Fat (g)	% Cal. Fat	Sat. Fat (g)	Chol. (mg)	Sod. (mg)	Carb. (g)	Fiber (g)	Pro. (g)	Servings/Exchanges
BAGELS											
✔Banana Nut	1	300	5	15	1	0	520	55	3	10	3 1/2 starch, 1 fat
✔Blueberry	1	270	1	3	0	0	550	56	2	10	3 1/2 starch
✔Cheddar Cheese	1	270	2	7	1	5	560	51	2	11	3 1/2 starch, 1 fat
✔Chocolate Chip	1	280	2	6	1	0	510	58	3	10	4 starch
✔Cinnamon Raisin	1	270	1	3	0	0	520	56	3	10	3 1/2 starch
✔Egg	1	260	2	7	0	0	710	53	2	10	3 1/2 starch
✔Everything	1	260	1	3	0	0	510	53	2	10	3 1/2 starch
✔Garlic	1	260	1	3	0	0	510	54	2	10	3 1/2 starch

✔ = Healthiest Bets; n/a = not available

(Continued)

BAGELS (*Continued*)	Amount	Cal.	Fat (g)	% Cal. Fat	Sat. Fat (g)	Chol. (mg)	Sod. (mg)	Carb. (g)	Fiber (g)	Pro. (g)	Servings/Exchanges
✔Jalapeno Cheddar	1	260	2	7	0	0	280	52	3	10	3 1/2 starch
✔Marble	1	260	1	3	0	0	550	53	3	10	3 1/2 starch
✔Oat Goodness	1	280	3	10	0	0	390	55	3	10	3 1/2 starch
✔Onion	1	260	1	3	0	0	510	54	2	10	3 1/2 starch
✔Plain	1	270	1	3	0	0	540	55	2	11	3 1/2 starch
✔Poppy	1	270	2	7	0	0	510	53	3	10	3 1/2 starch
✔Pumpernickel	1	260	1	3	0	0	450	54	2	10	3 1/2 starch
✔Rye	1	260	1	3	0	0	550	53	3	10	3 1/2 starch
✔Salt	1	270	1	3	0	0	640	55	2	11	3 1/2 starch
✔Sesame	1	270	2	7	0	0	510	53	2	10	3 1/2 starch
✔Spinach	1	250	1	4	0	0	550	52	2	10	3 1/2 starch
✔Sun-Dried Tomato	1	260	1	3	0	0	320	53	3	11	3 1/2 starch

CREAM CHEESES

	Amount	Cal	Fat (g)	% Cal from Fat	Sat Fat (g)	Chol (mg)	Sod (mg)	Carb (g)	Fiber (g)	Pro (g)	Choices/Exchanges
✔ French Vanilla	2 T	100	7	63	4.5	20	85	8	0	1	1/2 carb, 1 fat
✔ Garlic and Herb	2 T	80	9	101	6	30	120	1	0	1	2 fat
✔ Honey Walnut	2 T	110	8	65	5	20	80	6	0	2	1/2 carb, 1 fat
✔ Lox	2 T	90	9	90	5	20	120	1	0	2	2 fat
✔ Olive and Pimento	2 T	80	8	90	4.5	20	180	1	0	1	2 fat
✔ Plain	2 T	90	9	90	6	30	120	1	0	1	2 fat
✔ Raisin Walnut	2 T	90	7	70	4	20	75	6	0	1	1/2 carb, 1 fat
✔ Scallion	2 T	90	9	90	5	20	100	2	0	1	2 fat
✔ Strawberry	2 T	80	6	68	3.5	15	60	6	0	1	1/2 carb, 1 fat
✔ Sun-Dried Tomato	2 T	80	7	79	4	15	110	2	0	1	1 1/2 fat
✔ Tijuana Hot	2 T	90	9	90	5	30	140	2	0	1	2 fat
✔ Vegetable	2 T	70	7	90	4	20	110	1	0	1	1 1/2 fat

✔ = Healthiest Bets; n/a = not available

(Continued)

CREAM CHEESES, LIGHT

	Amount	Cal.	Fat (g)	% Cal. Fat	Sat. Fat (g)	Chol. (mg)	Sod. (mg)	Carb. (g)	Fiber (g)	Pro. (g)	Servings/Exchanges
✔Lox	2 T	60	6	90	3.5	20	120	1	0	3	1 fat
✔Plain	2 T	70	6	77	4	20	105	1	0	3	1 fat
✔Raisin Walnut	2 T	80	5	56	3	15	75	6	0	2	1/2 carb, 1 fat
✔Scallion	2 T	60	6	90	3.5	20	100	1	0	2	1 fat
✔Vegetable	2 T	50	5	90	2.5	15	100	1	0	2	1 fat

✔ = Healthiest Bets; n/a = not available

Starbucks

❖Starbucks provided nutrition information only for some of its coffees.

Light 'n Lean Choice

Cappuccino (nonfat milk)

Calories......................80	Sodium (mg).............110
Fat (g) 0	Carbohydrate (g).........11
% calories from fat ...0	Fiber (g).................n/a
Saturated fat (g)........0	Protein (g) 7
Cholesterol (mg) 5	

Exchanges: 1 fat-free milk

Healthy 'n Hearty Choice

Caffè Latte (nonfat milk)

Calories......................120	Sodium (mg).............170
Fat (g) 1	Carbohydrate (g).........17
% calories from fat ...8	Fiber (g).................n/a
Saturated fat (g)........0	Protein (g) 12
Cholesterol (mg) 5	

Exchanges: 1 fat-free milk

(*Continued*)

Starbucks

BEVERAGES

	Amount	Cal.	Fat (g)	% Cal. Fat	Sat. Fat (g)	Chol. (mg)	Sod. (mg)	Carb. (g)	Fiber (g)	Pro. (g)	Servings/Exchanges
Caffè Americano	12 oz	10	0	0	0	0	10	2	n/a	0	free
✔Caffè Latte (nonfat milk)	12 oz	120	1	8	0	5	170	17	n/a	12	1 fat-free milk
Caffè Latte (whole milk)	12 oz	210	11	47	7	45	160	17	n/a	11	1 whole milk, 1 fat
Caffè Mocha w/ whipping cream (nonfat milk)	12 oz	260	12	42	7	40	170	32	n/a	12	1 fat-free milk, 1 carb, 2 fat
Caffè Mocha w/ whipping cream (whole milk)	12 oz	340	21	56	13	70	160	31	n/a	12	1 whole milk, 1 carb, 2 1/2 fat
✔Cappuccino (nonfat milk)	12 oz	80	0	0	0	5	110	11	n/a	7	1 fat-free milk
Cappuccino (whole milk)	12 oz	140	7	45	4.5	30	105	11	n/a	7	1 whole milk

| Coffee Frappuccino | 12 oz | 200 | 3 | 14 | 0 | 0 | 170 | 39 | n/a | 6 | 2 1/2 carb, 1/2 fat |
| Mocha Frappuccino | 12 oz | 230 | 3 | 12 | 0 | 0 | 180 | 44 | n/a | 6 | 3 carb, 1/2 fat |

✔ = Healthiest Bets; n/a = not available

12 oz—Tall; 16 oz—Grande; 20 oz—Venti

Tim Hortons

❖Tim Hortons provides nutrition information
for all their menu items on their website at
www.timhortons.com.

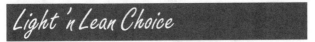

Light 'n Lean Choice

Multigrain Bagel
1/2 Package Light Plain Cream Cheese (*1 1/2 T*)

Calories 345
Fat (g) 7
  % calories from fat..18
  Saturated fat (g)........3
Cholesterol (mg) 10

Sodium (mg) 755
Carbohydrate (g).........60
  Fiber (g) 6
Protein (g) 14

Exchanges: 4 starch, 1 fat

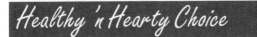

Healthy 'n Hearty Choice

Minestrone Soup (*10 oz*)
Chunky Chicken Salad Sandwich on Country Bun
Oatmeal Raisin Cookie (*1*)

Calories 655
Fat (g) 18
  % calories from fat..25
  Saturated fat (g)........3
Cholesterol (mg) 61

Sodium (mg) 1,820
Carbohydrate (g).........97
  Fiber (g) 6
Protein (g) 29

Exchanges: 6 starch, 1 vegetable, 2 lean meat, 1 fat

Tim Hortons

	Amount	Cal.	Fat (g)	% Cal. Fat	Sat. Fat (g)	Chol. (mg)	Sod. (mg)	Carb. (g)	Fiber (g)	Pro. (g)	Servings/Exchanges
BAGELS											
✔Blueberry	1	300	2	6	0	0	520	59	3	11	4 starch
✔Cinnamon Raisin	1	300	2	6	0	0	390	58	4	11	4 starch
✔Everything	1	300	2	6	0	0	560	57	3	12	4 starch
✔Multigrain	1	300	3	9	0	0	655	58	6	12	4 starch
✔Onion	1	295	2	6	0	0	530	58	3	11	4 starch
✔Plain	1	290	2	6	0	0	600	57	3	11	4 starch
✔Poppy Seed	1	300	3	9	0	0	500	58	4	11	4 starch
✔Sesame Seed	1	300	3	9	0	0	570	57	4	11	4 starch

(Continued)

✔ = Healthiest Bets; n/a = not available

BAGELS (Continued)	Amount	Cal.	Fat (g)	% Cal. Fat	Sat. Fat (g)	Chol. (mg)	Sod. (mg)	Carb. (g)	Fiber (g)	Pro. (g)	Servings/Exchanges
✔ Whole Wheat & Honey	1	300	2	6	0	0	590	59	6	11	4 starch
BEVERAGES											
✔ Apple Juice	9 oz	140	0	0	0	0	16	36	0	0	2 1/2 fruit
Café Mocha	10 oz	250	10	36	4	0	330	34	0	3	2 carb, 2 fat
Cappuccino Ice	16 oz	430	23	48	14	80	50	54	0	3	3 1/2 carb, 4 fat
Chocolate Milk (1%)	14 oz	280	5	16	3	15	270	46	0	15	2 fat-free milk, 1 carb, 1 fat
✔ English Toffee Cappuccino	10 oz	130	5	35	4	0	120	20	0	3	1 carb, 1 fat
Fruit Punch	10 oz	150	0	0	0	0	10	38	0	0	2 1/2 carb
Hot Chocolate	10 oz	200	6	27	2	0	370	44	0	2	3 carb
CAKE DONUTS											
Chocolate Glazed	1	350	22	57	7	10	340	35	1	3	2 carb, 4 fat
Old Fashion Glazed	1	270	12	40	4	15	260	39	0	3	2 1/2 carb, 2 fat

	Amount	Cal.	Fat (g)	% Fat	Sat. Fat (g)	Chol. (mg)	Sod. (mg)	Carb. (g)	Fiber (g)	Pro. (g)	Exchanges/Choices
Old Fashion Plain	1	220	12	49	4	15	260	24	0	3	1 1/2 carb, 2 fat
Sour Cream Plain	1	280	18	58	6	20	230	25	0	3	1 1/2 carb, 3 fat
CAKE TIMBITS											
✔Chocolate Glazed	1	70	3	39	1	5	95	9	0	1	1/2 carb, 1/2 fat
✔Old Fashion Plain	1	45	2	40	0	5	70	7	0	1	1/2 carb
CAKES											
Black Forest	1/8 cake	500	21	38	14	0	790	75	3	4	5 carb, 3 fat
Celebration (white)	1/8 cake	500	16	29	8	5	530	85	1	4	5 1/2 carb, 3 fat
Chocolate Fantasy	1/8 cake	420	15	32	7	35	630	72	3	5	5 carb, 2 fat
Shadow (chocolate & white)	1/8 cake	430	19	40	10	35	470	63	2	4	4 carb, 3 fat
COOKIES											
✔Chocolate Chip	1	150	7	42	3	20	140	21	1	2	1 1/2 carb, 1 fat

✔ = Healthiest Bets; n/a = not available

(Continued)

COOKIES (Continued)	Amount	Cal.	Fat (g)	% Cal. Fat	Sat. Fat (g)	Chol. (mg)	Sod. (mg)	Carb. (g)	Fiber (g)	Pro. (g)	Servings/Exchanges
✔Oatcakes	1	190	10	47	4	0	150	22	1	10	1 1/2 carb, 2 fat
✔Oatmeal Raisin	1	150	6	36	2	15	140	22	1	2	1 1/2 carb, 1 fat
✔Peanut Butter	1	170	10	53	3	20	190	17	1	3	1 carb, 2 fat
✔Peanut Butter Chocolate Chunk	1	170	10	53	1	15	150	18	1	3	1 carb, 2 fat
✔Plain Macaroon	1	140	8	51	7	0	60	14	3	1	1 carb, 1 1/2 fat
CREAM CHEESE											
✔Garden Vegetable	1.5 oz	150	13	78	9	40	230	3	0	3	3 fat
✔Plain	1.5 oz	140	14	90	10	45	140	1	0	3	3 fat
✔Plain Light	1.5 oz	90	7	70	5	20	200	3	0	4	1/2 fat
✔Strawberry	1.5 oz	150	12	72	8	35	150	7	0	1	1/2 carb, 2 fat
FANCIES											
Honey Stick	1	280	15	48	5	30	350	34	0	4	2 carb, 3 fat

✔Sugar Twist	1	230	10	39	3	0	280	32	0	5	2 carb, 2 fat
Walnut Crunch	1	320	18	51	5	10	410	36	2	5	2 1/2 carb, 3 fat

FILLED DONUTS

Angel Cream	1	280	13	42	4	0	280	36	0	4	2 1/2 carb, 2 fat
✔Blueberry	1	220	8	33	3	0	260	33	0	4	2 carb, 1 1/2 fat
✔Boston Cream	1	230	8	31	3	0	320	36	0	4	2 1/2 carb, 1 fat
✔Canadian Maple	1	230	8	31	3	0	320	36	0	4	2 1/2 carb, 1 fat
✔Strawberry	1	220	8	33	3	0	310	33	0	4	2 carb, 1 1/2 fat

FILLED TIMBITS

✔Banana Cream	1	45	1	20	0	0	70	8	0	1	1/2 carb
✔Lemon	1	50	2	36	0	0	75	9	0	1	1/2 carb
✔Spiced Apple	1	50	1	18	0	0	75	9	0	1	1/2 carb
✔Strawberry	1	50	1	18	0	0	80	9	0	1	1/2 carb

✔ = Healthiest Bets; n/a = not available

(Continued)

MUFFINS

	Amount	Cal.	Fat (g)	% Cal. Fat	Sat. Fat (g)	Chol. (mg)	Sod. (mg)	Carb. (g)	Fiber (g)	Pro. (g)	Servings/Exchanges
✔Blueberry Bran	1	300	9	27	2	10	690	51	5	5	3 1/2 carb, 1 fat
Carrot Whole Wheat	1	410	22	48	2	10	580	52	4	5	3 1/2 carb, 3 fat
Chocolate Chip Plain	1	390	15	35	4	20	550	62	2	5	4 carb, 2 fat
✔Low Fat Carrot	1	260	2	7	0	0	620	50	6	5	3 1/2 carb
✔Low Fat Cranberry	1	260	2	7	0	0	610	60	6	5	4 carb
✔Lowfat Honey	1	290	2	6	0	0	700	66	6	5	4 1/2 carb
Oatbran 'n Apple	1	350	12	31	3	0	430	58	4	5	4 carb, 1 fat
Oatbran Carrot 'n Raisin	1	340	11	29	2	0	390	57	4	5	4 carb, 1 fat
Oatmeal Raisin	1	430	11	23	2	20	520	80	3	6	5 carb, 1 fat
✔Raisin Bran	1	360	10	25	2	10	750	66	6	6	4 1/2 carb, 1 fat
Wild Blueberry	1	330	11	30	2	15	520	54	2	4	3 1/2 carb, 1 fat

PASTRIES

Butter Croissant	1	210	11	47	6	30	370	25	1	5	1 1/2 starch, 2 fat
Cheese Croissant	1	240	12	45	5	20	370	27	1	6	1 1/2 starch, 2 fat
Cherry Cheese Danish	1	380	23	54	9	45	410	33	1	7	2 carb, 4 fat
✔ Plain Tea Biscuit	1	220	6	25	6	0	590	36	1	5	2 1/2 starch, 1 fat
✔ Raisin Tea Biscuit	1	350	6	15	2	0	570	47	2	5	3 starch, 1 fat
Southern Country Cranberry Biscuit	1	470	19	36	5	0	1050	68	2	7	4 1/2 carb, 3 fat
Southern Country Raspberry Biscuit	1	470	19	36	5	0	1050	68	2	7	4 1/2 carb, 3 fat

PIES

Apple	1/4 pie	540	31	52	6	0	230	62	3	4	4 carb, 5 fat
Banana Cream	1/4 pie	440	26	53	13	0	135	50	1	2	3 carb, 4 1/2 fat

✔ = Healthiest Bets; n/a = not available

(Continued)

PIES *(Continued)*	Amount	Cal.	Fat (g)	% Cal. Fat	Sat. Fat (g)	Chol. (mg)	Sod. (mg)	Carb. (g)	Fiber (g)	Pro. (g)	Servings/Exchanges
Cherry	1/4 pie	570	31	49	6	0	320	70	2	4	4 1/2 carb, 4 fat
Chocolate Cream	1/4 pie	490	31	57	16	10	170	52	1	2	3 1/2 carb, 5 fat
SANDWICHES											
✔ Albacore Tuna Salad	1	350	8	21	1	15	1100	49	3	21	3 starch, 2 very lean meat, 1 fat
Black Forest Ham & Swiss	1	640	27	38	9	75	1540	53	2	33	3 1/2 starch, 3 lean meat, 5 fat
✔ Chunky Chicken Salad	1	380	10	24	1	45	770	50	3	23	3 starch, 2 lean meat, 1 fat
Fireside Roast Beef	1	470	19	36	3	35	1470	48	2	22	3 starch, 2 lean meat, 3 fat
Garden Vegetable	1	460	24	47	11	45	730	50	3	12	3 starch, 1 medium-fat meat, 3 fat
Harvest Turkey Breast	1	470	18	34	2	30	1460	53	2	22	3 starch, 2 lean meat, 3 fat

SOUPS

	Serving	Cal									Exchanges
✔ Chili	10 oz	320	9	25	3	65	960	32	8	29	2 starch, 3 lean meat
Cream of Broccoli	10 oz	190	7	33	2	5	1120	27	1	7	2 starch, 1 fat
✔ Cream of Mushroom	10 oz	195	10	46	3	5	950	21	1	4	1 1/2 starch, 2 fat
✔ Hearty Vegetable	10 oz	130	2	14	0	0	830	27	2	3	1 1/2 starch
✔ Minestrone	10 oz	125	2	14	0	1	910	25	2	4	1 1/2 starch
Potato Bacon	10 oz	195	7	32	2	5	1100	29	1	4	2 starch, 1 fat
✔ Tim's Own Chicken Noodle	10 oz	100	3	27	1	14	710	15	1	5	1 starch, 1/2 fat
✔ Turkey & Wild Rice	10 oz	120	2	15	0	6	330	22	1	22	1 1/2 starch, 2 very lean meat
✔ Vegetable Beef Barley	10 oz	110	2	16	0	9	840	18	2	5	1 starch

TARTS

	Serving	Cal									Exchanges
Fresh Strawberry	1	220	9	37	2	0	140	36	2	1	1 fruit, 1 carb, 2 fat

(Continued)

✔ = Healthiest Bets; n/a = not available

TARTS (*Continued*)	Amount	Cal.	Fat (g)	% Cal. Fat	Sat. Fat (g)	Chol. (mg)	Sod. (mg)	Carb. (g)	Fiber (g)	Pro. (g)	Servings/Exchanges
Raisin Butter	1	330	11	30	3	15	200	54	1	3	3 1/2 carb, 1 1/2 fat
YEAST DONUTS											
Apple Fritter	1	300	14	42	5	0	280	40	2	5	2 1/2 carb, 2 fat
✓Chocolate Dip	1	230	10	39	3	0	270	33	0	4	2 carb, 2 fat
Dutchie	1	280	13	42	4	0	240	39	1	4	2 1/2 carb, 2 fat
✓Honey Dip	1	230	10	39	3	0	250	32	0	4	2 carb, 2 fat
✓Maple Dip	1	250	10	36	3	0	280	36	0	4	2 1/2 carb, 2 fat
✓Dutchie (timbit)	1	60	2	30	0	0	60	10	0	1	1/2 carb
✓Honey Dip (timbit)	1	50	1	18	0	0	70	10	0	1	1/2 carb

✓ = Healthiest Bets; n/a = not available

Burgers, Fries, and More

RESTAURANTS

Burger King

Carl's Jr.

Dairy Queen/Brazier

Hardee's

Jack in the Box

McDonald's

Sonic, America's Drive-In

Wendy's

NUTRITION PROS

- Small portions are plentiful as long as you know and use the right words, such as regular, small, junior, and single.
- There's no waiting for food. You order, then eat.
- No foods greet you at the table. What you order is what you eat. This puts you in the driver's seat.
- You can fill up on fiber from multigrain buns and baked potatoes.
- It's easy to add to your 5-a-day (fruits and vegetables) with an entree or a side salad.
- Salad dressing is served on the side. There's no need for a special request.
- Healthier cold drinks flow freely: low-fat (1%) or fat-free milk, fruit juice, water, unsweetened ice tea, diet soft drinks.
- Low-fat and low-calorie or fat-free salad dressings are now common. Keep in mind that these salad

dressings are not calorie free. They can also be high in sodium.

- Healthier dessert options include low-fat frozen yogurt in a cone or dish, low-fat milkshakes, or fat-free muffins.
- Honesty is their policy. Full disclosure of nutrition information is there for the asking.
- You know the menu well. You can plan what to order before you walk in the door.

NUTRITION CONS

- Many menu items are high in fat. Cheese, cheese sauce, bacon, special sauce, and mayonnaise add fat.
- Large-portions are all too frequent: large, jumbo, double, and triple are a few words to watch out for.
- Sodium can skyrocket from the salt on french fries, in special sauces, and in salad dressings.
- Chicken and fish start off healthy, but they are often buried in a crisp, golden, high-fat coating.
- Several fast-food restaurants have said so long to healthier options such as lean hamburgers, grilled chicken without special sauce, and salads.
- Biscuits are loaded with fat to begin with. Tuck sausage, bacon, egg, and/or cheese in the middle and you've just downed your fat grams for the day in one fell swoop.
- Fruit is nowhere to be found—other than in juice and between the pie crust.
- Vegetables are few and far between, just salad and a few bits of lettuce and tomato on some sandwiches.
- French fries or onion rings—deep fried of course—are still the traditional side.

- Super-sized and "value" meals push you to eat larger portions because you can buy more food for less. Don't get caught up in this unhealthy mentality.

Healthy Tips

★ Zero in on the words regular, junior, small, or single. These mean small portions.

★ Try lower-calorie ketchup, mustard, or barbecue sauce as an option to higher-fat mayonnaise or special sauce.

★ Walk in rather than drive through. If you eat and drive, you hardly realize food has passed your lips.

★ Order less food to start. Remember, you can go back and get more in a flash.

★ Want fries? Go ahead, but split a small or medium order with your fast-food partner.

Get It Your Way

★ Avoid the busy times. This way you'll get your food your way with a smile on the order taker's face.

★ Be ready to wait. Fast-food restaurants are not set up for special requests.

★ Ask for simple changes: leave off the special sauce or mayonnaise; hold the pickles, bacon, or cheese; or hold the salt on the french fries.

Burger King

❖Burger King provides nutrition information for all of its menu items on their website at www.burgerking.com.

Light 'n Lean Choice

Whopper Jr (*without mayo*)
Barbecue Dipping Sauce (*2 T/ 1 pkg*)
2% milk (*8 oz*)

Calories	495	Sodium (mg)	990
Fat (g)	19	Carbohydrate (g)	53
% calories from fat	35	Fiber (g)	2
Saturated fat (g)	9	Protein (g)	28
Cholesterol (mg)	65		

Exchanges: 2 starch, 1 fat free milk, 2 medium-fat meats, 2 fat

Healthy 'n Hearty Choice

BK Broiler Chicken Sandwich (*without mayo*)
Barbecue Dipping Sauce (*2 T/ 1 pkg*)
French Fries (*small*)

Calories	655	Sodium (mg)	2,040
Fat (g)	19	Carbohydrate (g)	89
% calories from fat	26	Fiber (g)	5
Saturated fat (g)	5	Protein (g)	31
Cholesterol (mg)	90		

Exchanges: 5 1/2 starch, 2 lean meat, 2 fat

Burger King

BEVERAGES

	Amount	Cal.	Fat (g)	% Cal. Fat	Sat. Fat (g)	Chol. (mg)	Sod. (mg)	Carb. (g)	Fiber (g)	Pro. (g)	Servings/Exchanges
Frozen Coca Cola Classic (large)	18 oz	460	0	0	0	0	n/a	116	0	0	7 1/2 carb
Frozen Coca Cola Classic (medium)	15 oz	370	0	0	0	0	n/a	92	0	0	6 carb
Frozen Minute Maid Cherry (large)	18 oz	460	0	0	0	0	n/a	116	0	0	7 1/2 carb
Frozen Minute Maid Cherry (medium)	15 oz	370	0	0	0	0	n/a	92	0	0	6 carb

✔ = Healthiest Bets; n/a = not available

(*Continued*)

BREAKFAST

	Amount	Cal.	Fat (g)	% Cal. Fat	Sat. Fat (g)	Chol. (mg)	Sod. (mg)	Carb. (g)	Fiber (g)	Pro. (g)	Servings/Exchanges
Biscuit	1	300	15	45	3.5	0	830	35	1	6	2 starch, 3 fat
Biscuit with Egg	1	390	22	51	5	150	1020	37	1	11	2 1/2 starch, 1 medium-fat meat, 4 fat
Biscuit with Sausage	1	510	35	62	10	30	1190	35	1	13	2 starch, 1 high-fat meat, 6 fat
Biscuit with Sausage, Egg, & Cheese	1	650	46	64	14	190	1600	38	1	20	2 1/2 starch, 2 high-fat meat, 6 fat
Cini-minis-4 rolls (without icing)	1 order	440	15	31	4	25	710	51	1	6	3 1/2 starch, 4 fat
Croissan'wich w/ Sausage & Cheese	1	410	29	64	11	40	830	24	1	14	1 1/2 starch, 1 high-fat meat, 4 fat

Croissan'wich w/ Sausage, Egg, & Cheese	1	500	36	65	13	190	1020	26	1	19	1 1/2 starch, 2 high-fat meat, 4 fat
French Toast Sticks	1 order	390	20	46	4.5	0	440	46	2	6	3 starch, 3 1/2 fat
Hash Brown Rounds (large)	1 order	390	25	58	7	0	760	38	4	3	2 1/2 starch, 4 fat
Hash Browns (small)	1 order	240	15	56	5	0	450	23	2	2	1 1/2 starch, 3 fat

BURGERS

Bacon Double Cheeseburger	1	480	26	49	11	85	580	30	2	31	2 starch, 3 medium-fat meat, 3 fat
Bacon Double Cheeseburger	1	610	37	55	18	120	1170	32	2	38	2 starch, 4 medium-fat meat, 2 1/2 fat
✓ Bull's Eye BBQ Deluxe (w/out mayo)	1	310	14	41	7	45	370	30	2	17	2 starch, 2 medium-fat meat

(Continued)

✓ = Healthiest Bets; n/a = not available

BURGERS (*Continued*)	Amount	Cal.	Fat (g)	% Cal. Fat	Sat. Fat (g)	Chol. (mg)	Sod. (mg)	Carb. (g)	Fiber (g)	Pro. (g)	Servings/Exchanges
Bull's Eye BBQ Deluxe (with mayo)	1	400	23	52	7	50	420	30	2	18	2 starch, 2 medium-fat meat, 2 fat
✔Cheeseburger	1	370	18	44	9	55	750	31	2	22	2 starch, 2 medium-fat meat, 2 fat
Double Cheeseburger	1	570	34	54	17	110	1020	32	2	35	2 starch, 2 medium-fat meat, 2 1/2 fat
Double Hamburger	1	480	26	49	11	85	580	30	2	31	2 starch, 3 medium-fat meat, 3 fat
Double Whopper	1	920	57	56	20	150	1020	53	4	48	3 1/2 starch, 5 medium-fat meat, 6 fat
Double Whopper (w/out mayo)	1	760	40	47	17	135	920	53	4	48	3 1/2 starch, 6 medium-fat meat, 1 fat

	Amount	Cal	Fat (g)	% Fat Cal	Sat Fat (g)	Chol (mg)	Sod (mg)	Carb (g)	Fiber (g)	Pro (g)	Servings/Exchanges
Double Whopper with Cheese	1	1020	65	57	25	170	1460	55	4	53	3 1/2 starch, 6 medium-fat meat, 7 fat
Double Whopper with Cheese (w/out mayo)	1	860	48	50	23	160	1350	54	4	53	3 1/2 starch, 3 medium-fat meat, 3 fat
✔Hamburger	1	320	14	39	6	45	530	30	2	18	2 starch, 2 medium-fat meat, 1/2 fat
Whopper	1	680	39	52	12	80	940	53	4	29	3 1/2 starch, 3 medium-fat meat, 4 fat
Whopper (w/out mayo)	1	530	22	37	9	70	840	53	4	29	3 1/2 starch, 3 medium-fat meat, 1 fat
✔Whopper Jr (w/out mayo)	1	330	14	38	6	45	470	32	2	18	2 starch, 2 medium-fat meat, 1/2 fat

✔ = Healthiest Bets; n/a = not available

(Continued)

BURGERS (*Continued*)	Amount	Cal.	Fat (g)	% Cal. Fat	Sat. Fat (g)	Chol. (mg)	Sod. (mg)	Carb. (g)	Fiber (g)	Pro. (g)	Servings/Exchanges
✓Whopper Jr. with Cheese (w/out mayo)	1	370	18	44	9	55	680	32	2	21	2 starch, 3 medium-fat meat
Whopper Jr.	1	410	23	50	7	50	520	32	2	18	2 starch, 2 medium-fat meat, 3 fat
Whopper Jr. with Cheese	1	460	27	53	10	60	740	33	2	21	2 starch, 2 medium-fat meat, 4 fat
Whopper with Cheese	1	780	47	54	17	105	1350	55	4	34	3 1/2 starch, 3 medium-fat meat, 6 fat
Whopper with Cheese (w/out mayo)	1	620	30	44	14	90	1280	54	4	33	3 1/2 starch, 3 medium-fat meat, 3 fat

CHICKEN TENDERS

	Amount	Cal.	Fat (g)	% Cal. Fat	Sat. Fat (g)	Chol. (mg)	Sod. (mg)	Carb. (g)	Fiber (g)	Pro. (g)	Servings/Exchanges
✓4 pieces	1	170	9	48	3	25	420	10	0	11	1/2 starch, 1 lean meat, 1 fat

5 pieces		1	220	12	49	3	30	530	13	0	14	1 starch, 2 lean meat, 1 fat
6 pieces		1	250	14	50	4	35	630	15	0	15	1 starch, 2 lean meat, 2 fat
8 pieces		1	340	19	50	5	50	840	20	1	22	1 starch, 3 lean meat, 2 1/2 fat

CONDIMENTS

✔ Bacon	3 pieces	40	3	68	1	10	150	0	0	3	1/2 fat
✔ Barbecue Dipping Sauce	1 oz/2 T	35	0	0	0	0	400	9	0	0	1/2 carb
✔ Breakfast Syrup	1 oz/2 T	80	0	0	0	0	20	21	0	0	1 1/2 carb
✔ Bull's Eye Barbecue Sauce	1/2 oz/1 T	20	0	0	0	0	130	5	0	0	free
✔ Grape Jam	1/2 oz/1 T	30	0	0	0	0	0	7	0	0	1/2 carb
✔ Honey Dipping Sauce	1 oz/2 T	90	0	0	0	0	0	23	0	0	1 1/2 carb

✔ = Healthiest Bets; n/a = not available

(Continued)

CONDIMENTS (*Continued*)	Amount	Cal.	Fat (g)	% Cal. Fat	Sat. Fat (g)	Chol. (mg)	Sod. (mg)	Carb. (g)	Fiber (g)	Pro. (g)	Servings/Exchanges
✔Honey Mustard Dipping Sauce	1 oz/2 T	90	6	60	1	10	150	9	0	0	1/2 carb, 1 fat
✔Land O' Lakes Whipped Classic Blend	1 1/2 t	25	4	144	0.5	0	30	0	0	0	1 fat
✔Marinara Dipping Sauce	1 oz/2 T	20	0	0	0	0	280	5	0	0	free
Ranch Dipping Sauce	1 oz/2 T	120	13	98	2	5	85	1	0	1	3 fat
✔Strawberry Jam	1/2 oz/1 T	30	0	0	0	0	0	7	0	0	1/2 carb
✔Sweet & Sour Dipping Sauce	1 oz/2 T	40	0	0	0	0	65	10	0	0	1/2 carb
✔Tartar Sauce	1/2 oz/1 T	70	8	103	4	5	100	0	0	0	1 1/2 fat
Vanilla Icing (Cini-minis)	1 oz	110	3	25	0.5	0	0	20	n/a	0	1 1/2 carb

DESSERTS

Dutch Apple Pie	1	340	14	37	3	0	470	52	2	3	3 1/2 carb, 1 1/2 fat
Hershey's Sundae Pie	1 piece	310	18	52	13	10	135	33	1	3	2 carb, 3 fat

SANDWICHES

BK Big Fish Sandwich	1	710	38	48	14	50	1200	67	4	24	4 1/2 starch, 2 lean meat, 5 fat
✔BK Broiler (w/out mayo)	1	390	8	18	2	90	1010	51	3	29	3 1/2 starch, 2 lean meat
BK Broiler Chicken Sandwich	1	550	25	41	5	105	1110	52	3	30	3 1/2 starch, 3 lean meat, 2 1/2 fat
Chicken (fried) (w/out mayo)	1	460	17	33	5	55	1190	52	3	25	3 1/2 starch, 2 lean meat, 1 1/2 fat
Chicken Club	1	740	44	54	10	85	1530	55	4	30	3 1/2 starch, 3 lean meat, 7 fat

(Continued)

✔ = Healthiest Bets; n/a = not available

SANDWICHES (*Continued*)	Amount	Cal.	Fat (g)	% Cal. Fat	Sat. Fat (g)	Chol. (mg)	Sod. (mg)	Carb. (g)	Fiber (g)	Pro. (g)	Servings/Exchanges
Chicken Club (w/out mayo)	1	530	21	36	6	65	1390	54	4	30	3 1/2 starch, 3 lean meat, 2 fat
Chicken Sandwich (fried)	1	660	39	53	8	70	1330	53	3	25	3 1/2 starch, 3 lean meat, 5 fat
✔ Chicken Tenders (w/out mayo)	1	290	10	31	3	20	570	36	2	14	2 1/2 starch, 1 lean meat, 1 fat
Chicken Tenders	1	450	27	54	5	30	680	37	2	14	2 1/2 starch, 1 lean meat, 4 fat
SHAKES											
Chocolate Shake (medium)	13 oz	440	8	16	5	35	270	80	4	13	3 1/2 carb, 1 fat
Chocolate Shake (medium, syrup added)	14 oz	500	8	14	5	25	440	95	3	13	5 carb, 1 fat

	Amount										
Chocolate Shake (small)	10 oz	340	6	16	4	25	210	62	3	10	4 carb, 1 fat
Chocolate Shake (small, syrup added)	11 oz	400	6	14	4	20	360	77	2	10	5 carb, 1 fat
Strawberry Shake (medium, syrup added)	14 oz	500	8	14	5	25	350	95	2	12	6 carb, 1 1/2 fat
Strawberry Shake (small, syrup added)	11 oz	390	6	14	4	20	270	76	1	9	5 carb, 1 fat
Vanilla Shake (medium)	13 oz	430	8	17	5	25	340	79	2	12	5 carb, 1 fat
Vanilla Shake (small)	10 oz	330	6	16	4	20	260	61	1	9	4 carb, 1 fat

SIDES

	Amount										
French Fries (king size, salted)	1 order	600	30	45	8	0	1140	76	6	7	5 starch, 5 fat

✔ = Healthiest Bets; n/a = not available

(Continued)

SIDES (*Continued*)	Amount	Cal.	Fat (g)	% Cal. Fat	Sat. Fat (g)	Chol. (mg)	Sod. (mg)	Carb. (g)	Fiber (g)	Pro. (g)	Servings/Exchanges
French Fries (king size, unsalted)	1 order	600	30	45	8	0	620	76	6	7	5 starch, 5 fat
French Fries (large, salted)	1 order	500	25	45	7	0	940	53	5	6	3 1/2 starch, 5 fat
French Fries (large, unsalted)	1 order	500	25	45	7	0	510	63	5	6	3 1/2 starch, 5 fat
French Fries (medium, salted)	1 order	360	18	45	5	0	690	46	4	4	3 starch, 3 fat
French Fries (medium, unsalted)	1 order	360	18	45	5	0	370	46	4	4	3 starch, 3 fat
French Fries (small, salted)	1 order	230	11	43	3	0	630	29	2	3	2 starch, 2 fat
✔French Fries (small, unsalted)	1 order	230	11	43	3	0	240	29	2	3	2 starch, 2 fat

Jalapeno Poppers— 4 pieces	1 order	230	13	51	5	20	790	22	2	7	1 1/2 starch, 2 fat
Onion Rings (medium)	1 order	320	16	45	4	0	460	40	5	4	2 1/2 starch, 3 fat
Onion Rings (child size)	1 order	360	18	45	5	0	690	46	4	4	3 starch, 3 fat
Onion Rings (large)	1 order	480	23	43	6	0	690	60	5	7	4 starch, 3 fat
Onion Rings (king size)	1 order	550	27	44	7	0	800	70	5	8	4 1/2 starch, 4 fat

✔ = Healthiest Bets; n/a = not available

Carl's Jr.

❖Carl's Jr. provides nutrition information for all of its menu items on their website at www.carlsjr.com.

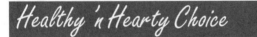
Light 'n Lean Choice

BBQ Chicken Sandwich
Garden Salad-To-Go
Fat-Free French Salad Dressing *(2 T)*
Milk, 1% fat *(10 oz)*

Calories	550	Sodium (mg)	1,740
Fat (g)	10	Carbohydrate (g)	79
% calories from fat	16	Fiber (g)	4
Saturated fat (g)	4	Protein (g)	42
Cholesterol (mg)	80		

Exchanges: 3 starch, 1 veg, 1/2 carb, 1 fat-free milk, 4 very lean meat, 1/2 fat

Healthy 'n Hearty Choice

Hamburger
Baked Potato *(plain)*
Sour Cream and Chives *(2 T)*

Calories	713	Sodium (mg)	560
Fat (g)	14	Carbohydrate (g)	119
% calories from fat	18	Fiber (g)	9
Saturated fat (g)	5	Protein (g)	22
Cholesterol (mg)	38		

Exchanges: 6 1/2 starch, 1 carb, 2 medium-fat meat, 1 fat

Carl's Jr.

	Amount	Cal.	Fat (g)	% Cal. Fat	Sat. Fat (g)	Chol. (mg)	Sod. (mg)	Carb. (g)	Fiber (g)	Pro. (g)	Servings/Exchanges
BAKERY											
Blueberry Muffin	1	340	14	37	2	40	340	49	1	5	2 1/2 starch, 3 fat
Bran Raisin Muffin	1	370	14	34	2	45	410	61	6	6	4 starch, 2 fat
Cheese Danish	1	400	23	52	6	15	390	49	1	5	3 carb, 4 fat
Cheesecake (Strawberry Swirl)	1	290	17	53	9	55	230	30	0	6	2 carb, 3 fat
Chocolate Cake	1	300	12	36	3	30	350	48	1	3	3 carb, 2 fat
Chocolate Chip Cookie	1	350	18	46	7	20	330	46	1	3	3 carb, 3 fa
BEVERAGES											
✔Hot Chocolate	12 oz	110	2	16	2	0	125	22	1	2	1 1/2 carb

(Continued)

✔ = Healthiest Bets; n/a = not available

	Amount	Cal.	Fat (g)	% Cal. Fat	Sat. Fat (g)	Chol. (mg)	Sod. (mg)	Carb. (g)	Fiber (g)	Pro. (g)	Servings/Exchanges
BREAKFAST											
Breakfast Burrito	1	550	32	52	11	495	980	26	1	29	1 1/2 starch, 3 medium-fat meat, 4 fat
✓Breakfast Quesadilla	1	370	17	41	5	240	910	38	1	16	2 1/2 starch, 1 medium-fat meat, 2 fat
✓English Muffin, w/ margarine	1	210	9	39	1	0	300	27	2	5	2 starch, 1 1/2 fat
French Toast Dips	1 order	370	20	49	2.5	0	430	42	1	6	3 starch, 3 fat
Scrambled Eggs	1 order	180	14	70	3	455	110	1	0	13	2 medium-fat meat, 1 fat
✓Sunrise Sandwich (no bacon or sausage)	1	360	21	53	6	245	470	28	2	12	2 starch, 1 medium-fat meat, 3 fat
BURGERS											
Carl's Famous Star Hamburger	1	590	32	49	9	70	910	50	3	24	3 starch, 2 medium-fat meat, 4 fat

Double Sourdough Bacon Cheeseburger	1	880	59	60	24	165	1010	37	2	50	2 1/2 starch, 6 medium-fat meat, 5 fat
Double Western Bacon Cheeseburger	1	920	50	49	21	155	1770	64	3	51	4 starch, 6 medium-fat meat, 4 fat
Famous Bacon Cheeseburger	1	700	41	53	13	95	1310	51	3	31	3 starch, 3 medium-fat meat, 5 fat
✔Hamburger	1	280	9	29	3.5	35	489	36	1	14	2 1/2 starch, 2 medium-fat meat
Sourdough Bacon Cheeseburger	1	640	40	56	15	95	690	37	2	30	2 1/2 starch, 3 medium-fat meat, 5 fat
Sourdough Ranch Bacon Cheeseburger	1	720	46	58	16	95	800	43	3	33	3 starch, 3 medium-fat meat, 6 fat

✔ = Healthiest Bets; n/a = not available

(Continued)

BURGERS *(Continued)*	Amount	Cal.	Fat (g)	% Cal. Fat	Sat. Fat (g)	Chol. (mg)	Sod. (mg)	Carb. (g)	Fiber (g)	Pro. (g)	Servings/Exchanges
Super Star Hamburger	1	790	47	54	15	130	980	51	3	41	3 starch, 3 medium-fat meat, 7 fat
CONDIMENTS											
✓BBQ Sauce	2 T	50	0	0	0	0	270	11	0	1	1/2 carb
✓Grape Jelly	1 T	40	0	0	0	0	15	9	0	0	1/2 carb
✓Honey Sauce	1 oz/2 T	90	0	0	0	0	0	22	0	0	1 1/2 carb
✓Mustard Sauce	1 oz/2 T	50	0	0	0	0	210	11	0	0	1 carb
✓Salsa	1/2 oz/1 T	10	0	0	0	0	160	2	0	0	free
Strawberry Jam	1/2 oz/1 T	40	0	0	0	0	15	9	0	0	1/2 carb
Sweet N' Sour Sauce	1 oz/2 T	50	0	0	0	0	80	12	0	0	1/2 carb
Table Syrup	1 oz/2 T	90	0	0	0	0	0	21	0	0	1 1/2 carb

POTATOES

Item	Amount	Cal.	Fat (g)	% Fat Cal.	Sat. Fat (g)	Chol. (mg)	Sod. (mg)	Carb. (g)	Fiber (g)	Pro. (g)	Exchanges
Bacon & Cheese Baked Potato	1	640	29	41	7	40	1660	75	6	21	5 starch, 1 high-fat meat, 4 fat
✔ Broccoli & Cheese Baked Potato	1	530	21	36	5	15	940	76	5	11	5 starch, 4 fat
✔ Plain Potato (no margarine)	1	290	0	0	0	0	20	68	6	6	4 1/2 starch
✔ Sour Cream & Chive Baked Potato	1	430	14	29	3	10	180	70	6	7	4 1/2 starch, 3 fat

DRESSINGS

Item	Amount	Cal.	Fat (g)	% Fat Cal.	Sat. Fat (g)	Chol. (mg)	Sod. (mg)	Carb. (g)	Fiber (g)	Pro. (g)	Exchanges
1000 Island	2 oz/4 T	230	23	90	4	20	420	5	0	1	4 1/2 fat
Blue Cheese	2 oz/4 T	320	35	98	7	25	370	1	0	2	7 fat
✔ Fat Free French	2 oz/4 T	60	0	0	0	0	660	16	1	0	1 carb
✔ Fat Free Italian	2 oz/4 T	15	0	0	0	0	770	4	0	0	free
House	2 oz/4 T	220	22	90	3.5	20	450	3	0	1	4 fat

✔ = Healthiest Bets; n/a = not available

(Continued)

	Amount	Cal.	Fat (g)	% Cal. Fat	Sat. Fat (g)	Chol. (mg)	Sod. (mg)	Carb. (g)	Fiber (g)	Pro. (g)	Servings/Exchanges
SALADS											
✔Chargrilled Chicken Salad-To-Go	1	200	7	32	3	76	440	12	4	25	2 veg, 3 lean meat
✔Garden Salad-To-Go	1	50	3	54	1.5	5	60	4	2	3	1 veg, 1/2 fat
SANDWICHES											
✔BBQ Chicken Sandwich	1	290	4	12	1	60	840	41	2	25	2 1/2 starch, 3 very lean meat
Carl's Bacon Swiss Crispy Chicken Sandwich	1	760	38	45	11	90	1550	72	3	31	5 starch, 2 lean meat, 5 fat
Carl's Catch Fish Sandwich	1	530	28	48	7	80	1030	55	2	18	3 1/2 starch, 2 lean meat, 3 fat
Carl's Ranch Crispy Chicken Sandwich	1	660	31	42	7	70	1180	71	3	24	4 starch, 2 lean meat, 5 fat

	Amount	Calories	Fat (g)	% Cal. Fat	Sat. Fat (g)	Chol. (mg)	Sodium (mg)	Carb. (g)	Fiber (g)	Protein (g)	Exchanges/Choices
Carl's Western Bacon Crispy Sandwich	1	750	28	34	11	80	1900	91	3	31	6 starch, 2 lean meat, 4 fat
Charbroiled Chicken Club Sandwich	1	470	23	44	7	95	1110	37	2	31	2 1/2 starch, 3 lean meat, 3 1/2 fat
Charbroiled Sante Fe Chicken Sandwich	1	540	31	52	8	95	1210	37	2	28	2 1/2 starch, 3 lean meat, 4 fat
Charbroiled Sirloin Steak Sandwich	1	550	24	39	4.5	80	1080	52	2	30	3 starch, 2 medium-fat meat, 3 fat
Southwest Spicy Chicken Sandwich	1	620	41	60	10	66	1640	48	2	18	3 starch, 2 lean meat, 6 fat
Spicy Chicken Sandwich	1	480	26	49	5	40	1220	47	2	14	3 starch, 1 lean meat, 4 fat
SHAKES											
Chocolate (regular)	32 oz	770	15	18	10	65	520	140	1	21	9 carb, 2 fat

✔ = Healthiest Bets; n/a = not available

(Continued)

SHAKES (*Continued*)	Amount	Cal.	Fat (g)	% Cal. Fat	Sat. Fat (g)	Chol. (mg)	Sod. (mg)	Carb. (g)	Fiber (g)	Pro. (g)	Servings/Exchanges
Chocolate (small)	21 oz	530	10	17	7	45	350	96	0	14	6 carb, 1 fat
Strawberry	32 oz	750	15	18	10	65	490	133	0	20	9 carb, 2 fat
Vanilla (regular)	32 oz	700	16	21	11	70	530	115	0	22	7 1/2 carb, 3 fat
Vanilla (small)	21 oz	470	11	21	7	90	350	78	0	15	5 carb, 2 fat
SIDES											
✔Breadsticks	1 order	35	1	26	0	0	60	7	1	1	1/2 starch
Chicken Stars	6 pieces	260	16	55	4.5	40	480	14	1	13	1 starch, 1 lean meat, 3 fat
CrissCut Fries (large)	1 order	410	24	53	5	0	950	43	4	5	3 starch, 5 fat
✔Croutons	1 T	30	1	30	0	0	105	5	0	1	free
✔French Fries (kids)	1 order	250	12	43	2.5	0	150	32	2	4	2 starch, 2 fat
French Fries (small)	1 order	290	14	43	3	0	180	37	3	5	2 1/2 starch, 3 fat

Hash Brown Nuggets	1 order	330	21	57	4.5	0	470	32	3	3	2 starch, 4 fat
Mozzarella Sticks—4 pieces	1 order	290	16	50	6	20	670	25	1	12	1 1/2 starch, 1 high-fat meat, 2 fat
Onion Rings	1 order	430	22	46	5	0	700	53	3	6	3 1/2 starch, 4 fat
Zucchini (fried)	1 order	320	19	53	5	0	860	31	2	6	2 starch, 4 fat

✔ = Healthiest Bets; n/a = not available

Dairy Queen/Brazier

❖Dairy Queen/Brazier provides nutrition information for all of its menu items on their website at www.dairyqueen.com.

Light 'n Lean Choice

DQ Homestyle Cheeseburger
Vanilla Cone (*small*)

Calories	570	Sodium (mg)	965
Fat (g)	24	Carbohydrate (g)	67
% calories from fat	38	Fiber (g)	2
Saturated fat (g)	13	Protein (g)	26
Cholesterol (mg)	75		

Exchanges: 2 starch, 2 1/2 carb, 3 medium-fat meat

Healthy 'n Hearty Choice

Grilled Chicken Breast Fillet Sandwich
1/2 French Fries (*small*)
DQ Chocolate Soft Serve (*1/2 cup*)

Calories	755	Sodium (mg)	1,275
Fat (g)	34	Carbohydrate (g)	80
% calories from fat	40	Fiber (g)	4
Saturated fat (g)	10	Protein (g)	30
Cholesterol (mg)	76		

Exchanges: 4 starch, 1 1/2 carb, 3 lean meat, 3 fat

Dairy Queen/Brazier

	Amount	Cal.	Fat (g)	% Cal. Fat	Sat. Fat (g)	Chol. (mg)	Sod. (mg)	Carb. (g)	Fiber (g)	Pro. (g)	Servings/Exchanges
BLIZZARD											
Chocolate Chip Cookie Dough (medium)	16 oz	950	36	34	19	75	660	143	2	17	9 1/2 carb, 7 fat
Chocolate Chip Cookie Dough (small)	12 oz	660	24	33	13	55	440	99	1	12	6 1/2 carb, 5 fat
Chocolate Sandwich Cookie (medium)	16 oz	640	23	32	11	45	500	97	1	12	6 1/2 carb, 4 1/2 fat
Chocolate Sandwich Cookie (small)	12 oz	520	18	31	9	40	380	79	1	10	5 carb, 3 1/2 fat

(Continued)

✔ = Healthiest Bets; n/a = not available

	Amount	Cal.	Fat (g)	% Cal. Fat	Sat. Fat (g)	Chol. (mg)	Sod. (mg)	Carb. (g)	Fiber (g)	Pro. (g)	Servings/Exchanges
BURGERS											
DQ Homestyle Bacon Double Cheeseburger	1	610	36	53	18	130	1380	31	2	41	2 starch, 5 medium-fat meat, 2 fat
✓DQ Homestyle Cheeseburger	1	340	17	45	8	55	850	29	2	20	2 starch, 2 medium-fat meat, 1 fat
DQ Homestyle Double Cheeseburger	1	540	31	52	16	115	1130	30	2	35	2 starch, 4 medium-fat meat, 2 fat
✓DQ Homestyle Hamburger	1	290	12	37	5	45	630	29	2	17	2 starch, 2 medium-fat meat
DQ Ultimate Burger	1	670	43	58	19	135	1210	29	2	40	2 starch, 5 medium-fat meat, 3 1/2 fat
FROZEN YOGURT											
✓Cup of Yogurt (medium)	1	230	1	4	0	5	150	48	0	8	3 carb

✔ DQ Nonfat Frozen Yogurt	1/2 cup	100	0	0	0	5	70	21	0	3	1 1/2 carb
Heath Breeze (medium)	16 oz	710	18	23	11	20	580	123	1	15	8 carb, 3 1/2 fat
Heath Breeze (small)	12 oz	470	10	19	6	10	380	85	1	11	5 1/2 carb, 1 fat
Strawberry Breeze (medium)	16 oz	460	1	2	1	10	270	99	1	13	6 1/2 carb
Strawberry Breeze (small)	12 oz	320	1	3	0.5	5	190	68	1	10	4 1/2 carb
✔ Yogurt Cone (medium)	1	260	1	3	0.5	5	160	56	0	9	4 carb

HOT DOGS

Chili 'n' Cheese Dog	1	330	21	57	9	45	1090	22	2	14	1 1/2 starch, 1 high-fat meat, 2 fat
✔ Hot Dog	1	240	14	53	5	25	730	19	1	9	1 starch, 1 high-fat meat, 1 fat

ICE CREAM

Chocolate Cone (medium)	1	340	11	29	7	30	160	53	0	8	3 1/2 carb, 2 fat

(Continued)

✔ = Healthiest Bets; n/a = not available

ICE CREAM *(Continued)*	Amount	Cal.	Fat (g)	% Cal. Fat	Sat. Fat (g)	Chol. (mg)	Sod. (mg)	Carb. (g)	Fiber (g)	Pro. (g)	Servings/Exchanges
✔Chocolate Cone (small)	1	240	8	30	5	20	115	37	0	6	2 1/2 carb, 1 1/2 fat
Dipped Cone (medium)	1	490	24	44	13	30	190	59	1	8	4 carb, 5 fat
Dipped Cone (small)	1	340	17	45	9	20	130	42	1	6	3 carb, 3 fat
✔DQ Chocolate Soft Serve	1/2 cup	150	5	30	3.5	15	75	22	0	4	1 1/2 carb, 1 fat
✔DQ Vanilla Soft Serve	1/2 cup	140	5	32	3	15	70	22	0	3	1 1/2 carb, 1 fat
Vanilla Cone (large)	1	410	12	26	8	40	200	65	0	10	4 carb, 2 fat
Vanilla Cone (medium)	1	330	9	25	6	30	160	53	0	8	3 1/2 carb, 2 fat
✔Vanilla Cone (small)	1	230	7	27	4.5	20	115	38	0	6	2 1/2 carb, 1 fat
ICE CREAM BARS											
Buster Bar	1	450	28	56	12	15	280	41	2	10	2 1/2 carb, 5 1/2 fat
Chocolate Dilly Bar	1	210	13	56	7	10	75	21	0	3	1 1/2 carb, 2 1/2 fat
✔DQ Fudge Bar, no sugar added	1	50	0	0	0	0	70	13	0	4	1 carb

	Amount	Cal.	Fat (g)	% Cal. Fat	Sat. Fat (g)	Chol. (mg)	Sod. (mg)	Carb. (g)	Fiber (g)	Pro. (g)	Choices/Exchanges
✓DQ Sandwich	1	200	6	27	3	10	140	31	1	4	2 carb, 1 fat
✓DQ Vanilla Orange Bar, no sugar added	1	60	0	0	0	0	40	17	0	2	1 carb
ICE CREAM CAKES											
DQ Frozen 8" Round Cake	1/8 cake	370	13	32	8	25	280	56	1	7	3 1/2 carb, 2 fat
DQ Layered 8" Round Cake	1/8 cake	330	12	33	6	15	350	49	0	6	3 carb, 2 fat
ICE CREAM PIZZAS											
✓Heath DQ Treatzza Pizza	1/8 pizza	180	7	35	3.5	5	160	28	1	3	2 carb, 1 fat
✓M&M DQ Treatzza Pizza	1/8 pizza	180	7	35	3.5	5	160	28	1	3	2 carb, 1 fat
MISCELLANEOUS											
✓DQ Lemon Freez'r	1/2 cup	80	0	0	0	0	10	20	0	0	1 carb
✓Starkiss	1	80	0	0	0	0	10	21	0	0	1 1/2 carb

✓ = Healthiest Bets; n/a = not available

(Continued)

	Amount	Cal.	Fat (g)	% Cal. Fat	Sat. Fat (g)	Chol. (mg)	Sod. (mg)	Carb. (g)	Fiber (g)	Pro. (g)	Servings/Exchanges
OTHER ENTREES											
Chicken Strip Basket w/ Gravy	1	1000	50	45	13	55	2510	102	5	35	7 starch, 2 lean meat, 9 fat
The Great Steakmelt Basket	1	770	38	44	13	75	2290	72	5	32	5 starch, 3 medium-fat meat, 3 fat
SANDWICHES											
Chicken Breast Fillet	1	430	20	42	4	55	760	37	2	24	2 1/2 starch, 2 lean meat, 3 fat
✔Grilled Chicken Sandwich	1	310	10	29	2.5	50	1040	30	3	24	2 starch, 3 lean meat
SHAKES AND MALTS											
Chocolate Malt (medium)	1	880	22	23	14	70	500	153	0	19	10 carb, 4 fat
Chocolate Malt (small)	1	650	16	22	10	55	370	111	0	15	7 carb, 3 fat
Chocolate Shake (medium)	1	770	20	23	13	70	420	130	0	17	8 carb, 4 fat

Chocolate Shake (small)	1	560	15	24	10	50	310	94	0	13	6 carb, 3 fat
Frozen Hot Chocolate	1	860	35	37	16	50	350	127	3	14	8 1/2 carb, 6 fat
Misty Slush (medium)	1	290	0	0	0	0	30	74	0	0	5 carb
Misty Slush (small)	1	220	0	0	0	0	20	56	0	0	4 carb

SIDES

French Fries (medium)	1 order	440	16	33	4	0	1110	53	4	5	3 1/2 starch, 3 fat
French Fries (small)	1 order	350	18	46	3.5	0	880	42	3	4	3 starch, 3 fat
Onion Rings	1 order	320	16	45	4	0	180	39	3	5	2 1/2 starch, 3 fat

SUNDAES

Banana Split	1	510	12	21	8	30	180	96	3	8	6 1/2 carb, 2 fat
Chocolate Sundae (medium)	1	410	10	22	6	30	210	71	0	8	4 1/2 carb, 2 fat
✔ Chocolate Sundae (small)	1	280	7	23	4.5	20	140	49	0	5	3 carb, 1 fat
Peanut Buster Parfait	1	730	31	38	17	35	400	99	2	16	6 1/2 carb, 6 fat

✔ = Healthiest Bets; n/a = not available

(Continued)

SUNDAES (*Continued*)	Amount	Cal.	Fat (g)	% Cal. Fat	Sat. Fat (g)	Chol. (mg)	Sod. (mg)	Carb. (g)	Fiber (g)	Pro. (g)	Servings/Exchanges
Pecan Mudslide Treat	1	650	30	42	12	35	420	85	2	11	5 1/2 carb, 6 fat
S'more Galore Parfait	1	720	30	38	10	30	340	111	3	11	7 1/2 carb, 6 fat
Strawberry Shortcake	1	430	14	29	9	60	360	70	1	7	4 1/2 carb, 3 fat
✔Yogurt Strawberry Sundae (medium)	1	280	1	3	0	5	160	61	1	8	4 carb

✔ = Healthiest Bets; n/a = not available

Hardee's

❖Hardee's provides nutrition information for all its menu items on their website at www.hardees.com.

Light 'n Lean Choice

**Grilled Chicken Sandwich
Mashed Potatoes, Small
Gravy** (*3 T*)
1/2 Chocolate Shake

Calories......................625	Sodium (mg)..........1,320
Fat (g) 18	Carbohydrate (g).........78
% calories from fat..26	Fiber (g)..................n/a
Saturated fat (g)........4	Protein (g) 32
Cholesterol (mg) 80	

Exchanges: 3 starch, 2 carb, 2 lean meat, 2 1/2 fat

Healthy 'n Hearty Choice

**Regular Roast Beef Sandwich
1/2 French Fries** (*regular*)
Cool Twist Cone

Calories......................660	Sodium (mg)..........1,115
Fat (g) 26	Carbohydrate (g).........83
% calories from fat..35	Fiber (g)..................n/a
Saturated fat (g)........8	Protein (g) 23
Cholesterol (mg) 50	

Exchanges: 3 1/2 starch, 2 carb, 2 medium-fat meat, 1 1/2 fat

(*Continued*)

Hardee's

	Amount	Cal.	Fat (g)	% Cal. Fat	Sat. Fat (g)	Chol. (mg)	Sod. (mg)	Carb. (g)	Fiber (g)	Pro. (g)	Servings/Exchanges
BREAKFAST											
Bacon, Egg and Cheese Biscuit	1	530	30	51	11	210	1420	45	n/a	20	3 starch, 2 medium-fat meat, 3 1/2 fat
Biscuit 'N' Gravy	1	520	30	52	11	210	1420	45	n/a	17	3 starch, 2 medium-fat meat, 3 fat
Chicken Biscuit	1	590	27	41	9	15	1550	56	n/a	10	4 starch, 5 fat
Country Ham Biscuit	1	440	22	45	7	30	1710	44	n/a	14	3 starch, 1 medium-fat meat, 3 fat
Frisco Breakfast Sandwich (ham)	1	450	22	44	8	30	1290	42	n/a	22	3 starch, 2 medium-fat meat, 2 fat

Item	Serving										Exchanges
Ham Biscuit	1	410	20	44	8	25	1200	45	n/a	13	3 starch, 1 medium-fat meat, 3 fat
✔ Jelly Biscuit	1	440	21	43	6	0	1000	57	n/a	6	3 starch, 1 carb, 3 fat
✔ Made from Scratch Biscuit	1	390	21	48	6	0	1000	44	n/a	6	3 starch, 4 fat
Omelet Biscuit	1	550	32	52	12	225	1350	45	n/a	20	3 starch, 2 medium-fat meat, 5 fat
Regular Hash Rounds 16 pieces		230	14	55	3	0	560	24	n/a	3	1 1/2 starch, 3 fat
Sausage and Egg Biscuit	1	620	41	60	13	225	1370	45	n/a	19	3 starch, 1 high-fat meat, 6 fat
Sausage Biscuit	1	550	36	59	11	25	1300	44	n/a	12	3 starch, 1 high-fat meat, 5 fat
Steak Biscuit	1	580	32	50	10	30	1580	56	n/a	15	3 1/2 starch, 1 medium-fat meat, 5 fat

(Continued)

✔ = Healthiest Bets; n/a = not available

BURGERS

	Amount	Cal.	Fat (g)	% Cal. Fat	Sat. Fat (g)	Chol. (mg)	Sod. (mg)	Carb. (g)	Fiber (g)	Pro. (g)	Servings/Exchanges
All-Star	1	660	43	59	14	100	1260	41	n/a	29	2 1/2 starch, 2 medium-fat meat, 7 fat
Famous Star	1	570	35	55	10	80	860	41	n/a	24	2 1/2 starch, 2 medium-fat meat, 5 fat
Frisco Burger	1	720	49	61	15	95	1180	37	n/a	31	3 starch, 3 medium-fat meat, 6 fat
✓Hamburger	1	270	11	37	4	35	550	29	n/a	13	2 starch, 1 medium-fat meat, 1 fat
Monster Burger	1	610	39	58	18	105	1940	26	n/a	35	2 1/2 starch, 4 medium-fat meat, 3 fat

Super Star	1	790	53	60	17	145	970	41	n/a	40	3 starch, 4 medium-fat meat, 7 fat

CHICKEN

Chicken Breast (fried)	1	370	15	36	4	75	1190	29	n/a	29	2 starch, 3 lean meat, 1 fat
Chicken Leg (fried)	1	170	7	37	2	45	570	15	n/a	13	1 starch, 1 lean meat, 1 fat
Chicken Thigh (fried)	1	330	15	41	4	60	1000	30	n/a	19	2 starch, 2 lean meat, 2 fat
Chicken Wing (fried)	1	200	8	36	2	30	740	23	n/a	10	1 1/2 starch, 1 medium-fat meat, 1/2 fat

DESSERTS

Apple Turnover	1	270	12	40	4	0	250	38	n/a	4	1 fruit, 1 1/2 carb, 2 fat
✔ Cool Twist Cone (vanilla or chocolate)	1	180	2	10	1	10	120	34	n/a	4	2 carb
✔ Peach Cobbler	1	310	7	20	1	0	360	60	n/a	2	4 carb, 1 fat

✔ = Healthiest Bets; n/a = not available

(Continued)

SANDWICHES

	Amount	Cal.	Fat (g)	% Cal. Fat	Sat. Fat (g)	Chol. (mg)	Sod. (mg)	Carb. (g)	Fiber (g)	Pro. (g)	Servings/Exchanges
Bacon Swiss Crispy Chicken	1	670	44	59	9	55	1600	45	n/a	24	3 starch, 3 lean meat, 6 fat
Big Roast Beef Sandwich	1	410	24	53	9	40	1140	26	n/a	24	1 1/2 starch, 3 medium-fat meat, 2 fat
Chicken Fillet Sandwich	1	480	18	34	3	55	1190	44	n/a	24	3 starch, 2 lean meat, 2 fat
Fisherman's Fillet Sandwich	1	560	28	45	7	75	1280	45	n/a	25	3 starch, 2 lean meat, 4 fat
✔ Grilled Chicken Sandwich	1	350	16	41	3	65	860	28	n/a	23	2 starch, 3 lean meat, 2 fat
Hot Dog	1	450	32	64	12	55	1240	25	n/a	15	1 1/2 starch, 2 medium-fat meat, 4 fat
Hot Ham 'N' Cheese	1	310	12	35	6	50	1390	34	n/a	16	2 starch, 1 medium-fat meat, 1 fat

	Amount										Exchanges
Monster Roast Beef	1	610	39	58	18	105	1940	26	n/a	35	1 1/2 starch, 4 medium-fat meat, 4 fat
✔Regular Roast Beef	1	320	16	45	6	40	800	26	n/a	17	1 1/2 starch, 2 medium-fat meat, 1 fat
SHAKES											
Chocolate	12 oz	370	5	12	3	30	270	67	n/a	13	4 1/2 carb, 1 fat
Vanilla	12 oz	350	5	13	3	20	300	65	n/a	12	4 carb, 1 fat
SIDES											
Cole Slaw	4 oz	240	20	75	3	10	340	13	n/a	2	1 veg, 1/2 carb, 4 fat
Crispy Curls (monster)	1 order	590	31	47	6	0	1640	70	n/a	8	4 1/2 starch, 6 fat
Crispy Curls (large)	1 order	520	28	48	5	0	1450	62	n/a	7	4 starch, 5 1/2 fat
Crispy Curls (medium)	1 order	340	18	48	4	0	950	41	n/a	5	3 starch, 3 1/2 fat

✔ = Healthiest Bets; n/a = not available

(Continued)

SIDES (*Continued*)	Amount	Cal.	Fat (g)	% Cal. Fat	Sat. Fat (g)	Chol. (mg)	Sod. (mg)	Carb. (g)	Fiber (g)	Pro. (g)	Servings/Exchanges
French Fries (monster)	1 order	510	24	42	3	0	590	67	n/a	6	4 1/2 starch, 5 fat
French Fries (large)	1 order	440	21	43	3	0	520	59	n/a	5	4 starch, 4 fat
French Fries (regular)	1 order	340	16	42	2	0	390	45	n/a	6	3 starch, 3 fat
✔Gravy	3 T	20	0	0	0	0	260	3	n/a	0	free
✔Mashed Potatoes	1/2 cup	70	0	0	0	0	330	14	n/a	2	1 starch

✔ = Healthiest Bets; n/a = not available

Jack in the Box

❖Jack in the Box provides nutrition information
for all its menu items on their website at
www.jackinthebox.com.

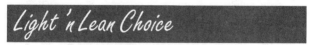

Chicken Fajita Pita
1/2 French Fries (*regular*)

Calories......................495	Sodium (mg)..........1,205
Fat (g) 18	Carbohydrate (g).........57
% calories from fat..33	Fiber (g) 5
Saturated fat (g)........7	Protein (g) 26
Cholesterol (mg) 55	

Exchanges: 3 1/2 starch, 2 lean meat, 2 fat

Healthy 'n Hearty Choice

2 Hamburgers with Cheese
Side Salad with Low Calorie Italian Dressing (*2 T*)

Calories......................662	Sodium (mg)..........2,085
Fat (g) 30	Carbohydrate (g).........66
% calories from fat..40	Fiber (g) 5
Saturated fat (g)......14	Protein (g) 31
Cholesterol (mg) 90	

Exchanges: 4 starch, 1 veg, 4 medium-fat meat, 4 fat

(*Continued*)

Jack in the Box

	Amount	Cal.	Fat (g)	% Cal. Fat	Sat. Fat (g)	Chol. (mg)	Sod. (mg)	Carb. (g)	Fiber (g)	Pro. (g)	Servings/Exchanges
BREAKFAST											
✓Biscuit	1	190	9	43	2.5	0	500	24	1	3	1 1/2 starch, 1 fat
✓Breakfast Jack	1	280	12	39	5	190	750	28	1	17	1 1/2 starch, 2 fat
✓French Toast Sticks	1 order	420	20	43	4	5	420	53	2	7	3 1/2 starch, 4 fat
Hash Browns	1 order	170	12	64	3	0	250	14	1	1	1 1/2 starch, 1 medium-fat meat, 1 fat
✓Pancakes with Bacon	1 order	370	9	22	2	30	1020	59	3	12	1 1/2 starch, 2 fat
Sausage Croissant	1	660	48	65	15	240	860	37	1	20	2 1/2 starch, 1 high-fat meat, 8 fat
Sausage, Egg & Cheese Biscuit	1	510	38	67	12	220	1050	27	2	19	2 starch, 2 high-fat meat, 3 fat

Sourdough Breakfast Sandwich	1	450	24	48	8	205	1040	36	1	21	2 starch, 1 high-fat meat, 4 fat
Supreme Croissant	1	530	34	58	10	225	1060	37	0	21	2 1/2 starch, 2 high-fat meat, 3 fat
Ultimate Breakfast Sandwich	1	600	34	51	10	410	1480	39	2	34	2 1/2 starch, 4 medium-fat meat, 3 fat

B U R G E R S

Bacon Bacon Burger	1	760	50	59	17	135	1570	39	2	39	2 1/2 starch, 3 medium-fat meat, 3 fat
Bacon Ultimate Cheeseburger	1	1020	71	63	26	210	1740	37	1	58	1 1/2 starch, 6 medium-fat meat, 12 fat
Double Cheeseburger	1	440	24	49	11	80	1100	31	2	24	2 starch, 3 medium-fat meat, 6 fat

(Continued)

✔ = Healthiest Bets; n/a = not available

BURGERS (Continued)	Amount	Cal.	Fat (g)	% Cal. Fat	Sat. Fat (g)	Chol. (mg)	Sod. (mg)	Carb. (g)	Fiber (g)	Pro. (g)	Servings/Exchanges
✔Hamburger	1	250	9	32	3.5	30	610	30	2	12	2 starch, 1 medium-fat meat, 1 fat
✔Hamburger with Cheese	1	300	13	39	6	31	840	31	2	14	2 starch, 2 medium-fat meat, 2 fat
Jumbo Jack	1	550	30	49	10	75	880	43	2	27	3 starch, 2 medium-fat meat, 4 fat
Jumbo Jack with Cheese	1	640	38	53	15	105	1340	44	2	31	3 starch, 3 medium-fat meat, 4 fat
Sourdough Jack	1	690	45	59	15	105	1180	37	2	34	2 1/2 starch, 4 medium-fat meat, 4 fat
Ultimate Cheeseburger	1	950	66	63	26	195	1370	37	1	52	3 1/2 starch, 6 medium-fat meat, 6 fat

CHICKEN

	Amount	Cal.	Fat (g)	% Cal. Fat	Sat. Fat (g)	Chol. (mg)	Sod. (mg)	Carb. (g)	Fiber (g)	Pro. (g)	Choices/Exchanges
Chicken Breast Pieces (breaded and fried)	5 pieces	360	17	43	3	80	970	24	1	27	1 1/2 starch, 3 lean meat, 3 fat
Chicken Teriyaki Bowl	1	670	4	5	1	15	1730	128	3	26	7 starch, 2 veg, 2 lean meat

CONDIMENTS

	Amount	Cal.	Fat (g)	% Cal. Fat	Sat. Fat (g)	Chol. (mg)	Sod. (mg)	Carb. (g)	Fiber (g)	Pro. (g)	Choices/Exchanges
✔Barbeque Dipping Sauce	1 oz/2 T	45	0	0	0	0	310	11	0	1	1/2 carb
Buttermilk House Dipping Sauce	1 oz/2 T	130	13	90	5	10	240	3	0	0	3 fat
✔Country Crock Spread	1 t	25	3	108	0.5	0	45	0	0	0	1/2 fat
✔Frank's Red Hot Buffalo Dipping Sauce	1 oz/2 T	10	0	0	0	0	840	2	0	0	free
✔Grape Jelly	1/2 oz/1 T	40	0	0	0	0	5	10	0	0	1/2 carb
Pancake Syrup	1.5 oz/3 T	130	0	0	0	0	5	30	0	0	2 starch

(Continued)

✔ = Healthiest Bets; n/a = not available

CONDIMENTS (Continued)	Amount	Cal.	Fat (g)	% Cal. Fat	Sat. Fat (g)	Chol. (mg)	Sod. (mg)	Carb. (g)	Fiber (g)	Pro. (g)	Servings/Exchanges
✓Salsa	1 oz/2 T	10	0	0	0	0	200	2	0	0	free
✓Sour Cream	1 oz/2 T	60	6	90	4	20	30	1	0	1	1 fat
✓Sweet & Sour Dipping Sauce	1 oz/2 T	45	0	0	0	0	160	11	0	0	1/2 carb
Tartar Dipping Sauce	1.5 oz/3 T	210	22	94	3	30	340	2	0	1	4 fat
DESSERTS											
Cheesecake	1	320	18	51	10	65	220	29	2	7	2 carb, 3 1/2 fat
✓Double Fudge Cake	1	300	10	30	2	50	320	50	1	3	3 carb, 2 fat
Hot Apple Turnover	1	340	18	48	4	0	510	41	2	4	3 carb, 3 1/2 fat
OTHER ENTREES											
Fish & Chips	1 order	780	39	45	9	45	1740	86	6	19	5 1/2 starch, 1 lean meat, 7 fat

	Serving	Cal	Fat (g)	% Fat Cal	Sat Fat (g)	Chol (mg)	Sod (mg)	Carb (g)	Fiber (g)	Prot (g)	Exchanges/Choices
Monster Taco	1	270	17	57	6	30	670	19	4	12	1 starch, 1 medium-fat meat, 2 fat
✔Taco	1	170	10	53	3.5	15	390	12	2	7	1/2 starch, 1 medium-fat meat, 1 fat

SALAD DRESSINGS

	Serving	Cal	Fat (g)	% Fat Cal	Sat Fat (g)	Chol (mg)	Sod (mg)	Carb (g)	Fiber (g)	Prot (g)	Exchanges/Choices
Blue Cheese	2 oz/4 T	210	15	64	2.5	25	750	11	0	1	1/2 carb, 3 fat
Buttermilk House	2 oz/4 T	290	30	93	11	20	560	6	0	1	1/2 carb, 6 fat
✔Low Calorie Italian	2 oz/4 T	25	2	72	0	0	670	2	0	0	free
Thousand Island	2 oz/4 T	250	24	86	4	35	570	10	0	1	1/2 carb, 5 fat

SALADS

	Serving	Cal	Fat (g)	% Fat Cal	Sat Fat (g)	Chol (mg)	Sod (mg)	Carb (g)	Fiber (g)	Prot (g)	Exchanges/Choices
✔Croutons	1 package	50	2	36	1.5	0	100	8	1	1	1/2 starch
✔Garden Chicken	1	200	9	41	4	65	420	8	3	23	1 veg, 3 lean meat
✔Side	1	50	3	54	1.5	10	75	3	1	2	1 veg, 1/2 fat

(Continued)

✔ = Healthiest Bets; n/a = not available

SANDWICHES

	Amount	Cal.	Fat (g)	% Cal. Fat	Sat. Fat (g)	Chol. (mg)	Sod. (mg)	Carb. (g)	Fiber (g)	Pro. (g)	Servings/Exchanges
Chicken	1	400	21	47	3	40	770	38	3	15	2 1/2 starch, 2 lean meat, 3 fat
✓Chicken Fajita Pita	1	280	10	32	4.5	55	850	34	3	24	1 1/2 starch, 3 lean meat
Chicken Supreme	1	830	49	53	7	65	2140	66	3	33	4 1/2 starch, 3 lean meat, 7 fat
Grilled Chicken Fillet	1	480	24	45	6	65	1110	39	4	27	2 1/2 starch, 3 lean meat, 4 fat
Jack's Spicy Chicken	1	570	29	46	2.5	50	1020	52	2	24	3 1/2 starch, 2 lean meat, 4 fat
Sourdough Grilled Chicken Club	1	520	27	47	6	80	1320	39	3	31	3 1/2 starch, 3 lean meat, 2 fat

SHAKES

	Amount	Cal.	Fat (g)	% Cal. Fat	Sat. Fat (g)	Chol. (mg)	Sod. (mg)	Carb. (g)	Fiber (g)	Prot. (g)	Exchanges
Cappuccino Classic	16 oz	630	29	41	17	90	320	80	0	11	5 carb, 5 fat
Chocolate Ice Cream Shake	16 oz	630	27	39	16	85	330	85	1	11	5 carb, 5 fat
Oreo Cookie Ice Cream Shake	16 oz	740	36	44	19	95	490	91	2	13	6 carb, 7 fat
Strawberry Ice Cream Shake	16 oz	640	28	39	15	85	300	85	0	10	5 1/2 carb, 5 1/2 fat
Vanilla Ice Cream Shake	16 oz	610	31	46	18	95	320	73	0	12	5 carb, 6 fat

SNACKS

	Amount	Cal.	Fat (g)	% Cal. Fat	Sat. Fat (g)	Chol. (mg)	Sod. (mg)	Carb. (g)	Fiber (g)	Prot. (g)	Exchanges
Bacon & Cheddar Potato Wedges	1 order	750	50	60	18	45	1510	55	0	20	3 starch, 2 high-fat meat, 2 1/2 fat
Chili Cheese Curly Fries	1 order	650	41	57	12	25	1760	60	4	14	4 starch, 8 fat
✔ Egg Rolls-1 piece	1 order	150	8	48	2	10	340	13	1	5	1 starch, 1 fat
Egg Rolls-3 piece	1 order	440	24	49	6	30	1020	40	4	15	2 1/2 starch, 1 medium-fat meat, 4 fat

✔ = Healthiest Bets; n/a = not available

(Continued)

SNACKS (Continued)	Amount	Cal.	Fat (g)	% Cal. Fat	Sat. Fat (g)	Chol. (mg)	Sod. (mg)	Carb. (g)	Fiber (g)	Pro. (g)	Servings/Exchanges
French Fries (super scoop)	1 order	610	28	41	6	0	1250	82	5	6	5 1/2 starch, 5 1/2 fat
French Fries (jumbo)	1 order	430	20	42	5	0	890	58	4	4	4 starch, 4 fat
French Fries (regular)	1 order	350	16	41	4	0	710	46	3	4	3 starch, 3 fat
Onion Rings	1 order	450	25	50	5	0	780	50	3	7	3 starch, 5 fat
Seasoned Curly Fries	1 order	410	23	50	5	0	1010	45	4	6	3 starch, 4 1/2 fat
Stuffed Jalapenos-3 piece	1 order	230	13	51	5	25	740	20	2	7	1 starch, 1 medium-fat meat, 2 fat
Stuffed Jalapenos-7 piece	1 order	530	31	53	12	60	1730	46	3	16	3 starch, 1 high-fat meat, 5 fat

✔ = Healthiest Bets; n/a = not available

McDonald's

❖McDonald's provides nutrition information
for all its menu items on their website at
www.mcdonalds.com.

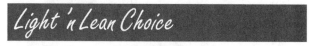
Light 'n Lean Choice

Hamburger
Garden Salad
Fat-Free Herb Vinaigrette (*1 pkt*)
Vanilla Reduced Fat Ice Cream Cone

Calories	565	Sodium (mg)	1,045
Fat (g)	21	Carbohydrate (g)	70
% calories from fat	33	Fiber (g)	n/a
Saturated fat (g)	10	Protein (g)	23
Cholesterol (mg)	125		

Exchanges: 2 starch, 1 veg, 2 carb, 2 medium-fat
meat, 1 1/2 fat

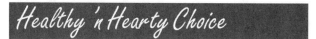
Healthy 'n Hearty Choice

Grilled Chicken Deluxe (*without mayonnaise*)
French Fries (*small*)
Garden Salad with Ranch Salad Dressing (*2 T*)

Calories	730	Sodium (mg)	1,375
Fat (g)	32	Carbohydrate (g)	77
% calories from fat	39	Fiber (g)	n/a
Saturated fat (g)	8	Protein (g)	36
Cholesterol (mg)	133		

Exchanges: 4 1/2 starch, 1 veg, 3 lean meat, 2 1/2 fat

(*Continued*)

McDonald's

	Amount	Cal.	Fat (g)	% Cal. Fat	Sat. Fat (g)	Chol. (mg)	Sod. (mg)	Carb. (g)	Fiber (g)	Pro. (g)	Servings/Exchanges
BREAKFAST											
Bacon, Egg & Cheese Biscuit	1	480	31	58	10	250	1410	36	2	20	2 1/2 starch, 2 medium-fat meat, 3 fat
✔Biscuit	1	240	11	41	2.5	0	640	30	n/a	4	2 starch, 1 1/2 fat
Breakfast Burrito	1	290	16	50	6	170	680	24	n/a	13	1 1/2 starch, 1 medium-fat meat, 3 fat
✔Egg McMuffin	1	290	12	37	4.5	235	790	27	n/a	17	2 starch, 2 medium-fat meat
✔English Muffin	1	140	2	13	0	0	210	25	n/a	4	1 1/2 starch
Ham, Egg and Cheese Bagel	1	550	23	38	8	255	1490	58	n/a	26	4 starch, 2 medium-fat meat, 2 fat

✔ Hash Browns	1 order	130	8	55	1.5	0	330	14	n/a	1	1 starch, 1 1/2 fat
✔ Hotcakes (2 pats margarine and syrup)	1 order	600	17	26	3	20	770	104	n/a	9	5 starch, 2 carb, 3 fat
✔ Hotcakes (plain)	1 order	340	8	21	1.5	20	630	58	n/a	9	4 starch, 1 fat
Sausage	1 order	170	16	85	5	35	290	0	0	6	1 high-fat meat, 1 fat
Sausage Biscuit	1	410	28	61	8	35	930	30	n/a	10	2 starch, 1 high-fat meat, 4 fat
Sausage Biscuit with Egg	1	490	33	61	10	245	1010	31	n/a	16	2 starch, 2 high-fat meat, 3 fat
Sausage McMuffin	1	360	23	58	8	45	740	26	n/a	13	1 1/2 starch, 1 high-fat meat, 3 fat
Sausage McMuffin with Egg	1	440	28	57	10	255	890	27	n/a	19	2 starch, 2 medium-fat meat, 3 1/2 fat

(Continued)

✔ = Healthiest Bets; n/a = not available

BREAKFAST (*Continued*)	Amount	Cal.	Fat (g)	% Cal. Fat	Sat. Fat (g)	Chol. (mg)	Sod. (mg)	Carb. (g)	Fiber (g)	Pro. (g)	Servings/Exchanges
✓ Scrambled Eggs (2)	1 order	160	11	62	3.5	425	170	1	n/a	13	2 medium-fat meat
Spanish Omelet Bagel	1	690	38	50	14	275	1570	60	n/a	27	4 starch, 2 medium-fat meat, 5 fat
Steak, Egg and Cheese Bagel	1	700	35	45	13	290	1290	57	n/a	38	4 starch, 4 medium-fat meat, 2 fat
BURGERS											
Big Mac	1	590	34	52	11	85	1090	47	n/a	24	3 starch, 2 medium-fat meat, 4 fat
Big N' Tasty	1	540	32	53	10	80	970	39	n/a	24	2 1/2 starch, 2 medium-fat meat, 2 fat
Big N' Tasty with Cheese	1	590	37	56	12	95	1210	40	n/a	27	2 1/2 starch, 2 medium-fat meat, 3 fat

✔Cheeseburger	1	330	14	38	6	45	830	36	n/a	15	2 1/2 starch, 1 medium-fat meat, 1 1/2 fat
✔Hamburger	1	280	10	32	4	30	590	35	n/a	12	2 starch, 1 medium-fat meat, 1 fat
✔Quarter Pounder	1	430	21	44	8	70	840	37	n/a	23	2 1/2 starch, 2 medium-fat meat, 2 fat
Quarter Pounder with Cheese	1	530	30	51	13	95	1310	38	n/a	28	2 1/2 starch, 3 medium-fat meat, 3 fat

CONDIMENTS

✔Barbeque Sauce (1 packet)	1 oz/2 T	45	0	0	0	0	250	10	n/a	0	1/2 carb
✔Honey (1 package)	1 oz/2T	45	0	0	0	0		12	n/a	0	1/2 carb

✔ = Healthiest Bets; n/a = not available

(Continued)

CONDIMENTS *(Continued)*	Amount	Cal.	Fat (g)	% Cal. Fat	Sat. Fat (g)	Chol. (mg)	Sod. (mg)	Carb. (g)	Fiber (g)	Pro. (g)	Servings/Exchanges
✓ Honey Mustard (1 packet)	1/2 oz/1 T	50	5	90	0.5	10	85	3	n/a	0	1 fat
✓ Hot Mustard (1 packet)	1 oz/2 T	60	4	60	0	5	240	7	n/a	1	1/2 carb, 1 fat
✓ Light Mayonnaise	1/2 oz/1 T	40	5	113	0.5	10	100	1	n/a	0	1 fat
✓ Sweet 'N Sour Sauce (1 packet)	1 oz/2 T	50	0	0	0	0	140	11	n/a	0	1 carb

DANISHES/MUFFINS

	Amount	Cal.	Fat (g)	% Cal. Fat	Sat. Fat (g)	Chol. (mg)	Sod. (mg)	Carb. (g)	Fiber (g)	Pro. (g)	Servings/Exchanges
Apple Danish	1	340	15	40	3	20	340	47	n/a	5	3 carb, 3 fat
Cheese Danish	1	400	21	47	5	40	400	45	n/a	7	3 carb, 4 fat
Cinnamon Roll	1	390	18	42	5	65	310	50	n/a	6	3 carb, 3 1/2 fat
✓ Lowfat Apple Bran Muffin	1	300	3	9	0.5	0	380	61	n/a	6	4 starch, 1/2 fat

DESSERTS

Baked Apple Pie	1	260	13	45	3.5	0	200	34	n/a	3	2 carb, 3 fat
Butterfinger McFlurry	1	620	22	32	14	70	260	90	n/a	16	6 carb, 3 fat
Chocolate Chip Cookie	1 pkg	280	14	45	8	40	170	37	n/a	3	2 1/2 carb, 2 fat
Fruit n' Yogurt Parfait	1	380	5	12	2	15	240	76	n/a	10	5 carb, 1 fat
✔Fruit n' Yogurt Parfait (w/o granola)	1	280	4	13	2	15	115	53	n/a	8	3 1/2 carb, 1 fat
Hot Caramel Sundae	1	360	10	25	6	35	180	61	n/a	7	4 carb, 2 fat
Hot Fudge Sundae	1	340	12	32	9	30	170	52	n/a	8	3 1/2 carb, 2 fat
M&M McFlurry	1	630	26	37	15	75	210	90	n/a	16	5 carb, 5 fat
✔McDonaldland Cookies	1 pkg.	230	8	31	2	0	250	38	n/a	3	2 1/2 carb, 1 fat
Nestle's Crunch McFlurry	1	630	24	34	16	75	230	89	n/a	16	6 carb, 4 fat
Nuts (on sundaes)	1/2 T	40	4	90	0	0	55	2	n/a	2	1 fat

✔ = Healthiest Bets; n/a = not available

(Continued)

DESSERTS (*Continued*)	Amount	Cal.	Fat (g)	% Cal. Fat	Sat. Fat (g)	Chol. (mg)	Sod. (mg)	Carb. (g)	Fiber (g)	Pro. (g)	Servings/Exchanges
Oreo McFlurry	1	570	20	32	12	70	280	82	n/a	15	5 1/2 carb, 3 fat
✔ Strawberry Sundae	1	290	7	22	5	30	95	50	n/a	7	3 carb, 1 fat
✔ Vanilla Reduced Fat Ice Cream Cone	1	150	5	30	3	20	75	23	n/a	4	1 1/2 carb, 1 fat
OTHER ENTREES											
✔ Chicken McNuggets (4 piece)	1 order	190	11	52	2.5	35	360	13	n/a	10	1 starch, 1 lean meat, 1 fat
Chicken McNuggets (6 piece)	1 order	290	17	53	3.5	55	540	20	n/a	15	1 starch, 2 lean meat, 2 fat
Chicken McNuggets (9 piece)	1 order	430	25	52	5	80	810	29	n/a	23	2 starch, 3 lean meat, 2 fat

SALAD DRESSINGS

	Amount	Cal.	Fat (g)	% Fat Cal.	Sat. Fat (g)	Chol. (mg)	Sod. (mg)	Carb. (g)	Fiber (g)	Prot. (g)	Exchanges/Choices
1000 Island	1 oz/2 T	130	9	62	1.5	15	350	11	n/a	1	1/2 carb, 1 fat
Caesar (1 packet)	2 oz/4 T	150	13	78	2.5	10	400	5	n/a	1	3 fat
✔Fat-Free Herb Vinaigrette (1 packet)	2 oz/4 T	35	0	0	0	0	260	8	n/a	0	1 carb
Honey Mustard (1 packet)	2 oz/4 T	160	11	62	1.5	15	260	13	n/a	1	1 carb, 2 fat
Ranch (1 packet)	2 oz/4 T	170	18	95	2.5	15	460	3	n/a	0	1/2 carb, 4 fat
✔Red French Reduced Calorie (1 packet)	2 oz/4 T	130	6	42	1	0	360	18	n/a	0	1 carb, 1 fat

SALADS

	Amount	Cal.	Fat (g)	% Fat Cal.	Sat. Fat (g)	Chol. (mg)	Sod. (mg)	Carb. (g)	Fiber (g)	Prot. (g)	Exchanges/Choices
✔Chef Salad	1	150	8	48	3.5	95	740	5	n/a	17	1 veg, 2 lean meat, 1/2 fat
✔Croutons	1 pkg.	50	1	18	0	0	105	9	n/a	1	1/2 starch

✔ = Healthiest Bets; n/a = not available

(Continued)

SALADS *(Continued)*	Amount	Cal.	Fat (g)	% Cal. Fat	Sat. Fat (g)	Chol. (mg)	Sod. (mg)	Carb. (g)	Fiber (g)	Pro. (g)	Servings/Exchanges
✔Garden Salad	1	100	6	54	3	75	120	4	n/a	7	1 veg, 1 lean meat, 1 fat
✔Grilled Chicken Caesar	1	100	3	27	1.5	40	240	3	n/a	17	1 veg, 2 lean meat
SANDWICHES											
✔Chicken McGrill	1	450	18	36	3	60	970	46	n/a	26	3 starch, 3 lean meat, 2 fat
✔Chicken McGrill (w/o mayonnaise)	1	340	7	19	1.5	50	890	45	n/a	26	3 starch, 3 lean meat
Crispy Chicken (fried)	1	550	27	44	4.5	50	1180	54	n/a	23	3 1/2 starch, 2 lean meat, 4 fat
Filet-o-Fish	1	470	26	50	5	50	890	45	n/a	15	3 starch, 1 lean meat, 4 fat
SHAKES											
Chocolate Shake (small)	1	360	9	23	6	40	250	60	n/a	11	4 carb, 2 fat
Strawberry Shake (small)	1	360	9	23	6	40	180	60	n/a	11	4 carb, 2 fat

Vanilla Shake (small)	1	360	9	23	6	40	250	59	n/a	11	4 carb, 2 fat

SIDES

French Fries (super size)	1 order	610	29	43	5	0	390	77	n/a	9	5 starch, 6 fat
French Fries (large)	1 order	540	26	43	4.5	0	350	68	n/a	8	4 1/2 starch, 5 fat
French Fries (medium)	1 order	450	22	44	4	0	290	57	n/a	6	4 starch, 4 fat
✔French Fries (small)	1 order	210	10	43	1.5	0	135	26	n/a	3	1 1/2 starch, 2 fat

✔ = Healthiest Bets; n/a = not available

Sonic, America's Drive-In

❖Sonic, America's Drive-In, provides nutrition
information for all its menu items on their website
at www.sonicdrivein.com.

Light 'n Lean Choice

Jr. Burger
1/2 Regular French Fries
1 Fat-Free Milk (*8 oz*)

Calories	539	
Fat (g)	20	
% calories from fat	43	
Saturated fat (g)	7	
Cholesterol (mg)	49	
Sodium (mg)	580	
Carbohydrate (g)	50	
Fiber (g)	3	
Protein (g)	23	

Exchanges: 2 1/2 starch, 1 fat-free milk, 2 medium-fat
meat, 2 fat

Healthy 'n Hearty Choice

No. 2 Burger
1/2 Onion Rings
1/2 Vanilla Shake

Calories	871	
Fat (g)	37	
% calories from fat	38	
Saturated fat (g)	10	
Cholesterol (mg)	29	
Sodium (mg)	1,140	
Carbohydrate (g)	91	
Fiber (g)	6	
Protein (g)	23	

Exchanges: 5 starch, 1 carb, 2 medium fat meat, 4 fat

Sonic, America's Drive-In

	Amount	Cal.	Fat (g)	% Cal. Fat	Sat. Fat (g)	Chol. (mg)	Sod. (mg)	Carb. (g)	Fiber (g)	Pro. (g)	Servings/Exchanges
ADD-ONS											
Bacon	1 strip	80	7	79	3	15	350	0	0	5	1 1/2 fat
Chocolate Cone Coat	1 oz	143	8	50	7	0	40	16	1	1	1 carb, 1 1/2 fat
Honey Mustard Dressing	1 oz	110	9	74	1	10	300	9	0	0	1/2 carb, 2 fat
✔Hot Fudge Topping	1 oz	101	4	36	3	0	39	16	0	1	1 carb, 1 fat
✔Marinara Sauce	1 oz	15	0	0	0	0	260	3	0	0	free
Ranch Dressing	1 oz	147	16	98	2	5	215	2	0	0	3 fat
Shredded Cheddar Cheese	1 oz	104	9	78	6	28	491	1	0	6	2 fat
✔Slaw	1 oz	45	3	60	0	0	45	4	1	0	1/2 fat
✔Sonic Chili	1 oz	52	4	69	2	8	59	1	0	2	1 fat

✔ = Healthiest Bets; n/a = not available

(Continued)

ADD-ONS (Continued)	Amount	Cal.	Fat (g)	% Cal. Fat	Sat. Fat (g)	Chol. (mg)	Sod. (mg)	Carb. (g)	Fiber (g)	Pro. (g)	Servings/Exchanges
✓Sonic Green Chiles	1 oz	10	0	0	0	0	24	3	0	0	free
✓Sonic Hickory BBQ Sauce	1 oz	41	0	0	0	0	429	10	n/a	n/a	1/2 carb
✓Strawberry Topping	1 oz	38	0	0	0	0	0	10	1	0	1/2 carb
✓Sweet Pickle Relish	1 oz	40	0	0	0	0	248	11	0	0	1/2 carb
Thousand Island Dressing	1 oz	150	15	90	2	10	170	3	0	0	3 carb

BURGERS

	Amount	Cal.	Fat (g)	% Cal. Fat	Sat. Fat (g)	Chol. (mg)	Sod. (mg)	Carb. (g)	Fiber (g)	Pro. (g)	Servings/Exchanges
Bacon Cheeseburger	1	727	49	61	13	67	1433	44	2	23	3 starch, 2 medium-fat meat, 7 fat
Jr. Burger	1	353	21	54	6	45	1294	27	1	14	2 starch, 1 medium-fat meat, 3 fat
No. 1 Burger	1	577	36	56	7	37	753	43	2	14	3 starch, 1 medium-fat meat, 6 fat

No. 1 Cheeseburger	1	647	42	58	11	52	1103	44	2	18	3 starch, 2 medium-fat meat, 6 fat
No. 2 Burger	1	481	25	47	5	29	761	43	2	14	3 starch, 1 medium-fat meat, 4 fat
No. 2 Cheeseburger	1	551	31	51	9	44	1110	44	2	18	3 starch, 2 medium-fat meat, 3 1/2 fat
Super Sonic No. 2	1	839	55	59	17	88	1571	46	3	28	3 starch, 3 medium-fat meat, 8 fat
Super Sonic No.1	1	929	66	64	19	96	1476	45	2	28	3 starch, 3 medium-fat meat, 10 fat

CHICKEN

Breaded Chicken Sandwich	1	582	23	36	4	427	427	66	2	28	4 1/2 starch, 3 lean meat, 1 fat

✔ = Healthiest Bets; n/a = not available

(Continued)

CHICKEN (Continued)	Amount	Cal.	Fat (g)	% Cal. Fat	Sat. Fat (g)	Chol. (mg)	Sod. (mg)	Carb. (g)	Fiber (g)	Pro. (g)	Servings/Exchanges
Chicken Strip Dinner	1 order	749	32	38	5	47	1973	86	5	32	5 1/2 starch, 3 lean meat, 3 fat
✓Chicken Strip Snack	1 order	272	13	43	2	35	760	22	0	19	1/2 starch, 3 lean meat, 1 fat
✓Grilled Chicken Sandwich	1	343	13	34	2	70	829	31	2	27	2 starch, 3 lean meat, 1 fat
CONEYS											
Corn Dog	1	262	17	58	5	15	480	23	1	6	1 1/2 starch, 1 high-fat meat, 1 fat
Extra Long Cheese Coney Plain	1	666	42	57	17	87	1648	47	2	23	3 starch, 2 high-fat meat, 5 fat
Extra Long Plain Coney	1	483	27	50	10	50	1162	44	1	14	3 starch, 1 high-fat meat, 3 fat

Regular Cheese Coney	1	366	24	59	10	52	962	24	1	13	1 1/2 starch, 2 high-fat meat, 2 fat
✔ Regular Coney Plain	1	262	16	55	5	30	657	22	1	8	1 1/2 starch, 1 high-fat meat, 1 fat

FAVES & CRAVES

✔ Ched 'R' Peppers	1 order	256	12	42	5	28	1056	29	4	8	2 starch, 2 fat
Large Cheese Fries	1 order	322	19	53	6	15	1108	31	5	7	2 starch, 4 fat
Large Cheese Tots	1 order	435	27	56	8	15	1708	41	4	4	2 1/2 starch, 5 fat
Large Chili Cheese Fries	1 order	357	22	55	7	22	1062	32	5	8	2 starch, 4 fat
Large Chili Cheese Tots	1 order	547	36	59	11	37	1844	43	5	9	3 starch, 5 fat
Large French Fries	1 order	252	13	46	2	0	758	30	5	3	2 starch, 3 fat
Large Onion Rings	1 order	507	7	12	1	0	486	102	10	12	7 starch, 1 fat
Large Tater Tots	1 order	365	21	52	4	0	1358	40	4	0	2 1/2 starch, 4 fat

✔ = Healthiest Bets; n/a = not available

(Continued)

FAVES & CRAVES (*Continued*)	Amount	Cal.	Fat (g)	% Cal. Fat	Sat. Fat (g)	Chol. (mg)	Sod. (mg)	Carb. (g)	Fiber (g)	Pro. (g)	Servings/Exchanges
Mozzarella Sticks	1 order	382	19	45	11	50	1300	35	0	20	2 starch, 2 high-fat meat, 1/2 fat
Regular Cheese Fries	1 order	265	17	58	6	15	998	23	4	6	1 1/2 starch, 3 fat
Regular Cheese Tater Tots	1 order	329	22	60	7	15	1396	28	3	4	2 starch, 4 fat
Regular Chili Cheese Fries	1 order	299	19	57	6	22	952	24	4	8	1 1/2 starch, 4 fat
Regular Chili Cheese Tater Tots	1 order	363	25	62	7	22	1350	28	3	5	2 starch, 5 fat
✔ Regular French Fries	1 order	195	11	51	2	0	648	22	4	2	1 1/2 starch, 2 fat
Regular Onion Rings	1 order	331	5	14	1	0	311	66	7	8	4 1/2 starch, 1 fat
Regular Tater Tots	1 order	259	16	56	3	0	1046	27	3	0	2 starch, 3 fat
Super Sonic Fries	1 order	358	18	45	3	53	963	44	7	5	3 starch, 3 fat
Super Sonic Onion Rings	1 order	611	44	65	13	0	816	36	3	18	2 1/2 starch, 9 fat

	1 order	485	28	52	5	0	1670	53	5	0	3 1/2 starch, 5 fat
Super Sonic Tots											

FOUNTAIN FAVORITES

Large Blue Coconut Slush	1	521	0	0	0	0	27	134	0	0	9 carb
Large Cherry Limeade	1	361	0	0	0	0	69	98	2	0	6 1/2 carb
Large Cherry Slush	1	517	0	0	0	0	17	131	0	0	9 carb
Large Grape Slush	1	520	0	0	0	0	24	134	0	0	9 carb
Large Lemon Berry Slush	1	519	0	0	0	0	14	134	1	0	9 carb
Large Lemon Slush	1	491	0	0	0	0	14	127	0	0	9 carb
Large Lime Slush	1	497	0	0	0	0	13	129	1	0	9 carb
Large Limeade	1	303	0	0	0	0	69	83	2	0	5 1/2 carb
Large Ocean Water	1	336	0	0	0	0	86	90	0	0	6 carb
Large Orange Slush	1	519	0	0	0	0	10	134	0	0	9 carb
Large Strawberry Limeade	1	341	0	0	0	0	69	93	2	0	6 carb

✔ = Healthiest Bets; n/a = not available

(Continued)

FOUNTAIN FAVORITES (*Continued*)	Amount	Cal.	Fat (g)	% Cal. Fat	Sat. Fat (g)	Chol. (mg)	Sod. (mg)	Carb. (g)	Fiber (g)	Pro. (g)	Servings/Exchanges
Large Strawberry Slush	1	531	0	0	0	0	10	137	1	0	9 carb
Large Watermelon Slush	1	526	0	0	0	0	31	136	0	0	9 carb
Regular Blue Coconut Slush	1	329	0	0	0	0	18	85	0	0	5 1/2 carb
Regular Cherry Limeade	1	220	0	0	0	0	40	60	1	0	4 carb
Regular Cherry Slush	1	327	0	0	0	0	11	84	0	0	5 1/2 carb
Regular Grape Slush	1	327	0	0	0	0	11	84	0	0	5 1/2 carb
Regular Lemon Berry Slush	1	331	0	0	0	0	11	86	1	0	5 1/2 carb
Regular Lemon Slush	1	313	0	0	0	0	11	81	0	0	5 1/2 carb
Regular Lime Slush	1	319	0	0	0	0	9	83	1	0	5 1/2 carb
Regular Limeade	1	178	0	0	0	0	40	49	1	0	3 1/2 carb
Regular Ocean Water	1	200	0	0	0	0	52	54	0	0	3 1/2 carb
Regular Orange Slush	1	328	0	0	0	0	6	85	0	0	5 1/2 carb

Item											
Regular Strawberry Limeade	1	207	0	0	0	0	40	57	1	0	4 carb
Regular Strawberry Slush	1	334	0	0	0	0	6	86	1	0	5 1/2 carb
Regular Watermelon Slush	1	332	0	0	0	0	21	86	0	0	5 1/2 carb
Route 44 Blue Coconut Slush	1	718	0	0	0	0	37	185	0	0	12 carb
Route 44 Cherry Limeade	1	454	0	0	0	0	86	123	2	0	8 carb
Route 44 Cherry Slush	1	713	0	0	0	0	24	184	0	0	12 carb
Route 44 Grape Slush	1	717	0	0	0	0	33	185	0	0	12 carb
Route 44 Lemon Berry Slush	1	710	0	0	0	0	20	184	1	0	12 carb
Route 44 Lemon Slush	1	673	0	0	0	0	20	175	1	0	11 1/2 carb
Route 44 Lime Slush	1	680	0	0	0	0	17	117	2	0	8 carb
Route 44 Limeade	1	380	0	0	0	0	86	105	2	0	7 carb
Route 44 Orange Slush	1	714	0	0	0	0	14	184	0	0	12 carb
Route 44 Strawberry Limeade	1	428	0	0	0	0	86	117	3	0	8 carb

✔ = Healthiest Bets; n/a = not available

(Continued)

FOUNTAIN FAVORITES (Continued)	Amount	Cal.	Fat (g)	% Cal. Fat	Sat. Fat (g)	Chol. (mg)	Sod. (mg)	Carb. (g)	Fiber (g)	Pro. (g)	Servings/Exchanges
Route 44 Strawberry Slush	1	728	0	0	0	0	14	188	1	0	12 carb
Route 44 Watermelon Slush	1	724	0	0	0	0	42	187	0	0	12 carb
Small Blue Coconut Slush	1	224	0	0	0	0	10	58	0	0	4 carb
Small Cherry Limeade	1	169	0	0	0	0	33	46	1	0	3 carb
Small Cherry Slush	1	223	0	0	0	0	7	58	0	0	4 carb
Small Grape Slush	1	224	0	0	0	0	9	58	0	0	4 carb
Small Lemon Berry Slush	1	233	0	0	0	0	9	60	0	0	4 carb
Small Lemon Slush	1	224	0	0	0	0	9	58	0	0	4 carb
Small Lime Slush	1	225	0	0	0	0	7	56	0	0	4 carb
Small Limeade	1	143	0	0	0	0	33	39	1	0	3 1/2 carb
Small Ocean Water	1	154	0	0	0	0	39	41	0	0	3 1/2 carb

	✓										
Small Orange Slush	✓	223	0	0	0	0	5	58	0	0	4 carb
Small Strawberry Limeade	✓	172	0	0	0	0	33	47	1	0	3 carb
Small Strawberry Slush	✓	227	0	0	0	0	5	59	0	0	4 carb
Small Watermelon Slush	✓	225	0	0	0	0	12	58	0	0	4 carb
Wacky Pack Watermelon Slush	✓	196	0	0	0	0	11	51	0	0	3 1/2 carb
Wacky Pack Blue Coconut Slush	✓	194	0	0	0	0	10	50	0	0	3 1/2 carb
Wacky Pack Cherry Limeade	✓	139	0	0	0	0	26	38	1	0	2 1/2 carb
Wacky Pack Cherry Slush	✓	193	0	0	0	0	6	50	0	0	3 1/2 carb
Wacky Pack Grape Slush	✓	194	0	0	0	0	9	50	0	0	3 1/2 carb
Wacky Pack Lemon Berry Slush	✓	194	0	0	0	0	8	50	0	0	3 1/2 carb
Wacky Pack Lemon Slush	✓	194	0	0	0	0	8	50	0	0	3 1/2 carb
Wacky Pack Lime Slush	✓	195	0	0	0	0	7	51	1	0	3 1/2 carb
Wacky Pack Limeade	✓	113	0	0	0	0	26	31	1	0	2 carb

✓ = Healthiest Bets; n/a = not available

(Continued)

FOUNTAIN FAVORITES (*Continued*)	Amount	Cal.	Fat (g)	% Cal. Fat	Sat. Fat (g)	Chol. (mg)	Sod. (mg)	Carb. (g)	Fiber (g)	Pro. (g)	Servings/Exchanges
Wacky Pack Ocean Water	1	124	0	0	0	0	32	33	0	0	2 carb
Wacky Pack Orange Slush	1	193	0	0	0	0	4	50	0	0	3 1/2 carb
Wacky Pack Strawberry Limeade	1	132	0	0	0	0	26	36	1	0	2 1/2 carb
Wacky Pack Strawberry Slush	1	188	0	0	0	0	4	48	0	0	3 carb
FROZEN FAVORITES											
Add 1 oz Malt to any Shake	1 oz	104	1	9	0	0	23	22	n/a	4	1 1/2 carb
Banana Cream Pie Shake Large	1	1058	35	30	28	63	636	130	3	16	8 1/2 carb, 7 fat
Banana Cream Pie Shake Regular	1	775	27	31	21	47	474	92	2	12	6 carb, 5 fat
Banana Shake Large	1	713	76	96	25	60	485	70	3	13	4 1/2 carb, 5 fat
Banana Shake Regular	1	508	52	92	18	45	363	46	1	10	3 carb, 3 fat
Banana Split	1	467	72	139	10	23	224	75	3	6	5 carb, 2 fat

Blue Coconut Float or Flurry Drink Large	1	609	17	25	17	43	367	75	0	9	3 carb, 2 fat
Blue Coconut Float or Flurry Drink Regular	1	424	12	25	12	30	255	52	0	6	3 1/2 carb, 2 fat
Butterfinger Blast Large	1	924	37	36	32	61	613	85	2	20	5 1/2 carb, 5 fat
Butterfinger Blast Regular	1	636	26	37	23	46	436	56	1	13	3 1/2 carb, 5 fat
Cherry Slush Float or Flurry Drink Large	1	605	17	25	17	43	358	74	0	9	5 carb, 3 fat
Cherry Slush Float or Flurry Drink Regular	1	421	12	26	12	30	249	52	0	6	3 1/2 carb, 2 fat
Chocolate Covered Banana Shake Large	1	831	31	34	29	61	515	85	3	14	5 1/2 carb, 6 fat

✔ = Healthiest Bets; n/a = not available

(Continued)

FROZEN FAVORITES (*Continued*)	Amount	Cal.	Fat (g)	% Cal. Fat	Sat. Fat (g)	Chol. (mg)	Sod. (mg)	Carb. (g)	Fiber (g)	Pro. (g)	Servings/Exchanges
Chocolate Covered Banana Shake Regular	1	625	25	36	23	46	393	60	2	10	4 carb, 5 fat
Chocolate Covered Cherry Shake Large	1	825	35	38	33	61	534	73	1	13	5 carb, 7 fat
Chocolate Covered Cherry Shake Regular	1	587	24	37	23	46	393	51	1	10	3 1/2 carb, 5 fat
Chocolate Covered Peanut Butter Shake Large	1	1007	54	48	36	61	687	72	2	17	5 carb, 10 fat
Chocolate Covered Peanut Butter Shake Regular	1	678	34	45	25	46	469	50	1	12	3 carb, 7 fat
Chocolate Covered Strawberry Shake Large	1	868	35	36	33	61	534	84	2	14	5 1/2 carb, 5 fat

Item											
Chocolate Covered Strawberry Shake Regular	1	608	24	36	23	46	393	56	1	10	3 1/2 carb, 4 fat
Chocolate Cream Pie Shake Large	1	1151	35	27	28	63	739	151	1	16	14 carb, 7 fat
Chocolate Cream Pie Shake Regular	1	795	27	31	21	47	525	96	1	12	6 1/2 carb, 5 fat
Chocolate Shake Large	1	752	25	30	24	60	587	77	0	13	5 carb, 5 fat
Chocolate Shake Regular	1	564	18	29	18	45	440	58	0	10	4 carb, 3 fat
Chocolate Sundae	1	362	11	27	11	26	270	41	0	6	2 1/2 carb, 2 fat
Coca Cola Float or Flurry Drink Large	1	544	17	28	17	43	353	59	0	9	4 carb, 3 fat
Coca Cola Float or Flurry Drink Regular	1	379	12	28	12	30	246	41	0	6	3 1/2 carb, 2 fat

✔ = Healthiest Bets; n/a = not available

(*Continued*)

FROZEN FAVORITES (Continued)	Amount	Cal.	Fat (g)	% Cal. Fat	Sat. Fat (g)	Chol. (mg)	Sod. (mg)	Carb. (g)	Fiber (g)	Pro. (g)	Servings/Exchanges
Coconut Cream Pie Shake Large	1	1004	35	31	27	63	636	116	1	15	7 1/2 carb, 5 fat
Coconut Cream Pie Shake Regular	1	721	26	32	21	47	474	79	1	11	5 carb, 4 fat
✓Dish of Vanilla	1	265	11	37	11	26	212	19	0	5	1 1/2 carb, 2 fat
Dr Pepper Float or Flurry Drink Large	1	541	17	28	17	43	385	59	0	9	4 carb, 3 fat
Dr Pepper Float or Flurry Drink Regular	1	377	12	29	12	30	268	41	0	6	3 carb, 2 fat
Grape Slush Float or Flurry Drink Large	1	608	17	25	17	43	365	75	0	9	5 carb, 3 fat
Grape Slush Float or Flurry Drink Regular	1	423	12	26	12	30	253	52	0	6	3 1/2 carb, 2 fat

Item											
Hot Fudge Sundae	1	392	15	34	15	27	255	40	0	6	2 1/2 carb, 3 fat
✔ Ice Cream Cone	1	285	11	35	11	26	223	23	0	6	1 1/2 carb, 2 fat
M&M's Blast Large	1	931	39	38	34	69	525	89	2	15	6 carb, 6 fat
M&M's Blast Regular	1	641	27	38	24	50	387	58	1	11	4 carb, 5 fat
Orange Slush Float or Flurry Drink Large	1	606	17	25	17	43	350	75	0	9	5 carb, 3 fat
Orange Slush Float or Flurry Drink Regular	1	422	12	26	12	30	244	52	0	6	3 1/2 carb, 2 fat
Oreo Blast Large	1	927	39	38	28	60	912	88	2	16	6 carb, 5 fat
Oreo Blast Regular	1	638	27	15	21	45	602	57	1	11	4 carb, 4 fat
Pineapple Shake Large	1	820	24	26	24	60	537	99	1	12	6 1/2 carb, 5 fat
Pineapple Shake Regular	1	615	18	26	18	45	403	74	1	9	5 carb, 3 fat
Pineapple Sundae	1	399	11	25	11	26	242	53	0	5	3 1/2 carb, 2 fat

✔ = Healthiest Bets; n/a = not available

(Continued)

FROZEN FAVORITES (*Continued*)	Amount	Cal.	Fat (g)	% Cal. Fat	Sat. Fat (g)	Chol. (mg)	Sod. (mg)	Carb. (g)	Fiber (g)	Pro. (g)	Servings/Exchanges
Reese's Blast Large	1	963	45	42	32	64	689	78	2	19	5 carb, 9 fat
Reese's Blast Regular	1	658	30	41	23	47	478	52	1	13	3 1/2 carb, 6 fat
Rootbeer Float or Flurry Drink Large	1	553	17	28	17	43	373	62	0	9	4 carb, 3 fat
Rootbeer Float or Flurry Drink Regular	1	386	12	28	12	30	260	44	0	6	3 carb, 2 fat
Strawberry Shake Large	1	680	24	32	24	60	484	61	1	13	4 carb, 5 fat
Strawberry Shake Regular	1	510	18	32	18	45	363	46	1	9	3 carb, 3 fat
Strawberry Sundae	1	322	11	31	11	26	213	32	1	6	2 carb, 2 fat
Vanilla Shake Large	1	605	24	36	24	60	484	42	0	12	3 carb, 5 fat
Vanilla Shake Regular	1	454	18	36	18	45	363	32	0	9	2 carb, 3 fat

	Amount	Cal	Fat (g)	% Cal. Fat	Sat. Fat (g)	Chol (mg)	Sod (mg)	Carb (g)	Fiber (g)	Pro (g)	Servings/Exchanges
Watermelon Slush Float or Flurry Drink Large	1	613	17	25	17	43	372	76	0	9	5 carb, 3 fat
Watermelon Slush Float or Flurry Drink Regular	1	427	12	25	12	30	258	53	0	6	3 1/2 carb, 2 fat
KIDS' MEALS											
✔Chicken Strips	2 strips	184	9	44	1	23	507	15	0	13	1 starch, 1 lean meat, 1 fat
Corn Dog	1	262	17	58	5	15	480	23	1	6	1 1/2 starch, 1 high-fat meat, 1 fat
✔Grilled Cheese	1	282	12	38	5	15	830	39	2	12	2 1/2 starch, 1 high-fat meat
Hot Dog Plain	1	262	16	55	5	30	657	22	1	8	1 1/2 starch, 1 high-fat meat, 1 fat
Jr. Burger	1	353	21	54	6	45	1294	27	1	14	2 starch, 1 medium-fat meat, 2 fat

✔ = Healthiest Bets; n/a = not available

(Continued)

KIDS' MEALS (*Continued*)	Amount	Cal.	Fat (g)	% Cal. Fat	Sat. Fat (g)	Chol. (mg)	Sod. (mg)	Carb. (g)	Fiber (g)	Pro. (g)	Servings/Exchanges
✔Regular French Fries	1	195	11	51	2	0	648	22	4	2	1 1/2 starch, 2 fat
Regular Tots	1	259	16	56	3	0	1046	27	3	0	2 starch, 3 fat
SANDWICHES											
Country Fried Steak Sandwich	1	748	47	57	12	60	804	56	2	24	3 1/2 starch, 2 lean meat, 8 fat
TOASTER SANDWICHES											
Bacon Cheddar Burger	1	675	38	51	11	59	1786	60	4	26	4 starch, 2 medium-fat meat, 5 fat
BLT	1	581	41	64	9	47	1307	42	3	19	3 starch, 2 medium-fat meat, 6 fat
Chicken Club	1	675	29	39	8	85	1458	75	3	39	5 starch, 3 lean meat, 3 fat
✔Grilled Cheese	1	282	12	38	5	15	830	39	2	12	2 1/2 starch, 1 high-fat meat

✔ = Healthiest Bets; n/a = not available

Wendy's

❖Wendy's provides nutrition information for all its
menu items on their website at www.wendys.com.

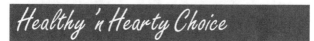

Light 'n Lean Choice

Plain Baked Potato
Chili (*small*)
Side Salad
Hidden Valley Ranch Salad Dressing
(*reduced fat and calories, 1 T*)

Calories	640	Sodium (mg)	1,215
Fat (g)	16	Carbohydrate (g)	100
% calories from fat	23	Fiber (g)	13
Saturated fat (g)	4	Protein (g)	27
Cholesterol (mg)	40		

Exchanges: 6 starch, 1 veg, 1 medium-fat meat,
1 1/2 fat

Healthy 'n Hearty Choice

Jr. Cheeseburger Deluxe
Jr. Frosty
Caesar Side Salad
Fat-Free French (*1 pkt*)

Calories	700	Sodium (mg)	1,640
Fat (g)	25	Carbohydrate (g)	86
% calories from fat	32	Fiber (g)	3
Saturated fat (g)	11	Protein (g)	31
Cholesterol (mg)	85		

Exchanges: 2 1/2 starch, 2 1/2 carb, 2 medium-fat
meat, 1 veg, 3 fat

(*Continued*)

Wendy's

	Amount	Cal.	Fat (g)	% Cal. Fat	Sat. Fat (g)	Chol. (mg)	Sod. (mg)	Carb. (g)	Fiber (g)	Pro. (g)	Servings/Exchanges
BAKED POTATOES											
✓Baked Potato w/ Bacon & Cheese	1	530	17	29	4	25	820	78	7	16	5 starch, 3 fat
✓Baked Potato w/ Broccoli & Cheese	1	470	14	27	3	5	470	80	9	9	5 starch, 2 fat
Baked Potato w/ Cheese	1	570	23	36	8	30	640	78	7	14	5 starch, 4 fat
✓Baked Potato w/ Sour Cream & Chives	1	370	5	12	4	15	75	72	7	7	5 starch
✓Plain Baked Potato	1	310	0	0	0	0	25	72	6	7	5 starch

BEVERAGES

Hot Chocolate	6 oz	80	3	34	0	0	135	15	0	1	1 carb

BURGERS

Big Bacon Classic	1	580	30	47	12	100	1460	46	3	34	3 starch, 4 medium-fat meat, 1 fat
✔ Classic Single with Everything	1	420	19	41	7	70	920	37	2	25	2 1/2 starch, 3 medium-fat meat, 1 fat
✔ Jr. Bacon Cheeseburger	1	380	19	45	7	55	870	34	2	20	2 starch, 2 medium-fat meat, 1 1/2 fat
✔ Jr. Cheeseburger	1	310	12	35	6	45	800	34	2	17	2 starch, 2 medium-fat meat
✔ Jr. Cheeseburger Deluxe	1	350	16	41	6	50	860	36	2	18	2 1/2 starch, 2 medium-fat meat, 1 fat

(Continued)

✔ = Healthiest Bets; n/a = not available

BURGERS (*Continued*)	Amount	Cal.	Fat (g)	% Cal. Fat	Sat. Fat (g)	Chol. (mg)	Sod. (mg)	Carb. (g)	Fiber (g)	Pro. (g)	Servings/Exchanges
✔Jr. Hamburger	1	270	9	30	3	30	620	34	2	14	2 starch, 1 medium-fat meat, 1 fat
CHICKEN NUGGET SAUCE											
✔Barbecue	1 pkt/2 T	45	0	0	0	0	160	10	0	1	1/2 carb
Honey Mustard	1 pkt/2 T	130	12	83	2	10	220	6	0	0	1/2 carb, 2 fat
✔Sweet & Sour	1 pkt/2 T	50	0	0	0	0	120	12	0	0	1 carb
CHICKEN SANDWICHES											
✔Breast Fillet (fried)	1	430	16	33	3	55	750	46	2	27	3 starch, 3 lean meat, 2 fat
Club (fried)	1	470	20	38	4.5	65	940	47	2	30	3 starch, 3 lean meat, 3 fat
✔Grilled	1	300	7	21	1.5	55	740	36	2	24	2 starch, 3 lean meat
✔Spicy (fried)	1	410	14	31	2.5	65	1280	43	2	28	3 starch, 3 lean meat, 1 fat

CONDIMENTS

	Serving	Cal.	Fat (g)	% Cal. Fat	Sat. Fat (g)	Chol. (mg)	Sod. (mg)	Carb. (g)	Fiber (g)	Pro. (g)	Exchanges
✔ Cheddar Cheese (shredded)	1 oz/2 T	70	6	77	3.5	15	110	1	0	4	1/2 high-fat meat
✔ Salad Oil	1/2 oz/1 T	120	14	105	2	0	0	0	0	0	2 1/2 fat
✔ Sour Cream	2 T	60	6	90	3.5	10	15	1	0	1	1 fat
✔ Whipped Margarine	1 pkt/1 T	60	7	105	1.5	0	115	0	0	0	1 fat
✔ Wine Vinegar	1/2 oz/1 T	0	0	0	0	0	0	0	0	0	free

DESSERTS

	Serving	Cal.	Fat (g)	% Cal. Fat	Sat. Fat (g)	Chol. (mg)	Sod. (mg)	Carb. (g)	Fiber (g)	Pro. (g)	Exchanges
Frosty (large)	20 oz	540	14	23	9	60	320	91	0	14	6 carb, 3 fat
Frosty (medium)	16 oz	440	11	23	7	50	260	73	0	11	5 carb, 2 fat
✔ Frosty (small)	12 oz	330	8	22	5	35	200	56	0	8	4 carb, 1 1/2 fat

KIDS' MEALS

	Serving	Cal.	Fat (g)	% Cal. Fat	Sat. Fat (g)	Chol. (mg)	Sod. (mg)	Carb. (g)	Fiber (g)	Pro. (g)	Exchanges
✔ Cheeseburger	1	310	12	35	6	45	800	33	2	17	2 starch, 2 medium-fat meat

✔ = Healthiest Bets; n/a = not available

(Continued)

KIDS' MEALS (*Continued*)	Amount	Cal.	Fat (g)	% Cal. Fat	Sat. Fat (g)	Chol. (mg)	Sod. (mg)	Carb. (g)	Fiber (g)	Pro. (g)	Servings/Exchanges
✓Chicken Nuggets	4 pieces	190	13	62	2.5	25	380	9	0	9	1/2 starch, 1 lean meat, 2 fat
✓Hamburger	1	270	9	30	3	30	620	33	1	14	2 starch, 1 medium-fat meat, 1 fat
OTHER ENTREES											
Chicken Nuggets	5 pieces	230	16	63	3	30	470	11	0	11	1 starch, 1 lean meat, 2 fat
Chili (large)	12 oz	310	10	29	3.5	45	1190	32	7	23	2 starch, 2 medium-fat meat
✓Chili (small)	8 oz	210	7	30	2.5	30	800	21	5	15	1 1/2 starch, 1 medium-fat meat
SALAD DRESSINGS											
Blue Cheese (w/ garden sensations)	1 pkt/4 T	290	30	93	6	45	870	3	0	2	6 fat
Caesar	1 pkt/2 T	150	16	96	2.5	20	240	1	0	1	3 fat

Creamy Ranch (w/ garden sensations)		1 pkt/4 T	250	25	90	4.5	15	640	5	0	1	5 fat
Creamy Ranch, reduced fat (w/ garden sensations)		1 pkt/4 T	110	9	74	1.5	15	61	7	1	1	2 fat
French, fat free (w/ garden sensations)		1 pkt/4 T	90	0	0	0	0	240	21	1	0	1 1/2 carb
Honey Mustard		1 pkt/4 T	310	29	84	4.5	25	410	12	0	1	6 fat
Honey Mustard, low fat (w/ garden sensations)		1 pkt/4 T	120	4	30	0	0	370	23	0	0	1 1/2 carb, 1 fat
House Vinaigrette		1 pkt/4 T	220	20	82	3	0	830	9	0	0	1/2 carb, 4 fat
Oriental Sesame		1 pkt/4 T	280	21	68	3	0	620	21	0	2	1 1/2 carb, 4 fat

SALADS

Caesar Side Salad	✔	1	70	4	51	2	15	240	2	2	6	1 veg, 1 lean meat

✔ = Healthiest Bets; n/a = not available

(Continued)

SALADS (Continued)	Amount	Cal.	Fat (g)	% Cal. Fat	Sat. Fat (g)	Chol. (mg)	Sod. (mg)	Carb. (g)	Fiber (g)	Pro. (g)	Servings/Exchanges
Chicken BLT	1	310	16	46	8	60	1140	10	4	33	2 veg, 4 lean meat, 1 fat
Mandarin Chicken	1	160	2	11	0	10	660	17	3	20	2 veg, 1/2 carb, 2 very lean meat
Side Salad	1	35	0	0	0	0	20	7	3	2	1 veg
Spring Mix	1	180	11	55	6	30	240	12	5	11	2 veg, 1 high-fat meat
Taco Supreme	1	360	17	43	9	65	1090	29	8	27	1 starch, 2 veg, 3 medium-fat meat

SALAD TOPPINGS

	Amount	Cal.	Fat (g)	% Cal. Fat	Sat. Fat (g)	Chol. (mg)	Sod. (mg)	Carb. (g)	Fiber (g)	Pro. (g)	Servings/Exchanges
Crispy Rice Noodles	1 pkt	60	2	30	0.5	0	180	10	0	1	1/2 starch
Garlic Croutons	1 pkt	70	3	39	0	0	120	9	0	1	1/2 starch, 1/2 fat
Honey Roasted Pecans	1 pkt	130	13	90	1	0	65	5	2	2	2 1/2 fat
Roasted Almonds	1 pkt	130	12	83	1	0	70	4	2	4	1 high-fat meat

	Amount										Exchanges
Salsa	1	30	0	0	0	0	440	6	0	1	1 veg
Sour Cream	1 pkt/2 T	60	6	90	3.5	15	15	1	0	1	1 fat
Taco Chips	1 pkt	220	11	45	2	0	150	25	2	3	1 1/2 starch, 2 fat

SIDES

	Amount										Exchanges
French Fries (Great Biggie)	1	570	27	43	4	0	180	73	7	8	5 starch, 5 fat
French Fries (Biggie)	1	470	23	44	3.5	0	150	61	6	7	4 starch, 4 1/2 fat
French Fries (medium)	1	420	20	43	3	0	130	55	5	6	3 1/2 starch, 4 fat
✔ French Fries (small)	1	270	13	43	2	0	85	35	3	4	2 starch, 2 1/2 fat
✔ Saltine Crackers	2	25	1	36	0	0	80	4	0	1	free
✔ Soft Breadstick	1	130	3	21	0.5	5	250	23	1	4	1 1/2 starch, 1/2 fat
Taco Chips	15	210	9	39	1.5	0	160	28	2	3	2 starch, 2 fat

✔ = Healthiest Bets; n/a = not available

Chicken—Fried, Roasted, or Grilled

RESTAURANTS

Chick-fil-A

Church's Chicken

El Pollo Loco

KFC

Popeyes Chicken & Biscuits

NUTRITION PROS

- No foods greet you at the table. What you order is what you eat. This puts you in the driver's seat.
- There's no waiting for food. You order, then eat.
- You can be in the know. Most large chicken chains provide full disclosure of nutrition information.
- You know the menu well, so you can plan what to order before you walk in the door.
- Order à la carte. That makes it easier for you to order and eat smaller quantities.
- Fried is not the only option in most chicken chains. They've mastered roasting or grilling. A couple of them don't fry at all.
- Healthier side items can fill your plate— corn, green beans, baked beans, rice, potatoes— but make sure they're not swimming in butter or gravy.
- You can sometimes get a salad. But take control: You pour the dressing.

Healthy Tips

★ You are better off skinless. If the chicken is served with skin, take the skin off and save some fat grams. You'll also lighten up on cholesterol and saturated fat.

★ If there's enough for two meals, ask for a take-out container and split the meal into two before you dig in.

★ To keep fat grams and calories down, go with the quarter white meat. Wings and thighs have the most fat.

★ If you are going to eat the meal at home, a better buy (price and healthwise) is a whole chicken and several sides. That way you—rather than the server—can decide on your portions.

★ Split a quarter of a chicken meal and add an extra side or two. This keeps the protein portion where it should be, about 2–3 ounces.

NUTRITION CONS

■ Portions are often enough for two people or two meals.

■ Some chicken chains stick to the tried and true, high-fat battered and fried chicken.

■ Some side items are sure candidates for the high-fat column: french fries, fried okra, potato salad, coleslaw, and biscuits.

- Some side items hide their fat grams: baked beans, mashed potatoes, and pasta salad.
- Unadulterated cooked vegetables don't appear often.
- Fruit is usually not available unless it's part of a high-fat, high-sugar dessert.

Get It Your Way

- ★ Ask to have the skin removed if you can't trust yourself to do it.
- ★ Ask the server to take the wing off the breast.
- ★ Ask for the gravy, butter, or salad dressing on the side.

Chick-fil-A

❖Chick-fil-A provides nutrition information for all its menu items on their website at www.chickfila.com.

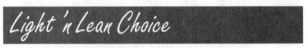

Light 'n Lean Choice

Hearty Breast of Chicken Soup
Chick-fil-A Chargrilled Chicken Garden Salad
Icedream (*small cone*)

Calories......................420	Sodium (mg)..........1,650
Fat (g) 8	Carbohydrate (g).........36
% calories from fat..17	Fiber (g) 6
Saturated fat (g)........2	Protein (g) 53
Cholesterol (mg) 110	

Exchanges: 1 starch, 2 veg, 1 carb, 5 very lean meat, 1 fat

Healthy 'n Hearty Choice

Chargrilled Chicken Deluxe Sandwich
Carrot & Raisin Salad
1/2 Chick-fil-A Waffle Potato Fries (*small order*)

Calories......................585	Sodium (mg)..........1,770
Fat (g) 10	Carbohydrate (g).........91
% calories from fat..15	Fiber (g) 4
Saturated fat (g)........3	Protein (g) 34
Cholesterol (mg) 49	

Exchanges: 3 1/2 starch, 2 veg, 1 carb, 3 very lean meat, 1 fat

Chick-fil-A

	Amount	Cal.	Fat (g)	% Cal. Fat	Sat. Fat (g)	Chol. (mg)	Sod. (mg)	carb (g)	Fiber (g)	Pro. (g)	Servings/Exchanges
BEVERAGES											
✔Diet Lemonade	9 oz	5	0	0	0	0	4	2	0	0	free
CHICKEN ITEMS											
✔Chargrilled Chicken (no bun, no pickles)	1	130	3	21	1	30	630	0	0	27	3 very lean meat
✔Chick-fil-A Chick-n-Strips (4 count)	1 order	230	8	31	2	20	380	10	0	29	1/2 starch, 4 very lean meat, 1 fat
✔Chick-fil-A Nuggets (8 pack)	1 order	290	14	43	3	60	770	12	0	28	1 starch, 3 lean meat, 1 fat
✔Chicken (no bun, no pickles)	1	160	8	45	2	45	690	1	0	21	3 lean meat

(Continued)

✔ = Healthiest Bets; n/a = not available

	Amount	Cal.	Fat (g)	% Cal. Fat	Sat. Fat (g)	Chol. (mg)	Sod. (mg)	carb (g)	Fiber (g)	Pro. (g)	Servings/Exchanges
DESSERTS											
Cheesecake	1 slice	270	21	70	9	10	510	7	0	13	1/2 carb, 2 high-fat meat
Cheesecake with Blueberry Topping	1 slice	290	23	71	10	10	550	9	0	14	1/2 carb, 2 high-fat meat, 1/2 fat
Cheesecake with Strawberry Topping	1 slice	290	23	71	10	10	580	8	0	14	1/2 carb, 2 high-fat meat, 1/2 fat
Fudge Nut Brownie	1	350	16	41	3	30	650	41	0	10	3 carb, 3 fat
✔Icedream (small cone)	1	140	4	26	1	40	240	16	0	11	1 carb, 1 fat
✔Icedream (small cup)	1	350	10	26	3	70	390	50	0	16	3 carb, 2 fat
Lemon Pie	1 slice	320	16	45	5	135	280	40	1	7	2 1/2 carb, 3 fat
SALADS											
✔Chick-fil-A Chargrilled Chicken Garden Salad	1	170	3	16	1	25	650	10	5	26	2 veg, 3 very lean meat

✔Chick-fil-A Chick-n-Strips Salad	1	290	9	28	2	20	430	21	5	32	1 starch, 1 veg, 4 very lean meat, 1 fat
✔Chick-fil-A Chicken Salad Plate	1	290	5	16	0	35	570	40	6	21	2 starch, 2 veg, 2 lean meat
✔Tossed Salad	1	70	0	0	0	0	0	13	1	5	2 veg

SANDWICHES

✔Chargrilled Chicken Club (no dressing)	1	390	12	28	5	70	980	38	2	33	2 starch, 1 veg, 3 lean meat
✔Chargrilled Chicken Deluxe	1	290	3	9	1	40	640	38	2	28	2 1/2 starch, 3 very lean meat
✔Chick-fil-A Chargrilled Chicken Sandwich	1	280	3	10	1	40	640	36	1	27	2 1/2 starch, 3 very lean meat
✔Chick-fil-A Chicken Salad Sandwich (whole wheat)	1	320	5	14	2	10	810	42	1	25	3 starch, 2 lean meat

✔ = Healthiest Bets; n/a = not available

(Continued)

SANDWICHES (*Continued*)	Amount	Cal.	Fat (g)	% Cal. Fat	Sat. Fat (g)	Chol. (mg)	Sod. (mg)	carb (g)	Fiber (g)	Pro. (g)	Servings/Exchanges
✔Chick-fil-A Chicken Sandwich	1	290	9	28	2	50	870	29	1	24	2 starch, 2 lean meat, 1/2 fat
✔Chicken Deluxe	1	300	9	27	2	50	870	31	2	25	2 starch, 3 lean meat, 1/2 fat
SIDES											
✔Carrot & Raisin Salad (small)	1	150	2	12	0	6	650	28	2	5	1 carb, 2 veg
✔Chick-fil-A Waffle Potato Fries (small/salted)	1 order	290	10	31	4	5	960	49	0	1	3 starch, 2 fat
✔Chick-fil-A Waffle Potato Fries (small/unsalted)	1 order	290	10	31	4	5	80	49	0	1	3 starch, 2 fat
✔Cole Slaw (small)	1	130	6	42	1	15	430	11	1	6	1 carb, 1 veg, 1 fat
SOUP											
✔Hearty Breast of Chicken Soup (cup)	7.6 oz	110	1	8	0	45	760	10	1	16	1 starch, 2 very lean meat

✔ = Healthiest Bets; n/a = not available

Church's Chicken

❖Church's Chicken provides nutrition information
for all of its menu items on its website at
www.churchs.com.

Light 'n Lean Choice

2 Tender Strips (*fried chicken*)
Corn on the Cob
Cajun Rice
Cole Slaw

Calories	521	Sodium (mg)	785
Fat (g)	24	Carbohydrate (g)	56
% calories from fat	41	Fiber (g)	12
Saturated fat (g)	n/a	Protein (g)	21
Cholesterol (mg)	35		

Exchanges: 3 starch, 1 veg, 2 medium-fat meat, 2 fat

Healthy 'n Hearty Choice

Chicken Breast (*fried*)
Potatoes & Gravy (*2 orders*)
Corn on the Cob
Cole Slaw

Calories	611	Sodium (mg)	1,795
Fat (g)	27	Carbohydrate (g)	64
% calories from fat	40	Fiber (g)	13
Saturated fat (g)	n/a	Protein (g)	29
Cholesterol (mg)	65		

Exchanges: 3 starch, 1 veg, 3 lean meat, 1 1/2 fat

(*Continued*)

Church's Chicken

	Amount	Cal.	Fat (g)	% Cal. Fat	Sat. Fat (g)	Chol. (mg)	Sod. (mg)	carb (g)	Fiber (g)	Pro. (g)	Servings/Exchanges
DESSERTS											
✔Apple Pie	1 slice	280	12	39	n/a	5	340	41	1	2	2 1/2 carb, 2 fat
FRIED CHICKEN											
Breast	1	200	12	54	n/a	65	510	4	0	19	3 lean meat, 1/2 fat
Leg	1	140	9	58	n/a	45	160	2	0	13	2 lean meat, 1/2 fat
Tender Strip	1 strip	80	4	45	n/a	15	140	5	0	6	1 medium-fat meat
Thigh	1	230	16	63	n/a	80	520	5	0	16	2 lean meat, 2 fat
Wing	1	250	16	58	n/a	60	540	8	0	18	1/2 starch, 3 medium-fat meat

SIDES

Cajun Rice	1	130	7	48	n/a	5	260	16	1	1	1 starch, 1 fat
Cole Slaw	1	92	6	59	n/a	0	230	8	2	4	1 veg, 1 fat
✔Corn on the Cob	1	139	3	19	n/a	0	15	24	9	4	1 1/2 starch, 1/2 fat
✔French Fries	1 order	210	11	47	n/a	0	60	28	2	3	1 1/2 starch, 2 fat
Jalapeno Bombers	1	300	12	36	n/a	35	1210	36	4	10	2 starch, 1 veg, 2 1/2 fat
✔Mashed Potatoes & Gravy	1 order	90	3	30	0	0	520	14	1	1	1 starch
Okra (fried)	1 order	210	16	69	n/a	0	520	19	4	3	1 starch, 1 veg, 3 fat

✔ = Healthiest Bets; n/a = not available

El Pollo Loco

❖El Pollo Loco provides nutrition information
for all its menu items on its website at
www.elpolloloco.com.

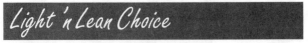

Light 'n Lean Choice

Chicken Tostada Salad (*w/o shell & sour cream*)
Pinto Beans

Calories.....................489	Sodium (mg) 1,919
Fat (g) 15	Carbohydrate (g).........57
% calories from fat..28	Fiber (g) 12
Saturated fat (g)........3	Protein (g) 41
Cholesterol (mg) 57	

Exchanges: 3 starch, 2 veg, 4 lean meat

Healthy 'n Hearty Choice

Taco al Carbon, Chicken (*2*)
Corn Cobette
Spanish Rice
Guacamole (*2 T*)
Pico de Gallo (*4 T*)

Calories.....................622	Sodium (mg) 1,133
Fat (g) 23	Carbohydrate (g).........88
% calories from fat..33	Fiber (g) 6
Saturated fat (g)........3	Protein (g) 19
Cholesterol (mg) 38	

Exchanges: 5 1/2 starch, 2 veg, 1 lean meat, 2 fat

El Pollo Loco

	Amount	Cal.	Fat (g)	% Cal. Fat	Sat. Fat (g)	Chol. (mg)	Sod. (mg)	carb (g)	Fiber (g)	Pro. (g)	Servings/Exchanges
BOWLS											
✔ Flame-Broiled Chicken	1	357	13	33	2	42	1079	39	4	25	2 starch, 2 veg, 2 very lean meat, 2 fat
BURRITOS											
BRC Burrito	1	503	16	29	6	17	1263	73	10	17	5 starch, 3 fat
Chicken Lover's	1	476	19	36	6	143	1373	47	8	29	3 starch, 3 medium-fat meat, 1 fat
Classic	1	580	22	34	7	108	1595	66	9	31	4 1/2 starch, 4 fat
Mexican Chicken Caesar	1	734	35	43	8	79	1214	65	2	36	4 starch, 3 lean meat, 5 1/2 fat

(Continued)

✔ = Healthiest Bets; n/a = not available

BURRITOS (*Continued*)	Amount	Cal.	Fat (g)	% Cal. Fat	Sat. Fat (g)	Chol. (mg)	Sod. (mg)	Carb (g)	Fiber (g)	Pro. (g)	Servings/Exchanges
Ranch	1	616	30	44	13	127	1356	45	7	40	3 starch, 4 lean meat, 3 fat
Spicy	1	633	21	30	8	69	1495	80	10	31	5 starch, 2 lean meat, 3 fat
Ultimate	1	633	23	33	8	89	1237	66	5	39	4 1/2 starch, 4 lean meat, 1 fat

CONDIMENTS

	Amount	Cal.	Fat (g)	% Cal. Fat	Sat. Fat (g)	Chol. (mg)	Sod. (mg)	Carb (g)	Fiber (g)	Pro. (g)	Servings/Exchanges
✔Avocado Salsa	1 oz/2 T	12	1	75	0	0	204	1	0	0	free
✔Chipotle Salsa	1 oz/2 T	7	0	0	0	0	180	1	0	0	free
✔Guacamole	1 oz/2 T	30	2	60	0	0	160	3	0	0	1/2 fat
✔House Salsa	1 oz/2 T	6	0	0	0	0	96	1	0	0	free
✔Jalapeno Hot Sauce (1 packet)	0.5 oz/1 T	5	0	0	0	0	110	1	0	0	free
✔Pico de Gallo Salsa	1 oz/2 T	11	1	82	0	0	131	2	0	0	free

	Amount	Cal.	Fat (g)	% Fat Cal.	Sat. Fat (g)	Chol. (mg)	Sod. (mg)	Carb. (g)	Fiber (g)	Pro. (g)	Exchanges
✔ Sour Cream	1 oz/2 T	60	5	75	3.5	20	15	1	0	1	1 fat
DESSERTS											
Banana Split	1	717	28	35	11	56	310	107	3	12	7 carb, 5 fat
Berry Banana Smoothie	11 oz	367	7	17	3	23	136	68	2	27	4 1/2 carb, 1 fat
✔ Churro	1	179	11	55	3	5	221	18	1	3	1 carb, 2 fat
✔ Fosters Freeze w/o cone	4.6 oz	180	5	25	3	20	100	30	0	4	2 carb, 1 fat
Kiwi Strawberry Smoothie	9.5 oz	357	7	18	3	23	141	66	2	5	4 1/2 carb, 1 fat
GRILLED CHICKEN											
✔ Breast	1	160	6	34	2	110	390	0	0	26	4 very lean meat
✔ Leg	1	90	5	50	1.5	75	150	0	0	11	2 lean meat
✔ Thigh	1	180	12	60	4	130	230	0	0	16	2 lean meat, 1 fat
✔ Wing	1	110	6	49	2	80	220	0	0	12	2 medium-fat meat

✔ = Healthiest Bets; n/a = not available

(Continued)

	Amount	Cal.	Fat (g)	% Cal. Fat	Sat. Fat (g)	Chol. (mg)	Sod. (mg)	carb (g)	Fiber (g)	Pro. (g)	Servings/Exchanges
OTHER ENTREES											
✓Chicken Soft Taco	1	237	12	46	4	74	629	15	1	17	1 starch, 2 lean meat, 1 fat
✓Chicken Taquito	1	370	17	41	4	25	690	43	3	15	3 starch, 1 medium-fat meat, 2 fat
✓Pollo Bowl	1	469	11	21	2	42	1868	66	8	30	3 starch, 3 veg, 2 lean meat, 1 fat
✓Taco al Carbon, Chicken	1	180	8	40	1	19	152	20	2	7	1 1/2 starch, 1 fat
SALAD BOWLS											
Mexican Chicken Caesar	1	494	30	55	6	55	1175	32	3	26	2 veg, 1 1/2 starch, 2 lean meat, 5 fat
Nacho Pollo	1	766	33	39	10	87	1358	64	11	37	4 starch, 4 lean meat, 5 fat
Smokey Black Bean Pollo	1	604	23	34	7	54	1955	75	6	29	5 starch, 2 lean meat, 2 fat

✓Tostada Salad, Chicken (w/o shell & sour cream)	1	304	11	33	3	57	1175	28	4	29	2 starch, 2 lean meat, 1 fat
SALAD DRESSINGS											
1,000 Island	1.5 oz/3 T	220	21	86	3	30	360	7	0	1	1/2 carb, 4 fat
Blue Cheese	1.5 oz/3 T	230	24	94	5	30	450	2	0	2	5 fat
Creamy Cilantro	1.75 oz/3 1/2 T	266	29	98	4	13	306	1	0	1	6 fat
✓Hidden Valley Ranch	1.5 oz/3 T	110	11	90	1.5	10	250	1	0	1	2 fat
✓Light Italian	1.5 oz/3 T	20	1	45	0	0	780	2	0	0	free
Ranch	1.5 oz/3 T	222	24	97	4	10	420	2	0	1	5 fat
SALADS											
✓Barbecue Chicken	1	543	24	40	3	55	1650	55	5	27	3 veg, 2 1/2 starch, 2 lean meat, 3 fat
✓Garden Salad	1	105	7	60	3	15	99	7	1	5	1 veg

✓ = Healthiest Bets; n/a = not available

(Continued)

	Amount	Cal.	Fat (g)	% Cal. Fat	Sat. Fat (g)	Chol. (mg)	Sod. (mg)	carb (g)	Fiber (g)	Pro. (g)	Servings/Exchanges
SIDES											
Cole Slaw	1 order	206	16	70	3	11	358	12	2	2	2 veg, 3 fat
✓Corn on the Cob, 3"	1	80	1	11	0	0	10	18	1	3	1 starch
French Fries	1 order	444	19	39	5	0	604	61	0	6	4 starch, 3 fat
✓Gravy	1 oz/2 T	14	1	64	0	1	1	2	0	0	free
Macaroni & Cheese	1 order	244	12	44	4	22	950	24	3	10	1 1/2 starch, 1 high-fat meat
✓Mashed Potatoes	1 order	97	1	9	0	0	369	21	2	3	1 1/2 starch
✓Pinto Beans	1 order	185	4	19	0	0	744	29	8	11	2 starch, 1 lean meat
Potato Salad	1 order	256	14	49	2	15	527	30	3	3	2 starch, 2 fat
Smokey Black Beans	1 order	306	16	47	6	13	731	35	5	7	2 starch, 3 fat
✓Spanish Rice	1 order	130	3	21	1	0	397	24	1	2	1 1/2 starch, 1/2 fat

TORTILLAS

✔11" Flour	1	260	7	24	2	0	583	42	6	7	3 starch
✔4.5" Corn	1	32	1	28	0	0	21	6	0	1	1/2 starch
✔6" Corn	1	70	1	13	0	0	35	14	1	1	1 starch
✔6.5" Flour	1	90	2	20	0	0	224	13	0	3	1 starch
✔Spicy Tomato	1	254	6	21	1	0	577	42	2	7	3 starch

✔ = Healthiest Bets; n/a = not available

KFC

❖KFC provides nutrition information for all its
menu items on their website at www.kfc.com.

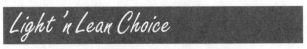

Light 'n Lean Choice

Honey BBQ Sandwich with Sauce
Mashed Potatoes with Gravy

Calories......................430	Sodium (mg)..........1,000
Fat (g) 12	Carbohydrate (g).........54
% calories from fat..25	Fiber (g) 4
Saturated fat (g)........3	Protein (g) 29
Cholesterol (mg) 125	

Exchanges: 3 1/2 starch, 3 lean meat

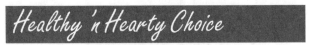

Healthy 'n Hearty Choice

Hot & Spicy Drumsticks (2)
Corn on the Cob
BBQ Baked Beans
1/2 Cole Slaw

Calories......................806	Sodium (mg)..........1,642
Fat (g) 30	Carbohydrate (g).........99
% calories from fat..33	Fiber (g) 11
Saturated fat (g)........8	Protein (g) 38
Cholesterol (mg) 163	

Exchanges: 5 1/2 starch, 1 carb, 1 veg, 3 lean meat,
2 fat

KFC

	Amount	Cal.	Fat (g)	% Cal. Fat	Sat. Fat (g)	Chol. (mg)	Sod. (mg)	carb (g)	Fiber (g)	Pro. (g)	Servings/Exchanges
CRISPY STRIPS											
Colonel's Crispy Strips (3)	1 order	300	16	48	4	56	1165	18	1	26	1 starch, 3 lean meat, 2 1/2 fat
Spicy Buffalo Crispy Strips (3)	1 order	335	15	40	4	70	1140	23	1	25	1 1/2 starch, 3 lean meat, 2 fat
DESSERTS											
Apple Pie	1 piece	310	14	41	3	0	280	44	0	2	2 carb, 1 fruit, 3 fat
Double Choc. Chip Cake	1 piece	320	16	45	4	55	230	41	1	4	2 1/2 carb, 3 fat
Little Bucket Parfait— Chocolate Cream	1	290	15	47	11	15	330	37	2	3	2 1/2 carb, 3 fat

(Continued)

✔ = Healthiest Bets; n/a = not available

DESSERTS (*Continued*)	Amount	Cal.	Fat (g)	% Cal. Fat	Sat. Fat (g)	Chol. (mg)	Sod. (mg)	carb (g)	Fiber (g)	Pro. (g)	Servings/Exchanges
Little Bucket Parfait—Fudge Brownies	1	280	10	32	3.5	145	190	44	1	3	3 carb, 2 fat
Little Bucket Parfait—Lemon Crème	1	410	14	31	8	62	290	62	4	7	4 carb, 3 fat
Little Bucket Parfait—Strawberry Shortcake	1	200	7	32	6	10	220	33	1	1	2 carb, 1 fat
Pecan Pie	1 piece	490	23	42	5	65	510	66	2	5	4 1/2 carb, 4 fat
Strawberry Crème Pie	1 piece	280	15	48	8	15	130	32	2	4	2 carb, 3 fat
Twister	1 order	600	34	51	7	50	1430	52	4	22	2 1/2 carb, 6 fat
EXTRA CRISPY FRIED CHICKEN											
Breast	1	470	28	54	8	160	874	17	1	39	1 starch, 5 lean meat, 2 1/2 fat

	Amount	Cal	Fat (g)	% Cal Fat	Sat Fat (g)	Chol (mg)	Sod (mg)	Carb (g)	Fiber (g)	Pro (g)	Exchanges/Choices
Drumstick	1	195	12	55	3	77	375	7	1	15	1/2 starch, 2 lean meat, 1 fat
Thigh	1	380	27	64	7	118	625	14	2	21	1 starch, 3 lean meat, 3 fat
Whole Wing	1	220	15	61	4	55	415	10	1	10	1/2 starch, 1 medium-fat meat, 2 fat

HOT & SPICY FRIED CHICKEN

	Amount	Cal	Fat (g)	% Cal Fat	Sat Fat (g)	Chol (mg)	Sod (mg)	Carb (g)	Fiber (g)	Pro (g)	Exchanges/Choices
Breast	1	505	29	52	8	162	1170	23	1	38	1 1/2 starch, 5 lean meat, 2 fat
✔Drumstick	1	175	10	51	3	77	360	9	1	13	1/2 starch, 2 lean meat, 1 fat
Thigh	1	335	26	70	7	126	630	13	1	19	1 starch, 2 lean meat, 3 fat
Whole Wing	1	210	25	107	4	55	350	9	0	10	1/2 starch, 1 medium-fat meat, 2 fat

ORIGINAL RECIPE FRIED CHICKEN

	Amount	Cal	Fat (g)	% Cal Fat	Sat Fat (g)	Chol (mg)	Sod (mg)	Carb (g)	Fiber (g)	Pro (g)	Exchanges/Choices
Breast	1	400	24	54	6	135	1116	16	1	29	1 starch, 3 lean meat, 3 fat

(Continued)

✔ = Healthiest Bets; n/a = not available

ORIGINAL RECIPE FRIED CHICKEN (*Continued*)	Amount	Cal.	Fat (g)	% Cal. Fat	Sat. Fat (g)	Chol. (mg)	Sod. (mg)	carb (g)	Fiber (g)	Pro. (g)	Servings/Exchanges
✔Drumstick	1	140	9	58	2	75	422	4	0	13	2 lean meat, 1/2 fat
Thigh	1	250	18	65	4.5	95	747	6	1	16	1/2 starch, 2 lean meat, 2 fat
Whole Wing	1	140	10	64	2.5	55	414	5	0	9	1 medium-fat meat, 1 fat
OTHER ENTREES											
Chunky Chicken Pot Pie (seasonal entree)	1	770	42	49	13	70	2160	69	5	29	4 starch, 1 veg, 2 lean meat, 7 fat
Honey BBQ Crunch Melt	1	556	26	42	5	60	1010	48	2	33	3 starch, 3 lean meat, 3 fat
✔Honey BBQ Flavored Chicken Sandwich	1	310	6	17	2	125	560	37	2	28	2 1/2 starch, 3 lean meat
Honey BBQ Pieces (6 pieces)	1 order	607	38	56	10	193	1145	33	1	33	2 starch, 4 lean meat, 5 fat

Item	Serving	Cal.								Exchanges
Hot Wings (6)	1 order	471	33	63	8	150	1230	18	2	27	1 starch, 3 medium-fat meat, 3 1/2 fat
Original Recipe Chicken Sandwich w/sauce	1	450	22	44	5	70	940	33	2	29	2 starch, 3 lean meat, 2 1/2 fat
✔Original Recipe Sandwich w/o sauce	1	360	13	33	3.5	60	890	21	1	29	1 1/2 starch, 3 lean meat, 2 fat
Popcorn Chicken (large)	1 order	620	40	58	10	73	1046	36	0	30	2 1/2 starch, 3 lean meat, 6 fat
Popcorn Chicken (small)	1 order	362	23	57	6	43	610	21	0	17	1 1/2 starch, 2 lean meat, 3 fat
✔Tender Roast Sandwich w/o sauce	1	270	5	17	1.5	65	690	23	1	31	1 1/2 starch, 3 lean meat
✔Tender Roast Sandwich w/sauce	1	350	15	39	3	75	880	26	1	32	1 1/2 starch, 4 lean meat

✔ = Healthiest Bets; n/a = not available

(Continued)

OTHER ENTREES (*Continued*)	Amount	Cal.	Fat (g)	% Cal. Fat	Sat. Fat (g)	Chol. (mg)	Sod. (mg)	carb (g)	Fiber (g)	Pro. (g)	Servings/Exchanges
Triple Chicken Zinger Sandwich w/sauce	1	550	32	52	7	85	830	39	2	28	2 1/2 starch, 3 lean meat, 4 fat
✓Triple Crunch Sandwich w/o sauce	1	390	15	35	4.5	50	650	29	2	25	2 starch, 3 lean meat, 1 fat
Triple Crunch Sandwich w/sauce	1	490	29	53	6	70	710	39	2	28	2 1/2 starch, 3 lean meat, 3 fat
✓Triple Crunch Zinger Sandwich w/o sauce	1	390	15	35	4.5	50	650	36	2	25	2 1/2 starch, 3 lean meat, 1 fat
SIDES											
✓BBQ Baked Beans	1 order	190	3	14	1	5	760	33	6	6	2 starch, 1/2 fat
✓Biscuit	1	180	10	50	2.5	0	560	20	0	4	1 starch, 2 fat
Cole Slaw	1 order	232	14	54	2	8	284	26	3	2	1 carb, 2 veg, 2 fat

✔ Corn on the Cob (1)	1 order	150	2	12	0	0	20	35	2	5	2 starch
✔ Mashed Potatoes with Gravy	1 order	120	6	45	1	1	440	17	2	1	1 starch, 1 fat
Potato Salad	1 order	230	14	55	2	15	540	23	3	4	1 1/2 starch, 3 fat
Potato Wedges	1 order	280	13	42	4	5	750	28	5	5	2 starch, 2 1/2 fat

✔ = Healthiest Bets; n/a = not available

Popeyes Chicken & Biscuits

❖Popeyes Chicken & Biscuits provided nutrition
information for all its menu items.

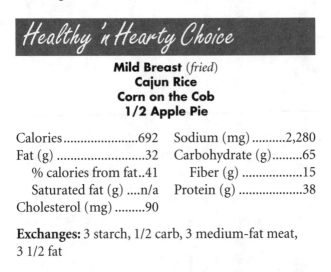

Light 'n Lean Choice

Spicy Leg (*fried*)
Cajun Rice
Corn on the Cob

Calories	397	Sodium (mg)	1,520
Fat (g)	15	Carbohydrate (g)	42
% calories from fat	34	Fiber (g)	12
Saturated fat (g)	n/a	Protein (g)	24
Cholesterol (mg)	65		

Exchanges: 2 starch, 3 lean meat, 1/2 fat

Healthy 'n Hearty Choice

Mild Breast (*fried*)
Cajun Rice
Corn on the Cob
1/2 Apple Pie

Calories	692	Sodium (mg)	2,280
Fat (g)	32	Carbohydrate (g)	65
% calories from fat	41	Fiber (g)	15
Saturated fat (g)	n/a	Protein (g)	38
Cholesterol (mg)	90		

Exchanges: 3 starch, 1/2 carb, 3 medium-fat meat,
3 1/2 fat

Popeyes Chicken & Biscuits

	Amount	Cal.	Fat (g)	% Cal. Fat	Sat. Fat (g)	Chol. (mg)	Sod. (mg)	carb (g)	Fiber (g)	Pro. (g)	Servings/Exchanges
DESSERTS											
Apple Pie	1 order	290	16	50	n/a	10	820	37	2	3	1 1/2 carb, 1 fruit, 2 fat
ENTREES											
Nuggets (fried chicken)	1 order	410	32	70	n/a	55	660	18	3	17	1 starch, 2 lean meat, 5 fat
Shrimp (fried)	1 order	250	16	58	n/a	110	650	13	3	13	1 starch, 2 very lean meat, 3 fat
FRIED CHICKEN											
Mild Breast	1	270	16	53	n/a	60	660	9	2	23	1/2 starch, 3 lean meat, 1 fat
✔ Mild Leg	1	120	7	53	n/a	40	240	4	0	10	1 lean meat, 1 fat
Mild Thigh	1	300	23	69	n/a	70	620	9	0	15	1/2 starch, 2 lean meat, 3 fat

(Continued)

✔ = Healthiest Bets; n/a = not available

FRIED CHICKEN (*Continued*)	Amount	Cal.	Fat (g)	% Cal. Fat	Sat. Fat (g)	Chol. (mg)	Sod. (mg)	carb (g)	Fiber (g)	Pro. (g)	Servings/Exchanges
Mild Wing	1	160	11	62	n/a	40	290	7	0	9	1/2 starch, 1 medium-fat meat, 1 fat
Spicy Breast	1	270	16	53	n/a	60	590	9	2	23	1/2 starch, 3 lean meat, 1 fat
✓Spicy Leg	1	120	7	53	n/a	40	240	4	0	10	1 lean meat, 1 fat
Spicy Thigh	1	300	23	69	n/a	70	450	9	0	15	1/2 starch, 2 lean meat, 3 fat
Spicy Wing	1	160	11	62	n/a	40	290	7	0	9	1/2 starch, 1 medium-fat meat, 1 fat
OTHER ENTREE ITEMS											
Mild Tender (fried chicken strip)	1 strip	110	7	57	n/a	15	160	6	0	6	1/2 starch, 1 lean meat, 1 fat

SIDES

✔Cajun Rice	1 order	150	5	30	n/a	25	1260	17	3	10	1 starch, 1 lean meat
✔Cole Slaw	1 order	149	11	66	n/a	3	271	14	3	1	1/2 carb, 1 veg, 2 fat
✔Corn on the Cob	1 order	127	3	21	n/a	0	20	21	9	4	1 1/2 starch, 1/2 fat
✔French Fries	1 order	240	12	45	n/a	10	610	31	4	4	2 starch, 2 fat
✔Potatoes & Gravy	1 order	100	6	54	n/a	0	460	10	3	5	1/2 starch, 1 fat
Red Beans & Rice	1 order	270	17	57	n/a	10	680	30	7	8	2 starch, 1 lean meat, 3 fat

✔ = Healthiest Bets; n/a = not available

Pizza, Pasta, and All Else Italian

RESTAURANTS

Chuck E. Cheese's

Domino's Pizza

Fazoli's

Godfather's Pizza

Little Caesars

Olive Garden Italian Restaurant

Papa John's Pizza

Pizza Hut

Round Table Pizza

Sbarro

NUTRITION PROS

- Surprisingly, pizza and pasta—as long as you top them wisely—can be healthy restaurant choices.
- Pizza and pasta can hold the line on fat and calories better than some burger and french fry meals.
- Pizza and pasta meals can match today's diabetes nutrition goals: low in fat, moderate in protein, and full of grains.
- You can eat vegetables, both raw and cooked, in most pizza and pasta restaurants. That's an accomplishment in a fast-food restaurant. Raw vegetables come as salads. Cooked vegetables come as pizza sauce and toppings, or as tomato-based sauces and toppings on pasta.

- Splitting and sharing is the way to go in most pizza restaurants.
- You can design your own pizza with healthier toppings (see list on page 260). Pizza parlors are used to made-for-you orders.
- Most pizza chains offer a veggie combination pizza.
- Pizza chains are slowly but surely divulging their nutrition information, so you can pick and choose with nutrition facts in hand.
- Several pizza chains have gone uptown. You might even call them yuppie, but that's good news for health-focused pizza lovers. They bake their pizzas in brick ovens, and they offer novel and healthy toppings. Pineapple, spinach, feta cheese, roasted red peppers, and grilled chicken are just a few.
- Pizza and pasta are served not only in pizza or Italian restaurants, but also in family-style and dinner house restaurants.
- Taking home leftovers is a snap. Boxes are ready.

NUTRITION CONS

- It's hard to eat just two or three slices. There's always just one more piece of pizza begging you to eat it.
- High-fat pizza toppings—extra cheese, three kinds of cheese, pepperoni, and sausage—can quickly add fat and calories.
- These high-fat toppings also add more sodium.
- Some pizza chains now promote more toppings, extra cheese, and bigger pizzas. That all adds up to more fat and calories.

- Restaurant combination pizzas often add high-fat and high-calorie toppers.
- Pasta with high-fat and high-calorie toppings—cream sauce, creamy cheese sauce, butter sauce—is easy to find.

Healthy Tips

★ If you count calories carefully, stick with the thin crust and load up on the veggies.

★ If your favorite chain does not publish nutrition information, check the nutrition information for similar items from two other pizza chains. That gives you ballpark figures to base your choice on.

★ If your dining partner wants not-so-healthy pizza toppings, order healthier toppings on one half and let your partner handle the other.

★ Order just enough for everyone at the table, to avoid that just-one-more-piece syndrome.

★ If you know a few extra pieces will be left over, package them up before you take your first bite.

★ Try an appetizer side portion of pasta, split an order with your dining partner, or stash a portion in a take-home container before you lift your fork to your mouth.

★ Along with pizza or pasta, crunch on a healthy garden salad to fill you up and not out.

(Continued)

★ Don't leave the crust for the birds; that's the healthy part. Eat it and count your grams of fiber.
★ The red pepper flakes you'll probably find sitting right on your table add zip to your pizza, pasta, or salad without adding calories.

■ Pasta portions are often heavy-handed.
■ Breadsticks and garlic bread sound healthy, but they are often drenched in fat. Check their nutrition numbers.

HEALTHY PIZZA TOPPINGS

part-skim cheese	sliced tomatoes	chicken
green peppers	spinach	ham
onions	broccoli	Canadian bacon
mushrooms	pineapple	

NOT-SO-HEALTHY PIZZA TOPPINGS

extra cheese	pepperoni	anchovies
several types of cheese	sausage	bacon

Get It Your Way

★ Ask your pizza maker to go light on the cheese and heavy on the veggies.
★ Request a half-order of pasta if you don't have someone to split it with.
★ Remember to order your salad dressing on the side.

Chuck E. Cheese's

❖Chuck E. Cheese's provides nutrition
information for all its menu items on its
website at www.chuckecheeses.com.

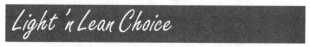

Medium BBQ Chicken Pizza (2 slices)

Calories 410	Sodium (mg) 640
Fat (g) 13	Carbohydrate (g).........51
% calories from fat..29	Fiber (g) 3
Saturated fat (g)........7	Protein (g) 22
Cholesterol (mg) 50	

Exchanges: 3 1/2 starch, 1 high-fat meat, 1 fat

Healthy 'n Hearty Choice

Cheese Pizza (4 slices)

Calories......................660	Sodium (mg) 920
Fat (g) 26	Carbohydrate (g).........86
% calories from fat..35	Fiber (g) 6
Saturated fat (g)........6	Protein (g) 30
Cholesterol (mg) 46	

Exchanges: 5 1/2 starch, 2 high-fat meat

(Continued)

Chuck E. Cheese's

	Amount	Cal.	Fat (g)	% Cal. Fat	Sat. Fat (g)	Chol. (mg)	Sod. (mg)	Carb. (g)	Fiber (g)	Pro. (g)	Servings/Exchanges
APPETIZERS											
✔Bread Sticks	1	370	12	29	4	5	480	51	3	14	3 starch, 1 medium-fat meat, 1 fat
✔Buffalo Wings	4	220	15	61	3.5	110	560	1	0	20	3 medium-fat meat
✔French Fries	1	283	10	32	2.5	0	433	43	3	5	3 starch, 2 fat
Mozzarella Sticks	2	380	24	57	7	40	380	26	2	13	1 1/2 starch, 2 high-fat meat, 1 fat
BIRTHDAY CAKES											
✔8" Chocolate/Whip Cream	1/12	208	11	48	8	21	200	25	1	2	1 1/2 carb, 2 fat
✔8" White/Whip Cream	1/12	208	11	48	8	25	167	26	0	2	1 1/2 carb, 2 fat

BREAKFAST

Item											
Banana Loaf Cake	1	350	11	28	4.4	30	320	50	2	5	3 carb, 2 fat
✔Cinnamon Blast	1 pkg	140	5	32	1	0	210	24	1	2	1 1/2 starch, 1 fat
Cinnamon Crumb Pound Cake	1	386	17	40	3	38	236	55	1	4	3 1/2 carb, 3 fat
✔Fruit Loops	1 pkg	120	1	8	1	0	160	28	1	2	2 starch
✔Rice Krispies	1 pkg	130	1	7	1	0	200	26	0	2	1 1/2 starch

DESSERTS

Item											
Brownie	1	382	18	42	4.4	60	143	51	1	4	3 1/2 carb, 3 1/2 fat
Chocolate Chunk Cookie	1	410	19	42	6	20	390	56	0	5	3 1/2 carb, 4 fat
Original Crispy Treat	1	340	9	24	2	0	250	50	1	3	3 carb, 2 fat

PIZZA

Item											
✔BBQ Chicken	2 slices	410	13	29	7	50	640	51	3	22	3 1/2 starch, 1 medium-fat meat, 1 1/2 fat

(Continued)

✔ = Healthiest Bets; n/a = not available

PIZZA (*Continued*)	Amount	Cal.	Fat (g)	% Cal. Fat	Sat. Fat (g)	Chol. (mg)	Sod. (mg)	Carb. (g)	Fiber (g)	Pro. (g)	Servings/Exchanges
✔Beef	2 slices	411	17	37	9	36	607	43	3	18	3 1/2 starch, 1 medium-fat meat, 2 fat
✔Cheese	2 slices	330	10	27	6	20	460	43	3	15	3 starch, 1 medium-fat meat, 1 fat
✔Pepperoni	2 slices	371	14	34	7	28	619	43	3	17	3 1/2 starch, 1 medium-fat meat, 1 1/2 fat
✔Sausage	2 slices	387	15	35	8	31	662	44	3	18	3 1/2 starch, 1 medium-fat meat, 2 fat
SALAD DRESSINGS											
Bleu Cheese	2 T	170	18	95	3	15	120	1	0	1	3 1/2 fat
✔Kraft Catalina	2 T	35	0	0	0	0	320	8	0	0	1/2 carb
✔Lite Ranch	2 T	80	8	90	1	5	240	2	0	1	1 1/2 fat

✔Olive Oil & Vinegar	2 T	90	9	90	1	0	170	2	0	0	2 fat
✔Thousand Island	2 T	110	10	82	2	10	170	4	0	0	2 fat

SANDWICHES

Grilled Chicken Sub	1	740	39	47	12	110	1080	57	5	41	4 starch, 5 lean meat, 5 fat
Ham & Cheese	1	770	41	48	9	85	1490	60	6	39	4 starch, 4 medium-fat meat, 4 fat
Hot Dog	1	430	29	61	13	50	710	27	2	15	1 1/2 starch, 1 high-fat meat, 4 fat
Italian Sub	1	770	47	55	16	80	1560	52	4	35	3 1/2 starch, 3 medium-fat meat, 6 fat

✔ = Healthiest Bets; n/a = not available

Domino's Pizza

❖Domino's provides nutrition information for all its menu items on their website at www.dominos.com.

Light 'n Lean Choice

Small Garden Salad
Light Italian Dressing (*3 T*)
14″ Hand-Tossed Crust Pizza with
Fresh Mushrooms (*3 slices*)

Calories......................567	Sodium (mg)..........1,874
Fat (g)...........................16	Carbohydrate (g).........83
% calories from fat..25	Fiber (g)....................7
Saturated fat (g)........7	Protein (g)...................23
Cholesterol (mg).........32	

Exchanges: 5 starch, 1 veg, 1 high-fat meat, 1 fat

Healthy 'n Hearty Choice

Large Garden Salad
Fat-Free Ranch Dressing (*3 T*)
12″ Thin-Crust Pizza with Pineapple Tidbits
(*1/2 pizza*)

Calories......................631	Sodium (mg)..........2,262
Fat (g)...........................24	Carbohydrate (g).........82
% calories from fat..34	Fiber (g)....................8
Saturated fat (g)......10	Protein (g)...................26
Cholesterol (mg).........38	

Exchanges: 4 starch, 2 veg, 1 carb, 2 medium-fat meat, 2 fat

Domino's Pizza

12" CLASSIC PIZZA W/TOPPINGS

	Amount	Cal.	Fat (g)	% Cal. Fat	Sat. Fat (g)	Chol. (mg)	Sod. (mg)	Carb. (g)	Fiber (g)	Pro. (g)	Servings/Exchanges
Anchovies	2 slices/1/4 pizza	408	13	29	5	36	1369	55	3	22	3 1/2 starch, 2 medium-fat meat, 1/2 fat
✔Bacon	2 slices/1/4 pizza	477	19	36	7.9	37	1059	54	3	21	3 1/2 starch, 2 medium-fat meat, 1 fat
✔Banana Peppers	2 slices/1/4 pizza	380	11	26	4.8	23	913	56	3	16	3 1/2 starch, 2 medium-fat meat, 1/2 fat
✔Cheddar Cheese	2 slices/1/4 pizza	432	16	33	7.8	37	864	55	3	19	3 1/2 starch, 2 medium-fat meat, 1 fat

(Continued)

✔ = Healthiest Bets; n/a = not available

12" CLASSIC PIZZA W/TOPPINGS *(Continued)*	Amount	Cal.	Fat (g)	% Cal. Fat	Sat. Fat (g)	Chol. (mg)	Sod. (mg)	Carb. (g)	Fiber (g)	Pro. (g)	Servings/Exchanges
✔Extra Cheese	2 slices/1/4 pizza	423	15	32	6.9	33	939	56	3	19	3 1/2 starch, 2 medium-fat meat, 1 fat
✔Fresh Mushrooms	2 slices/1/4 pizza	381	11	26	4.8	23	777	56	3	16	3 1/2 starch, 2 medium-fat meat
Green Olives	2 slices/1/4 pizza	393	13	30	5	23	1159	55	3	16	3 1/2 starch, 2 medium-fat meat, 1/2 fat
✔Green Peppers	2 slices/1/4 pizza	379	11	26	4.8	23	776	56	3	16	3 1/2 starch, 2 medium-fat meat
✔Ham	2 slices/1/4 pizza	398	12	27	5.1	32	990	55	3	19	3 1/2 starch, 2 medium-fat meat
✔Italian Sausage	2 slices/1/4 pizza	452	17	34	7.3	39	1015	57	3	19	3 1/2 starch, 2 medium-fat meat, 1 fat

✔Onion	2 slices/1/4 pizza	380	11	26	4.8	23	776	56	3	16	3 1/2 starch, 2 medium-fat meat
✔Pepperoni	2 slices/1/4 pizza	448	18	36	7.5	38	1049	55	3	19	3 1/2 starch, 2 medium-fat meat, 1 fat
✔Pineapple Tidbits	2 slices/1/4 pizza	387	11	26	4.8	23	777	58	3	16	3 1/2 starch, 2 medium-fat meat
✔Pre-Cooked Beef	2 slices/1/4 pizza	452	18	36	7.6	37	992	55	3	19	3 1/2 starch, 2 medium-fat meat, 1 1/2 fat
✔Ripe Olives	2 slices/1/4 pizza	395	13	30	5.1	23	883	56	4	16	3 1/2 starch, 2 medium-fat meat, 1/2 fat

12" MEDIUM CHEESE

Deep Dish	2 slices/1/4 pizza	482	22	41	8	30	1123	56	3	19	3 1/2 starch, 1 medium-fat meat, 3 fat

(Continued)

✔ = Healthiest Bets; n/a = not available

12" MEDIUM CHEESE (Continued)	Amount	Cal.	Fat (g)	% Cal. Fat	Sat. Fat (g)	Chol. (mg)	Sod. (mg)	Carb. (g)	Fiber (g)	Pro. (g)	Servings/Exchanges
✓Hand Tossed	2 slices/1/4 pizza	374	11	26	5	22	775	55	3	15	3 1/2 starch, 1 medium-fat meat, 1 fat
✓Thin Crust	2 slices/1/4 pizza	272	12	40	4.8	23	835	31	2	12	2 starch, 1 medium-fat meat, 1 fat
14" CLASSIC PIZZA W/TOPPINGS											
Anchovies	2 slices/1/4 pizza	561	17	27	7.3	50	1871	75	4	30	5 starch, 2 medium-fat meat, 1 fat
Bacon	2 slices/1/4 pizza	669	29	39	11	54	1504	75	4	29	5 starch, 2 medium-fat meat, 4 fat
Banana Peppers	2 slices/1/4 pizza	523	16	28	6.7	32	1263	76	4	22	5 starch, 2 medium-fat meat, 1 fat

Cheddar Cheese	2 slices/1/4 pizza	587	21	32	11	50	1190	75	4	26	5 starch, 2 medium-fat meat, 2 fat
Extra Cheese	2 slices/1/4 pizza	584	21	32	9.7	47	1308	76	4	26	5 starch, 2 medium-fat meat, 2 fat
✔Fresh Mushrooms	2 slices/1/4 pizza	525	16	27	7	32	1082	77	5	22	5 starch, 2 medium-fat meat, 1 fat
Green Olives	2 slices/1/4 pizza	540	18	30	7	32	1591	75	4	22	5 starch, 2 medium-fat meat, 1 fat
✔Green Peppers	2 slices/1/4 pizza	521	16	28	7	32	1081	76	4	22	5 starch, 2 medium-fat meat, 1 fat
Ham	2 slices/1/4 pizza	547	17	28	7.1	44	1372	76	4	26	5 starch, 2 medium-fat meat, 1 fat

✔ = Healthiest Bets; n/a = not available

(Continued)

14" CLASSIC PIZZA W/TOPPINGS (Continued)	Amount	Cal.	Fat (g)	% Cal. Fat	Sat. Fat (g)	Chol. (mg)	Sod. (mg)	Carb. (g)	Fiber (g)	Pro. (g)	Servings/Exchanges
Italian Sausage	2 slices/1/4 pizza	626	24	35	10.2	54	1421	78	5	26	5 starch, 2 medium-fat meat, 3 fat
✓Onion	2 slices/1/4 pizza	523	15	26	6.7	32	1081	77	4	22	5 starch, 2 medium-fat meat, 1 fat
Pepperoni	2 slices/1/4 pizza	614	24	35	10	52	1444	75	4	26	5 starch, 2 medium-fat meat, 3 fat
✓Pineapple Tidbits	2 slices/1/4 pizza	534	15	25	7	32	1082	80	4	21	5 starch, 2 medium-fat meat, 1 fat
Pre-Cooked Beef	2 slices/1/4 pizza	627	26	37	10.7	53	1389	75	4	27	5 starch, 2 medium-fat meat, 3 fat
Ripe Olives	2 slices/1/4 pizza	543	18	30	7	32	1223	76	5	22	5 starch, 2 medium-fat meat, 1 fat

14" LARGE CHEESE

	Amount										Exchanges
✔Deep Dish	2 slices/1/4 pizza	677	30	40	10.9	41	1576	80	5	27	5 starch, 2 medium-fat meat, 3 fat
✔Hand Tossed	2 slices/1/4 pizza	516	15	26	6.7	32	1080	75	4	21	5 starch, 2 medium-fat meat
Thin Crust	2 slices/1/4 pizza	382	17	40	6.7	32	1172	43	2	17	3 starch, 1 medium-fat meat, 2 fat

6" DEEP DISH PIZZA

	Amount										Exchanges
Cheese	whole pizza	598	27	41	9.9	36	1341	68	4	23	4 1/2 starch, 2 medium-fat meat, 3 fat

6" DEEP DISH PIZZA W/TOPPINGS

	Amount										Exchanges
Anchovies	whole pizza	643	30	42	11	55	2132	68	4	31	4 1/2 starch, 2 medium-fat meat, 4 fat

(Continued)

✔ = Healthiest Bets; n/a = not available

6" DEEP DISH PIZZA W/TOPPINGS (Continued)	Amount	Cal.	Fat (g)	% Cal. Fat	Sat. Fat (g)	Chol. (mg)	Sod. (mg)	Carb. (g)	Fiber (g)	Pro. (g)	Servings/Exchanges
Bacon	whole pizza	680	35	46	13	48	1568	68	4	27	4 1/2 starch, 2 medium-fat meat, 5 fat
Banana Peppers	whole pizza	601	28	42	10	36	1415	69	4	23	4 1/2 starch, 2 medium-fat meat, 3 1/2 fat
Cheddar Cheese	whole pizza	684	35	46	14	59	1474	69	4	28	4 1/2 starch, 2 medium-fat meat, 5 fat
Extra Cheese	whole pizza	656	32	44	13	50	1537	69	4	27	4 1/2 starch, 2 medium-fat meat, 4 fat
Fresh Mushrooms	whole pizza	600	28	42	9.9	36	1342	69	4	23	4 1/2 starch, 2 medium-fat meat, 3 1/2 fat
Green Olives	whole pizza	608	29	43	10	36	1546	68	4	23	4 1/2 starch, 2 medium-fat meat, 4 fat

Green Peppers	whole pizza	600	28	42	9.9	36	1342	69	4	23	4 1/2 starch, 2 medium-fat meat, 3 1/2 fat
Ham	whole pizza	615	28	41	10.1	43	1497	69	4	25	4 1/2 starch, 2 medium-fat meat, 3 1/2 fat
Italian Sausage	whole pizza	642	31	43	11.3	45	1478	70	4	25	4 1/2 starch, 2 medium-fat meat, 3 1/2 fat
Onion	whole pizza	601	28	42	9.9	36	1342	69	4	23	4 1/2 starch, 2 medium-fat meat, 4 fat
Pepperoni	whole pizza	647	32	45	11.7	47	1524	69	4	25	4 1/2 starch, 2 medium-fat meat, 4 fat
Pineapple Tidbits	whole pizza	602	28	42	9.9	36	1342	70	4	23	4 1/2 starch, 2 medium-fat meat, 4 fat

✔ = Healthiest Bets; n/a = not available

(Continued)

6" DEEP DISH PIZZA W/TOPPINGS (*Continued*)	Amount	Cal.	Fat (g)	% Cal. Fat	Sat. Fat (g)	Chol. (mg)	Sod. (mg)	Carb. (g)	Fiber (g)	Pro. (g)	Servings/Exchanges
Pre-Cooked Beef	whole pizza	642	32	45	11.6	45	1465	68	4	25	4 1/2 starch, 2 medium-fat meat, 4 fat
Ripe Olives	whole pizza	609	29	43	10.1	36	1340	69	4	23	4 1/2 starch, 2 medium-fat meat, 4 fat
SIDES											
✔Breadsticks	1 piece	116	4	31	.8	0	512	18	1	3	1 starch, 1/2 fat
Buffalo Wings	1 piece	50	2	36	0.6	26	175	2	0	6	1 lean meat
✔Double Cheesy Bread	1 piece	142	6	38	2	6	183	18	1	4	1 starch, 1 medium-fat meat

✔ = Healthiest Bets; n/a = not available

Fazoli's

❖Fazoli's provides some nutrition information for its menu items on their website at www.fazolis.com. They provided additional information for this book.

Light 'n Lean Choice

Baked Ziti
Garden Salad
Ranch Dressing (*1 T, dilute with vinegar*)

Calories......................520	Sodium (mg).............695
Fat (g) 25	Carbohydrate (g).........67
% calories from fat..42	Fiber (g) 6
Saturated fat (g)........8	Protein (g) 25
Cholesterol (mg) 38	

Exchanges: 3 1/2 starch, 1 veg, 2 medium-fat meat, 1 1/2 fat

Healthy 'n Hearty Choice

Minestrone Soup
Spaghetti with Meat Sauce
Garden Salad
Reduced Calorie Italian Dressing (*2 T*)

Calories......................680	Sodium (mg)..........1,690
Fat (g) 18	Carbohydrate (g).......106
% calories from fat..24	Fiber (g) 15
Saturated fat (g)........9	Protein (g) 17
Cholesterol (mg) 10	

Exchanges: 6 1/2 starch, 1 veg, 1 medium-fat meat, 1 fat

(Continued)

Fazoli's

	Amount	Cal.	Fat (g)	% Cal. Fat	Sat. Fat (g)	Chol. (mg)	Sod. (mg)	Carb. (g)	Fiber (g)	Pro. (g)	Servings/Exchanges
BREADS											
✔Breadstick (dry)	1	90	1	10	0	0	170	17	1	4	1 starch
✔Breadstick (regular)	1	140	6	39	1	0	310	18	1	4	1 starch, 1 fat
DESSERTS											
Cheesecake (plain)	1 slice	290	22	68	14	95	220	17	0	6	1 carb, 4 fat
Chocolate Chip Cheesecake	1 slice	300	22	66	14	85	200	22	1	7	1 1/2 carb, 4 fat
Lemon Italian Ice	12 oz	190	0	0	0	0	95	45	0	0	3 carb
Strawberry Topping	1 oz/2 T	35	0	0	0	0	40	8	0	0	1/2 carb
Turtle Cheesecake	1 piece	420	34	73	17	100	220	24	2	8	1 1/2 carb, 7 fat

OTHER ENTREES

Baked Ravioli with Meat Sauce	1	790	29	33	15	95	1190	87	6	37	6 starch, 3 medium-fat meat, 3 fat
✔ Broccoli Lasagna	1	420	18	39	5	140	750	45	5	21	3 starch, 2 medium-fat meat, 1 1/2 fat
Calzone Classic	1	880	40	41	17	95	2210	90	5	47	6 starch, 5 medium-fat meat, 3 fat
Calzone Pizzeria	1	910	41	41	18	90	2450	93	6	51	6 starch, 5 medium-fat meat, 3 fat
✔ Chicken Parmesan	1	460	9	18	2.5	85	680	47	3	42	3 starch, 4 lean meat,
✔ Lasagna	1	440	19	39	6	970	970	41	4	22	2 1/2 starch, 2 medium-fat meat, 2 fat

✔ = Healthiest Bets; n/a = not available

(Continued)

OTHER ENTREES (*Continued*)	Amount	Cal.	Fat (g)	% Cal. Fat	Sat. Fat (g)	Chol. (mg)	Sod. (mg)	Carb. (g)	Fiber (g)	Pro. (g)	Servings/Exchanges
Pizza Baked Spaghetti	1	750	31	37	15	75	1000	78	5	40	5 starch, 4 medium-fat meat, 2 fat
✔Sampler Platter	1	710	21	27	6	85	750	97	6	26	5 starch, 2 medium-fat meat, 2 fat
Submarino— Ham & Swiss	1/2	1000	37	33	11	75	2350	120	7	44	8 starch, 3 medium-fat meat, 4 fat
Submarino—Meatball	1/2	1260	59	42	23	125	2340	128	8	55	8 starch, 4 medium-fat meat, 8 fat
Submarino—Original	1/2	1160	55	43	17	105	230	124	8	45	8 starch, 3 medium-fat meat, 8 fat
Submarino— Pepperoni Pizza	1/2	1060	40	34	19	95	2700	133	6	55	9 starch, 4 medium-fat meat, 4 fat

											Exchanges
Submarino—Turkey	1/2	990	34	31	10	90	2440	121	7	43	8 starch, 3 medium-fat meat, 3 fat
Submarino—Veggie	1/2	1150	55	43	13	55	2085	128	8	37	8 1/2 starch, 1 medium-fat meat, 10 fat
Submarino Club	1/2	1100	44	36	14	120	2890	121	7	51	8 starch, 3 medium-fat meat, 6 fat
PANINI SANDWICHES											
Chicken Caesar Club	1	660	35	48	11	110	1670	51	3	39	3 1/2 starch, 3 medium-fat meat, 4 fat
Four Cheese & Tomato	1	720	43	54	16	75	1450	55	3	28	3 1/2 starch, 3 medium-fat meat, 5 fat
Ham & Swiss	1	600	30	45	9	70	2000	53	2	31	3 1/2 starch, 3 medium-fat meat, 3 fat

(Continued)

✔ = Healthiest Bets; n/a = not available

PANINI SANDWICHES (*Continued*)	Amount	Cal.	Fat (g)	% Cal. Fat	Sat. Fat (g)	Chol. (mg)	Sod. (mg)	Carb. (g)	Fiber (g)	Pro. (g)	Servings/Exchanges
Italian Club	1	670	37	50	11	85	1970	54	3	30	3 1/2 starch, 3 medium-fat meat, 4 fat
Italian Deli	1	660	35	48	13	90	2450	61	4	34	4 starch, 3 medium-fat meat, 4 fat
Smoked Turkey	1	710	38	48	12	110	2110	57	3	32	4 starch, 3 medium-fat meat, 3 1/2 fat
PASTA ENTREES											
Baked Spaghetti Parmesan	1	700	25	32	13	60	770	76	5	38	5 starch, 3 medium-fat meat, 2 fat
✔Baked Ziti	1	490	17	31	7	35	570	56	4	23	3 1/2 starch, 2 medium-fat meat, 1 fat

Baked Ziti (large)	1	750	26	31	11	55	860	87	6	36	6 starch, 3 medium-fat meat, 2 fat
✔Broccoli Fettuccine	1	560	15	24	4	15	190	85	6	19	5 1/2 starch, 3 fat
Broccoli Fettuccine (large)	1	830	23	25	6	20	250	125	8	27	8 starch, 4 1/2 fat
✔Cheese Ravioli with Meat Sauce	1	510	17	30	8	70	800	65	4	20	4 starch, 1 medium-fat meat, 2 fat
✔Cheese Ravioli with Tomato Sauce	1	480	15	28	7	65	530	65	4	21	4 starch, 1 medium-fat meat, 1 fat
✔Fettuccine Alfredo	1	530	15	25	4	15	170	80	3	17	5 starch, 3 fat
Fettuccine Alfredo (large)	1	800	22	25	6	20	230	119	5	25	8 starch, 4 fat
✔Manicotti with Alfredo Sauce	1	350	19	49	10	110	890	25	1	18	1 1/2 starch, 2 medium-fat meat, 2 fat

(Continued)

✔ = Healthiest Bets; n/a = not available

PASTA ENTREES (*Continued*)	Amount	Cal.	Fat (g)	% Cal. Fat	Sat. Fat (g)	Chol. (mg)	Sod. (mg)	Carb. (g)	Fiber (g)	Pro. (g)	Servings/Exchanges
✔Manicotti with Meat Sauce	1	310	16	46	8	105	990	22	2	17	1 1/2 starch, 2 medium-fat meat, 1 fat
✔Manicotti with Tomato Sauce	1	290	15	47	8	105	860	22	2	17	1 1/2 starch, 2 medium-fat meat, 1 fat
✔Peppery Chicken Alfredo	1	610	16	24	4	50	410	80	3	31	5 starch, 2 medium-fat meat, 5 fat
✔Shrimp & Scallop Fettuccine	1	610	16	24	4.5	95	590	81	3	32	5 1/2 starch, 2 lean meat, 2 fat
✔Spaghetti with Meat Sauce	1	450	8	16	2	10	370	74	5	14	5 starch, 1 1/2 fat
✔Spaghetti with Meat Sauce (large)	1	670	11	15	3	10	530	111	8	21	7 1/2 starch, 2 fat

(Continued)

	Amount	Cal	Fat (g)	% Cal Fat	Sat Fat (g)	Chol (mg)	Sod (mg)	Carb (g)	Fiber (g)	Pro (g)	Servings/Exchanges
Spaghetti with Meatballs	1	720	31	39	11	60	730	80	6	28	5 starch, 2 medium-fat meat, 4 fat
Spaghetti with Meatballs (large)	1	1020	42	37	14	80	970	119	8	39	8 starch, 3 medium-fat meat, 5 fat
✔Spaghetti with Tomato Sauce	1	420	6	13	1	0	105	74	5	15	5 starch, 1 fat
✔Spaghetti with Tomato Sauce (large)	1	620	8	12	1	0	140	111	7	21	7 1/2 starch, 1 1/2 fat

PIZZAS

	Amount	Cal	Fat (g)	% Cal Fat	Sat Fat (g)	Chol (mg)	Sod (mg)	Carb (g)	Fiber (g)	Pro (g)	Servings/Exchanges
✔Cheese	1	460	15	29	8	40	970	58	2	24	6 starch, 1 medium-fat meat, 2 fat
Combination	1	570	25	39	12	60	1360	63	3	29	4 starch, 2 medium-fat meat, 3 fat

✔ = Healthiest Bets; n/a = not available

PIZZAS *(Continued)*	Amount	Cal.	Fat (g)	% Cal. Fat	Sat. Fat (g)	Chol. (mg)	Sod. (mg)	Carb. (g)	Fiber (g)	Pro. (g)	Servings/Exchanges
Pepperoni	1	530	22	37	11	55	1230	61	2	27	4 starch, 2 medium-fat meat, 2 fat
SALAD DRESSINGS											
Honey French	1 oz/2 T	150	12	72	1.5	0	210	9	0	0	2 fat
✔House Italian	1 oz/2 T	110	9	74	1.5	0	510	5	0	0	2 fat
Ranch	1 oz/2 T	150	17	102	2.5	5	210	1	0	0	3 fat
✔Reduced Calorie Italian	1 oz/2 T	50	5	90	1	0	390	3	0	0	1 fat
Thousand Island	1 oz/2 T	130	13	90	2	15	220	4	0	0	2 1/2 fat
SALADS											
✔Chicken & Pasta Caesar Salad	1	370	13	32	2.5	45	920	33	3	24	2 starch, 2 veg, 2 medium-fat meat, 1/2 fat
✔Garden	1	30	0	0	0	0	20	6	2	2	1 veg

	Amount										Exchanges
Italian Chef	1	260	21	73	9	45	1450	13	3	15	2 veg, 2 medium-fat meat, 2 fat
Pasta	1	600	26	39	7	25	2020	69	5	19	4 1/2 starch, 1 medium-fat meat, 4 fat
SIDES											
Pasta Salad	1 order	240	10	38	3	5	580	29	2	7	2 starch, 2 fat
SOUPS											
✓Minestrone	1	120	1	8	0	0	910	23	8	1	1 1/2 starch

✓ = Healthiest Bets; n/a = not available

Godfather's Pizza

❖ Godfather's Pizza provides minimal nutrition
information for its menu on its website at
www.godfathers.com. They provided additional
information for this book.

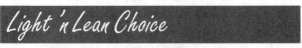

Light 'n Lean Choice

Large Original Veggie (*2 slices*)

Calories......................540	Sodium (mg)..........1,180
Fat (g) 16	Carbohydrate (g).........76
% calories from fat..27	Fiber (g) 2
Saturated fat (g)........7	Protein (g) 26
Cholesterol (mg) 50	

Exchanges: 4 1/2 starch, 1 veg, 2 medium-fat meat

Healthy 'n Hearty Choice

Large Golden Combo (*3 slices*)

Calories......................840	Sodium (mg)..........3,100
Fat (g) 33	Carbohydrate (g).........87
% calories from fat..35	Fiber (g) 3
Saturated fat (g)......14	Protein (g) 42
Cholesterol (mg) 90	

Exchanges: 5 1/2 starch, 1 veg, 3 medium-fat meat,
3 fat

Godfather's Pizza

	Amount	Cal.	Fat (g)	% Cal. Fat	Sat. Fat (g)	Chol. (mg)	Sod. (mg)	Carb. (g)	Fiber (g)	Pro. (g)	Servings/Exchanges
GOLDEN CRUST											
✔Golden Cheese Pizza (large)	1 slice	210	6	26	3	20	390	27	0	10	2 starch, 1 medium-fat meat
✔Golden Cheese Pizza (medium)	1 slice	200	7	32	2.5	15	380	26	0	9	1 1/2 starch, 1 medium-fat meat
Golden Combo Pizza (large)	1 slice	280	11	35	4.5	30	700	29	1	14	2 starch, 1 medium-fat meat
✔Golden Combo Pizza (medium)	1 slice	250	11	40	4	25	600	27	1	12	2 starch, 1 medium-fat meat
✔Golden Veggie (large)	1 slice	210	6	26	3	20	450	29	1	11	2 starch, 1 medium-fat meat
✔Golden Veggie (medium)	1 slice	210	7	30	2.5	15	410	27	1	9	2 starch, 1 medium-fat meat

✔ = Healthiest Bets; n/a = not available

(Continued)

ORIGINAL CRUST

	Amount	Cal.	Fat (g)	% Cal. Fat	Sat. Fat (g)	Chol. (mg)	Sod. (mg)	Carb. (g)	Fiber (g)	Pro. (g)	Servings/Exchanges
✔Cheese Pizza (large)	1 slice	260	7	24	3.5	25	500	35	0	13	2 starch, 1 medium-fat meat
✔Cheese Pizza (medium)	1 slice	230	6	23	2.5	20	440	34	0	11	2 starch, 1 medium-fat meat
Combo Pizza (large)	1 slice	350	14	36	6	35	890	38	1	18	2 1/2 starch, 2 medium-fat meat, 1 fat
Combo Pizza (medium)	1 slice	320	12	34	5	30	800	36	1	16	2 1/2 starch, 2 medium-fat meat
✔Veggie (large)	1 slice	270	8	27	3.5	25	590	28	1	13	2 starch, 1 medium-fat meat, 1/2 fat
✔Veggie (medium)	1 slice	250	6	22	3	20	520	36	1	12	2 1/2 starch, 1 medium-fat meat

✔ = Healthiest Bets; n/a = not available

Little Caesars

❖Little Caesars provides nutrition information
for all its menu items on its website at
www.littlecaesars.com.

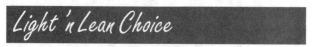
Light 'n Lean Choice

18" Round Cheese Pizza (*2 slices*)

Calories	480	Sodium (mg)	940
Fat (g)	16	Carbohydrate (g)	64
% calories from fat	30	Fiber (g)	4
Saturated fat (g)	7	Protein (g)	24
Cholesterol (mg)	40		

Exchanges: 4 starch, 2 medium-fat meat

Healthy 'n Hearty Choice

14" Round Veggie (*4 slices*)

Calories	760	Sodium (mg)	2,000
Fat (g)	28	Carbohydrate (g)	100
% calories from fat	33	Fiber (g)	8
Saturated fat (g)	12	Protein (g)	36
Cholesterol (mg)	60		

Exchanges: 6 starch, 2 veg, 2 medium-fat meat, 2 fat

(Continued)

Little Caesars

	Amount	Cal.	Fat (g)	% Cal. Fat	Sat. Fat (g)	Chol. (mg)	Sod. (mg)	Carb. (g)	Fiber (g)	Pro. (g)	Servings/Exchanges
COLD SANDWICHES											
Deli Ham & Cheese	1	600	22	33	9.5	55	1480	68	3	33	4 1/2 starch, 3 medium-fat meat, 8 fat
Deli Italian	1	690	32	42	13	75	1730	68	3	34	4 1/2 starch, 3 medium-fat meat, 12 fat
Deli Veggie	1	720	38	48	11.5	30	1240	71	4	26	4 1/2 starch, 2 medium-fat meat, 5 fat
DEEP DISH PIZZA											
✔12" Cheese	1 slice	140	5	32	2	10	280	19	1	7	1 starch, 1 medium-fat meat

✓12" Pepperoni	1 slice	160	6	34	2.5	15	350	19	1	8	1 starch, 1 medium-fat meat
✓14" Cheese	1 slice	140	5	32	2	10	280	19	1	7	1 starch, 1 medium-fat meat
✓14" Pepperoni	1 slice	160	7	39	2.5	15	350	19	1	8	1 starch, 1 medium-fat meat

MISCELLANEOUS

✓Baby Pan! Pan!	1 order	310	15	44	5.5	30	640	32	2	14	2 starch, 1 medium-fat meat, 2 fat
Chicken Wings	1 wing	50	4	72	1	15	640	0	0	4	1 medium-fat meat
✓Cinnamon Caesar Stick	1 order	340	9	24	1	0	440	57	1	8	4 starch, 2 fat
✓Crazy Bread (1 piece)	1	90	3	30	0.5	0	120	14	1	3	1 starch, 1/2 fat

✓ = Healthiest Bets; n/a = not available

(Continued)

MISCELLANEOUS (*Continued*)	Amount	Cal.	Fat (g)	% Cal. Fat	Sat. Fat (g)	Chol. (mg)	Sod. (mg)	Carb. (g)	Fiber (g)	Pro. (g)	Servings/Exchanges
✓Crazy Sauce	4 oz/8 T	45	0	0	0	0	250	9	3	1	1/2 carb
✓Italian Cheese Bread	1 piece	120	6	45	2	10	240	12	1	5	1 starch, 1 fat
PIZZA											
✓12" Cheese	1 slice	160	6	34	2.5	15	320	22	1	8	1 1/2 starch, 1 medium-fat meat
✓12" Pepperoni	1 slice	180	8	40	3	20	420	21	1	9	1 1/2 starch, 1 medium-fat meat, 1/2 fat
✓14" Cheese	1 slice	170	6	32	2.5	15	360	23	1	8	1 1/2 starch, 1 medium-fat meat
✓14" Cheese Thin Crust	1 slice	130	6	42	2.5	15	320	13	1	6	1 starch, 1 fat
✓14" Meatsa	1 slice	220	10	41	4	25	570	24	2	11	1 1/2 starch, 1 medium-fat meat, 1 fat

Item	Serving									Exchanges
✔ 14" Pepperoni	1 slice	200	8	36	3.5	20	460	23	1	9	1 1/2 starch, 1 medium-fat meat, 1/2 fat
✔ 14" Supreme	1 slice	230	10	39	4	25	550	25	2	11	1 1/2 starch, 1 medium-fat meat, 1 fat
✔ 14" Veggie	1 slice	110	7	57	3	15	500	25	2	9	1 1/2 starch, 1 medium-fat meat
✔ 16" Cheese	1 slice	230	8	31	3.5	20	470	32	2	12	1 1/2 starch, 1 medium-fat meat, 1/2 fat
✔ 16" Pepperoni	1 slice	260	11	38	4.5	25	570	31	2	12	2 starch, 1 medium-fat meat, 1 fat
✔ 18" Cheese	1 slice	240	8	30	3.5	20	470	32	2	12	1 1/2 starch, 1 medium-fat meat, 1/2 fat

(Continued)

✔ = Healthiest Bets; n/a = not available

PIZZA (*Continued*)	Amount	Cal.	Fat (g)	% Cal. Fat	Sat. Fat (g)	Chol. (mg)	Sod. (mg)	Carb. (g)	Fiber (g)	Pro. (g)	Servings/Exchanges
✓18" Pepperoni	1 slice	270	11	37	4.5	30	600	32	2	13	2 starch, 1 medium-fat meat, 1 fat
Deep Dish	1 slice	280	13	42	6	30	630	27	2	14	2 starch, 1 medium-fat meat, 2 fat
✓Deep Dish, Cheese Only (large)	1 slice	210	7	30	3.5	15	439	27	1	10	2 starch, 1 medium-fat meat
Stuffed Crust Cheese	1 slice	300	13	39	6	25	498	30	2	16	2 starch, 1 medium-fat meat 1 1/2 fat
Stuffed Crust Pepperoni	1 slice	340	17	45	7.5	35	678	30	2	18	2 starch, 2 medium-fat meat, 1 fat
PIZZA BY THE SLICE											
Cheese	1/6 of 14	290	10	31	4.5	25	570	39	2	14	1 1/2 starch, 1 medium-fat meat, 1 fat

Pepperoni	1/6 of 14	340	14	37	6	35	770	39	2	16	1 1/2 starch, 1 medium-fat meat, 2 fat

SALAD DRESSINGS

✔ Fat Free Italian	1.5 oz/3 T	25	0	0	0	0	390	5	0	0	free
Italian	1.5 oz/3 T	210	22	94	3	0	360	2	0	0	4 fat
Ranch	1.5 oz/3 T	270	29	97	5	4	380	1	0	0	1 fat

SALADS

✔ Antipasto	1	130	7	48	3.5	15	390	10	1	7	2 veg, 1 medium-fat meat
✔ Tossed Side	1	50	1	18	0	0	60	9	1	2	1/2 carb

THIN-CRUST PIZZA

✔ 12" Cheese	1 slice	120	6	45	2.5	15	280	12	1	6	1 starch, 1 medium-fat meat

(Continued)

✔ = Healthiest Bets; n/a = not available

THIN-CRUST PIZZA (*Continued*)	Amount	Cal.	Fat (g)	% Cal. Fat	Sat. Fat (g)	Chol. (mg)	Sod. (mg)	Carb. (g)	Fiber (g)	Pro. (g)	Servings/Exchanges
✔12″ Pepperoni	1 slice	150	8	48	3.5	20	380	12	1	7	1 starch, 1 medium-fat meat, 1/2 fat
✔14″ Pepperoni	1 slice	160	9	51	3.5	20	420	13	1	7	1 starch, 1 medium-fat meat, 1 fat

✔ = Healthiest Bets; n/a = not available

Olive Garden Italian Restaurant

❖Olive Garden provides no nutrition information for its menu on its website. They provided nutrition information only for their "garden-fare" menu items for this book. Meals are created from garden-fare offerings.

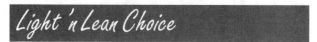

Light 'n Lean Choice

Minestrone Soup (*6 oz*)
Chicken Giardino (*lunch entree*)

Calories......................450	Sodium (mg) 1,790
Fat (g) 8	Carbohydrate (g).........58
% calories from fat..16	Fiber (g) ....n/a
Saturated fat (g)........3	Protein (g) 31
Cholesterol (mg) 50	

Exchanges: 4 starch, 3 lean meat

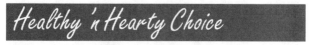

Healthy 'n Hearty Choice

Linguine Alla Marinara (*dinner entree*)
Plain Breadstick

Calories......................590	Sodium (mg) 1,040
Fat (g) 11	Carbohydrate (g).......105
% calories from fat..17	Fiber (g) ....n/a
Saturated fat (g)........2	Protein (g) 19
Cholesterol (mg) 0	

Exchanges: 7 starch, 1 fat

(*Continued*)

Olive Garden Italian Restaurant

	Amount	Cal.	Fat (g)	% Cal. Fat	Sat. Fat (g)	Chol. (mg)	Sod. (mg)	Carb. (g)	Fiber (g)	Pro. (g)	Servings/Exchanges
DINNER ENTREES											
✓Capellini Pomodoro	1	560	18	29	3	10	1130	84	n/a	17	4 1/2 starch, 2 veg, 3 1/2 fat
✓Chicken Giardino	1	460	8	16	3	60	1180	59	n/a	36	4 starch, 3 lean meat
✓Linguine Alla Marinara	1	450	9	18	1.5	0	770	79	n/a	44	5 starch, 1 veg, 2 fat
Shrimp Primavera	1	730	25	31	4	270	1220	84	n/a	44	6 starch, 2 veg, 3 very lean meat, 4 fat
LUNCH ENTREES											
✓Capellini Pomodoro	1	350	11	28	1.5	5	720	52	n/a	10	3 starch, 2 veg, 2 fat
✓Chicken Giardino	1	350	7	18	3	50	1180	40	n/a	26	2 1/2 starch, 2 lean meat
✓Linguine Alla Marinara	1	280	6	19	1	0	510	48	n/a	8	3 starch, 1 fat

✔Shrimp Primavera	1	490	15	28	2	140	820	65	n/a	26	3 1/2 starch, 2 veg, 2 lean meat, 2 fat

SIDES

✔Plain Breadstick	1	140	2	13	0	0	270	26	n/a	5	1 1/2 starch

SOUPS

✔Minestrone Soup	6 oz	100	1	9	0	0	610	18	n/a	5	1 starch

✔ = Healthiest Bets; n/a = not available

Papa John's Pizza

❖Papa John's provides nutrition information for all of its pizzas and side items on their website at www.papajohns.com.

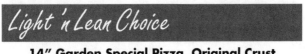

Light 'n Lean Choice

14" Garden Special Pizza, Original Crust
(2 slices)

Calories......................560	Sodium (mg)..........1,434
Fat (g) 20	Carbohydrate (g).........76
% calories from fat..32	Fiber (g) 4
Saturated fat (g)........8	Protein (g) 24
Cholesterol (mg) 40	

Exchanges: 4 1/2 starch, 2 veg, 1 medium-fat meat, 1 fat

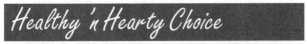

Healthy 'n Hearty Choice

14" Garden Special Pizza, Original Crust
(3 slices)

Calories......................840	Sodium (mg)..........2,139
Fat (g) 30	Carbohydrate (g) 114
% calories from fat..32	Fiber (g) 6
Saturated fat (g)........9	Protein (g) 36
Cholesterol (mg) 64	

Exchanges: 6 starch, 2 veg, 2 medium-fat meat, 3 fat

Papa John's Pizza

	Amount	Cal.	Fat (g)	% Cal. Fat	Sat. Fat (g)	Chol. (mg)	Sod. (mg)	Carb. (g)	Fiber (g)	Pro. (g)	Servings/Exchanges
ORIGINAL CRUST PIZZAS											
All the Meats	1 slice	390	19	44	7	41	1096	37	2	18	2 1/2 starch, 2 high-fat meat
✔Cheese	1 slice	283	10	32	4	20	717	37	2	13	2 1/2 starch, 1 high-fat meat
✔Garden Special	1 slice	280	10	32	3	16	713	38	2	12	2 starch, 1 veg, 1 high-fat meat
Pepperoni	1 slice	303	12	36	5	23	793	37	2	13	2 1/2 starch, 1 high-fat meat
Sausage	1 slice	322	19	53	7	41	1096	37	2	14	2 1/2 starch, 1 high-fat meat, 2 fat
The Works	1 slice	342	15	39	6	32	943	38	2	16	2 1/2 starch, 1 medium-fat meat, 2 fat

(Continued)

✔ = Healthiest Bets; n/a = not available

	Amount	Cal.	Fat (g)	% Cal. Fat	Sat. Fat (g)	Chol. (mg)	Sod. (mg)	Carb. (g)	Fiber (g)	Pro. (g)	Servings/Exchanges
SIDES											
✔Breadsticks	1 stick	140	2	13	0	0	260	26	1	4	2 starch
Cheesesticks	1 stick	180	8	40	3	13	380	20	1	8	1 starch, 1 1/2 fat
Garlic Sauce	1 T	75	9	108	1	0	115	0	n/a	0	2 fat
✔Nacho Cheese	1 T	30	2	60	1.5	8	115	0	n/a	2	free
✔Pizza Sauce	1 T	10	1	90	0	0	50	1	1	0	free
THIN-CRUST PIZZAS											
All the Meats	1 slice	393	26	60	9	50	183	22	1	19	1 1/2 starch, 2 medium-fat meat, 3 fat
Cheese	1 slice	233	13	50	4	20	496	22	1	11	1 1/2 starch, 1 high-fat meat, 1/2 fat

✔Garden Special	1 slice	226	12	48	4	16	496	24	2	10	1 starch, 1 veg, 1 high-fat meat
Pepperoni	1 slice	266	16	54	5	26	621	22	1	11	1 1/2 starch, 1 high-fat meat, 1 fat
Sausage	1 slice	283	17	54	6	30	697	22	1	12	1 1/2 starch, 1 high-fat meat, 1 fat
The Works	1 slice	322	20	56	7	37	871	24	2	15	1 1/2 starch, 1 high-fat meat, 2 fat

✔ = Healthiest Bets; n/a = not available

Pizza Hut

❖Pizza Hut provides nutrition information for all its menu items on their website at www.pizzahut.com.

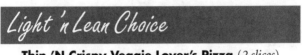

Light 'n Lean Choice

Thin 'N Crispy Veggie Lover's Pizza (*2 slices*)
Salad (*1 1/2 cups from salad bar*)
Reduced Calorie Italian Dressing (*2 T*)

Calories 445	Sodium (mg) 1,390
Fat (g) 17	Carbohydrate (g)........ 55
% calories from fat..34	Fiber (g) 5
Saturated fat (g)........6	Protein (g) 18
Cholesterol (mg) 10	

Exchanges: 3 starch, 2 veg, 1 1/2 medium-fat meat, 1 fat

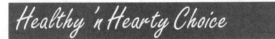

Healthy 'n Hearty Choice

Hand Tossed Chicken Supreme (*3 slices*)
Milk (*fat-free, 8 oz*)

Calories 780	Sodium (mg) 2,076
Fat (g) 21	Carbohydrate (g).........99
% calories from fat..24	Fiber (g) 6
Saturated fat (g)......11	Protein (g) 47
Cholesterol (mg) 45	

Exchanges: 5 starch, 2 veg, 1 milk, 3 medium-fat meat, 1 fat

Pizza Hut

	Amount	Cal.	Fat (g)	% Cal. Fat	Sat. Fat (g)	Chol. (mg)	Sod. (mg)	Carb. (g)	Fiber (g)	Pro. (g)	Servings/Exchanges
DESSERTS											
Apple Dessert Pizza	1 slice	250	5	18	1	0	230	48	2	3	3 carb, 1 fat
Cherry Dessert Pizza	1 slice	250	5	18	1	0	220	47	3	3	3 carb, 1 fat
HAND-TOSSED CRUST PIZZAS											
Beef Topping	1 slice	330	17	46	8	25	880	29	3	16	2 starch, 1 medium-fat meat, 2 fat
✔Cheese	1 slice	240	10	38	5	10	650	28	2	12	2 starch, 1 high-fat meat
✔Chicken Supreme	1 slice	230	7	27	3.5	15	650	29	2	13	2 starch, 1 lean meat, 1/2 fat
✔Ham	1 slice	260	10	35	5	20	800	28	2	14	2 starch, 1 lean meat, 1/2 fat

(Continued)

✔ = Healthiest Bets; n/a = not available

HAND-TOSSED CRUST PIZZAS (Continued)	Amount	Cal.	Fat (g)	% Cal. Fat	Sat. Fat (g)	Chol. (mg)	Sod. (mg)	Carb. (g)	Fiber (g)	Pro. (g)	Servings/Exchanges
Italian Sausage	1 slice	340	18	48	8	30	910	28	2	16	2 starch, 1 high-fat meat, 1/2 fat
Meat Lover's	1 slice	320	17	48	7	30	900	28	2	14	2 starch, 1 high-fat meat, 1 fat
Pepperoni	1 slice	280	13	42	6	20	790	28	2	13	2 starch, 1 high-fat meat, 1/2 fat
✓ Pepperoni Lover's	1 slice	250	11	40	4.5	15	730	27	2	11	2 starch, 1 medium-fat meat, 1 fat
Pork Topping	1 slice	320	16	45	7	25	920	29	3	16	2 starch, 1 high-fat meat, 1 fat
Super Supreme	1 slice	290	14	43	6	25	850	29	2	13	2 starch, 1 high-fat meat, 1 fat

	Amount										Exchanges/Choices
Supreme	1 slice	270	12	40	5	20	730	29	3	13	2 starch, 1 high-fat meat
✔Veggie Lover's	1 slice	220	8	33	3	5	580	29	2	9	1 1/2 starch, 1 veg, 1 1/2 fat
OTHER ENTREES											
✔Cavatini Pasta	1	480	14	26	6	8	1170	66	9	21	4 1/2 starch, 1 high-fat meat, 1 fat
Cavatini Supreme Pasta	1	560	19	31	8	10	1400	73	10	24	5 starch, 2 medium-fat meat, 2 fat
Ham & Cheese Sandwich	1	550	21	34	7	22	2150	57	4	33	4 starch, 3 medium-fat meat, 1 fat
✔Spaghetti w/ Marinara Sauce	1	490	6	11	1	0	730	91	8	18	5 starch, 1 fat
✔Spaghetti w/ Meat Sauce	1	600	13	20	5	8	910	98	9	23	6 1/2 starch, 1 medium-fat meat, 1 1/2 fat

✔ = Healthiest Bets; n/a = not available

(Continued)

OTHER ENTREES *(Continued)*	Amount	Cal.	Fat (g)	% Cal. Fat	Sat. Fat (g)	Chol. (mg)	Sod. (mg)	Carb. (g)	Fiber (g)	Pro. (g)	Servings/Exchanges
Spaghetti w/ Meatballs	1	850	24	25	10	17	1120	120	10	37	9 starch, 2 medium-fat meat, 3 fat
Supreme Sandwich	1	640	28	39	10	28	2150	62	4	34	4 starch, 3 lean meat, 3 fat
PAN PIZZAS											
Beef Topping	1 slice	330	18	49	7	20	690	29	3	14	2 starch, 1 medium-fat meat, 2 1/2 fat
Cheese	1 slice	290	14	43	6	10	590	28	2	12	2 starch, 1 high-fat meat, 1 fat
✔Chicken Supreme	1 slice	270	12	40	4	15	580	29	2	13	2 starch, 1 medium-fat meat, 1 fat
✔Ham	1 slice	260	12	42	4	15	610	28	2	11	2 starch, 1 medium-fat meat, 1 fat

Italian Sausage	1 slice	340	20	53	7	25	720	29	2	13	2 starch, 1 high-fat meat, 2 fat
Meat Lover's	1 slice	360	21	53	7	30	840	29	3	14	2 starch, 1 high-fat meat, 2 fat
Pepperoni	1 slice	280	14	45	5	15	610	28	2	11	2 starch, 1 high-fat meat, 1 fat
Pepperoni Lover's	1 slice	330	18	49	7	20	760	29	2	14	2 starch, 1 high-fat meat, 1 1/2 fat
Pork Topping	1 slice	320	17	48	6	20	760	29	3	13	2 starch, 1 high-fat meat, 1/2 fat
Super Supreme	1 slice	340	18	48	6	25	780	30	3	14	2 starch, 1 high-fat meat, 1 fat

✔ = Healthiest Bets; n/a = not available

(Continued)

PAN PIZZAS *(Continued)*	Amount	Cal.	Fat (g)	% Cal. Fat	Sat. Fat (g)	Chol. (mg)	Sod. (mg)	Carb. (g)	Fiber (g)	Pro. (g)	Servings/Exchanges
Supreme	1 slice	320	17	48	6	20	670	29	3	13	2 starch, 1 high-fat meat, 1 fat
Veggie Lover's	1 slice	270	12	40	4	5	510	30	3	10	1 1/2 starch, 1 veg, 2 fat
PERSONAL PAN PIZZAS											
Cheese	whole pizza	630	28	40	12	25	1370	71	6	28	4 1/2 starch, 2 high-fat meat, 1 1/2 fat
Pepperoni	whole pizza	620	28	41	11	30	1430	70	5	26	4 1/2 starch, 2 high-fat meat, 1 1/2 fat
PERSONAL PIZZA											
Beef	whole pizza	710	35	44	14	45	1580	71	6	31	5 starch, 2 high-fat meat, 5 fat

	Serving										Exchanges
Ham	whole pizza	580	23	36	9	35	1450	70	5	27	4 1/2 starch, 2 high-fat meat, 1/2 fat
Italian Sausage	whole pizza	740	39	47	14	55	1640	71	6	31	4 1/2 starch, 2 high-fat meat, 2 fat
Pork	whole pizza	700	34	44	13	40	1670	71	6	31	4 1/2 starch, 2 high-fat meat, 3 fat

SIDES

	Serving										Exchanges
✔ Bread Stick	1	130	4	28	1	0	170	20	1	3	1 starch, 1 fat
✔ Bread Stick Dipping Sauce	1 order	30	1	30	0	0	170	5	1	1	free
✔ Garlic Bread	1 slice	150	8	48	1.5	0	240	16	1	3	1 starch, 1 1/2 fat
✔ Hot Buffalo Wings	4 wings	210	12	51	3	130	900	4	1	22	3 medium-fat meat
✔ Mild Buffalo Wings	5 wings	200	12	54	3.5	150	510	1	1	23	3 medium-fat meat

✔ = Healthiest Bets; n/a = not available

(Continued)

STUFFED-CRUST PIZZAS

	Amount	Cal.	Fat (g)	% Cal. Fat	Sat. Fat (g)	Chol. (mg)	Sod. (mg)	Carb. (g)	Fiber (g)	Pro. (g)	Servings/Exchanges
Beef Topping	1 slice	466	22	42	10	30	1137	46	3	23	3 starch, 2 medium-fat meat, 2 fat
Cheese	1 slice	445	19	38	10	24	1090	46	3	22	3 starch, 2 medium-fat meat, 2 fat
Chicken Supreme	1 slice	432	17	35	8	32	1111	47	3	24	3 starch, 2 medium-fat meat, 1 fat
Ham	1 slice	404	22	49	12.3	39	1190	45	2	24	3 starch, 2 medium-fat meat, 2 fat
Italian Sausage	1 slice	478	23	43	10.3	35	1164	46	3	22	3 starch, 2 high-fat meat, 1/2 fat
Meat Lover's	1 slice	543	29	48	12.5	48	1427	46	3	26	3 starch, 2 high-fat meat, 2 fat

Pepperoni	1 slice	438	19	39	9.1	27	1116	45	2	21	3 starch, 2 medium-fat meat, 2 fat
Pepperoni Lover's	1 slice	525	26	45	12.5	40	1413	56	3	26	3 starch, 2 high-fat meat, 1 fat
Pork Topping	1 slice	461	21	41	9.7	29	1176	46	3	22	3 starch, 2 medium-fat meat, 2 fat
Super Supreme	1 slice	505	25	45	11	44	1371	46	3	25	3 starch, 2 high-fat meat, 1 fat
Supreme	1 slice	487	23	43	10.5	33	1227	47	3	24	3 1/2 starch, 2 high-fat meat, 1/2 fat
Veggie Lover's	1 slice	421	17	36	8	19	1039	48	3	20	3 starch, 1 veg, 1 high-fat meat, 1 fat

✔ = Healthiest Bets; n/a = not available

(Continued)

THE BIG NEW YORKER

	Amount	Cal.	Fat (g)	% Cal. Fat	Sat. Fat (g)	Chol. (mg)	Sod. (mg)	Carb. (g)	Fiber (g)	Pro. (g)	Servings/Exchanges
Beef Topping	1 slice	480	26	49	11	40	1380	42	8	24	4 starch, 2 high-fat meat, 1 fat
Cheese	1 slice	380	17	40	6	20	1140	41	7	19	3 1/2 starch, 2 medium-fat meat, 1 fat
Ham	1 slice	340	13	34	6	25	1160	41	7	18	3 1/2 starch, 2 medium-fat meat, 1/2 fat
Pepperoni	1 slice	370	16	39	7	20	1150	41	7	17	3 1/2 starch, 2 medium-fat meat, 1 fat
Pork	1 slice	470	25	48	10	35	1470	42	8	23	3 1/2 starch, 2 medium-fat meat, 3 fat
Sausage	1 slice	570	33	52	14	55	1620	42	8	27	3 1/2 starch, 2 medium-fat meat, 4 fat

Supreme	1 slice	450	23	46	10	35	1350	43	8	22	3 1/2 starch, 2 medium-fat meat, 2 fat
Veggie Lover's	1 slice	450	22	44	6	1	1340	52	9	18	3 1/2 starch, 1 veg, 2 medium-fat meat, 2 fat

THE EDGE PIZZA

✓Chicken Supreme	1 slice	90	4	40	1.5	15	290	9	3	7	1/2 starch, 1 medium-fat meat
✓Meat Lover's	1 slice	160	11	62	4.5	20	440	8	1	7	1/2 starch, 1 medium-fat meat, 1 fat
✓The Works	1 slice	110	6	49	2.5	10	270	9	1	5	1/2 starch, 1 medium-fat meat
✓Veggie Lover's	1 slice	70	3	39	1.5	5	180	9	1	2	1/2 starch, 1 fat

✓ = Healthiest Bets; n/a = not available

(Continued)

THE SICILIAN PIZZA

	Amount	Cal.	Fat (g)	% Cal. Fat	Sat. Fat (g)	Chol. (mg)	Sod. (mg)	Carb. (g)	Fiber (g)	Pro. (g)	Servings/Exchanges
Beef Topping	1 slice	260	11	38	4.5	15	640	31	2	11	2 starch, 1 medium-fat meat, 1 fat
Cheese	1 slice	290	13	40	6	10	630	31	2	12	2 starch, 1 medium-fat meat, 1 1/2 fat
Chicken Supreme	1 slice	270	11	37	4	15	620	32	2	12	2 starch, 1 medium-fat meat, 1 fat
✔ Ham	1 slice	257	10	35	5	14	745	30	3	11	2 starch, 1 medium-fat meat, 1 fat
Italian Sausage	1 slice	333	18	49	7.4	24	855	31	3	13	2 starch, 1 medium-fat meat, 2 1/2 fat
Meat Lover's	1 slice	350	19	49	7	25	830	31	2	14	2 starch, 1 medium-fat meat, 2 1/2 fat

	Amount	Cal	Fat (g)	% Fat Cal	Sat Fat (g)	Chol (mg)	Sod (mg)	Carb (g)	Fiber (g)	Pro (g)	Servings/Exchanges
Pepperoni	1 slice	320	16	45	7	20	780	31	2	13	2 starch, 1 medium-fat meat, 2 fat
Pepperoni Lover's	1 slice	320	16	45	7	20	780	31	2	13	2 starch, 1 medium-fat meat, 2 fat
Pork Topping	1 slice	320	16	45	6	20	890	31	3	13	2 starch, 1 medium-fat meat, 2 fat
Super Supreme	1 slice	340	18	48	6	20	780	32	2	13	2 starch, 1 medium-fat meat, 2 1/2 fat
Supreme	1 slice	310	15	44	6	15	690	32	3	12	2 starch, 1 medium-fat meat, 2 fat
Veggie Lover's	1 slice	270	11	37	4	15	620	32	2	12	2 starch, 1 medium-fat meat, 1 fat

(Continued)

✔ = Healthiest Bets; n/a = not available

THIN 'N CRISPY CRUST PIZZAS

	Amount	Cal.	Fat (g)	% Cal. Fat	Sat. Fat (g)	Chol. (mg)	Sod. (mg)	Carb. (g)	Fiber (g)	Pro. (g)	Servings/Exchanges
Beef Topping	1 slice	270	15	50	7	25	750	22	2	13	1 1/2 starch, 1 medium-fat meat, 2 fat
✔Cheese	1 slice	200	9	41	5	10	590	22	2	10	1 1/2 starch, 1 medium-fat meat, 1 fat
✔Chicken Supreme	1 slice	200	7	32	3.5	20	620	23	2	12	1 1/2 starch, 1 medium-fat meat
✔Ham	1 slice	170	7	37	3.5	15	610	21	2	9	1 1/2 starch, 1 medium-fat meat
Italian Sausage	1 slice	290	17	53	7	30	800	22	2	12	1 1/2 starch, 1 medium-fat meat, 2 fat

Meat Lover's	1 slice	310	19	55	8	65	910	22	2	14	1 1/2 starch, 2 medium-fat meat, 2 fat
✔ Pepperoni	1 slice	190	9	43	4	20	610	21	2	9	1 1/2 starch, 1 high-fat meat
Pepperoni Lover's	1 slice	250	13	47	6	20	760	22	2	12	1 1/2 starch, 2 medium-fat meat, 1/2 fat
Pork Topping	1 slice	270	14	47	6	25	820	22	2	13	1 1/2 starch, 1 medium-fat meat, 1 1/2 fat
Super Supreme	1 slice	280	15	48	5	25	840	23	2	13	1 1/2 starch, 2 medium-fat meat, 2 fat
Supreme	1 slice	250	13	47	6	20	710	23	2	12	1 1/2 starch, 1 medium-fat meat, 1 1/2 fat
✔ Veggie Lover's	1 slice	190	7	33	3	5	520	24	2	8	1 1/2 starch, 1 medium-fat meat

✔ = Healthiest Bets; n/a = not available

Round Table Pizza

❖Round Table Pizza provides nutrition information for all its menu items on their website at www.roundtablepizza.com.

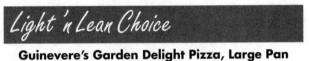

Light 'n Lean Choice

Guinevere's Garden Delight Pizza, Large Pan
(*2 slices*)

Calories......................580	Sodium (mg)..........1,380
Fat (g) 18	Carbohydrate (g)..........76
% calories from fat..28	Fiber (g) 4
Saturated fat (g)......10	Protein (g) 22
Cholesterol (mg).........50	

Exchanges: 4 1/2 starch, 2 veg, 4 medium-fat meat, 2 fat

Healthy 'n Hearty Choice

Western BBQ Chicken Supreme, Large Thin Crust
(*3 slices*)

Calories......................720	Sodium (mg)..........2,130
Fat (g) 27	Carbohydrate (g)..........69
% calories from fat..34	Fiber (g) 3
Saturated fat (g)......14	Protein (g) 33
Cholesterol (mg).......105	

Exchanges: 4 starch, 3 medium-fat meat, 3 1/2 fat

Round Table Pizza

	Amount	Cal.	Fat (g)	% Cal. Fat	Sat. Fat (g)	Chol. (mg)	Sod. (mg)	Carb. (g)	Fiber (g)	Pro. (g)	Servings/Exchanges
APPETIZERS											
Buffalo Wings	6	420	28	60	7	210	1060	2	0	38	5 medium-fat meat, 1 fat
Honey BBQ Wings	6	390	25	58	7	205	740	8	0	35	5 medium-fat meat
✔Honey BBQ Wings	3	190	13	62	3.5	100	370	4	0	17	2 medium-fat meat, 1 fat
Garlic Bread	1	470	21	40	4.5	5	910	59	2	11	4 starch, 3 fat
Garlic Bread w/ Cheese	1	630	33	47	13	45	1240	59	2	21	4 starch, 1 high-fat meat, 5 fat

(Continued)

✔ = Healthiest Bets; n/a = not available

APPETIZERS *(Continued)*	Amount	Cal.	Fat (g)	% Cal. Fat	Sat. Fat (g)	Chol. (mg)	Sod. (mg)	Carb. (g)	Fiber (g)	Pro. (g)	Servings/Exchanges
Garlic Parmesan Twists	1	510	14	25	5	25	1350	76	3	17	5 starch, 2 fat
PAN PIZZAS, PERSONAL SIZE											
Cheese	whole pizza	810	26	29	15	70	1880	106	4	33	7 starch, 2 high-fat meat, 1 fat
Chicken & Garlic Gourmet	whole pizza	850	27	29	13	85	2120	110	5	36	7 starch, 2 medium-fat meat, 3 fat
Chicken Rostadoro	whole pizza	910	31	31	16	85	2510	112	5	41	7 1/2 starch, 3 medium-fat meat, 2 fat
Gourmet Veggie	whole pizza	820	25	27	12	60	1790	114	7	32	7 starch, 2 veg, 1 high-fat meat, 2 fat
Guinevere's Garden Delight	whole pizza	760	21	25	11	50	1850	110	6	29	7 starch, 1 veg, 1 high-fat meat, 2 fat

	Amount									Servings/Exchanges
Hearty Bacon Supreme	whole pizza	940	37	35	16	85	2310	105	4	38	7 starch, 2 high-fat meat, 4 fat
Italian Garlic Supreme	whole pizza	990	43	39	19	95	2310	109	5	37	7 starch, 2 high-fat meat, 5 fat
King Arthur's Supreme	whole pizza	900	34	34	15	90	2340	109	5	36	7 starch, 2 high-fat meat, 3 fat
Maui Zaui	whole pizza	820	24	26	12	70	2160	111	5	35	7 1/2 starch, 2 high-fat meat
Pepperoni	whole pizza	840	29	31	15	70	2120	106	4	32	7 starch, 2 high-fat meat, 2 fat
Pepperoni Rostadoro	whole pizza	970	37	34	18	85	2610	116	5	39	8 starch, 2 high-fat meat, 3 fat
Western BBQ Chicken Supreme	whole pizza	840	25	27	19	85	2310	107	5	34	7 starch, 2 medium-fat meat, 3 fat

(Continued)

✔ = Healthiest Bets; n/a = not available

PAN PIZZAS, LARGE

	Amount	Cal.	Fat (g)	% Cal. Fat	Sat. Fat (g)	Chol. (mg)	Sod. (mg)	Carb. (g)	Fiber (g)	Pro. (g)	Servings/Exchanges
Cheese	1/12 pizza	290	10	31	6	25	680	37	2	12	2 1/2 starch, 1 high-fat meat
Chicken & Garlic Gourmet	1/12 pizza	320	11	31	6	35	780	38	2	14	2 1/2 starch, 1 high-fat meat, 1 fat
Chicken Rostadoro	1/12 slice	330	12	33	6	35	920	39	2	15	2 1/2 starch, 1 medium-fat meat, 1 fat
Gourmet Veggie	1/12 pizza	310	11	32	5	25	670	39	2	12	2 starch, 1 veg, 1 high-fat meat, 1/2 fat
Guinevere's Garden Delight	1/12 pizza	290	9	28	5	25	690	38	2	11	2 starch, 1 veg, 1 high-fat meat
Italian Garlic Supreme	1/12 pizza	360	16	40	7	35	820	37	2	14	2 starch, 1 high-fat meat, 2 fat

King Arthur's Supreme	1/12 pizza	340	14	37	6	35	840	38	2	13	2 1/2 starch, 1 high-fat meat, 1 fat
Montague's All Meat Marvel	1/12 slice	350	16	41	6	40	860	37	2	14	2 1/2 starch, 1 high-fat meat, 1 fat
Pepperoni	1/12 pizza	310	12	35	6	30	790	37	2	12	2 1/2 starch, 1 high-fat meat, 1 fat
Pepperoni Rostadoro	1/12 slice	350	14	36	7	35	930	40	2	15	1 starch, 1 veg, 1 high-fat meat, 1 fat
Roastin' Toastin' Chicken Club	1/12 slice	350	14	36	7	35	840	39	2	15	2 starch, 1 medium-fat meat, 2 1/2 fat
Western BBQ Chicken Supreme	1/12 pizza	320	11	31	6	40	900	37	2	14	2 starch, 1 medium-fat meat, 1 fat

(Continued)

✔ = Healthiest Bets; n/a = not available

	Amount	Cal.	Fat (g)	% Cal. Fat	Sat. Fat (g)	Chol. (mg)	Sod. (mg)	Carb. (g)	Fiber (g)	Pro. (g)	Servings/Exchanges
SANDWICHES											
Gourmet Chicken Club	1	820	39	43	14	125	2540	75	3	38	5 starch, 3 lean meat, 6 fat
Gourmet Ham Club	1	810	37	41	13	90	2710	76	3	36	5 starch, 3 lean meat, 5 fat
Gourmet Turkey Club	1	800	37	42	14	85	2290	75	3	39	5 starch, 3 lean meat, 6 fat
RT Pizza	1	690	34	44	15	90	2070	65	4	30	4 starch, 3 medium-fat meat, 3 fat
RT Veggie	1	680	29	38	11	55	1650	79	5	23	5 starch, 1 veg, 1 high-fat meat, 3 fat
THIN CRUST PIZZAS, PERSONAL											
Cheese	whole pizza	580	24	37	15	70	1410	60	3	26	4 starch, 2 high-fat meat, 1 fat
Chicken & Garlic Gourmet	whole pizza	620	25	36	13	85	1600	64	3	29	4 starch, 2 medium-fat meat, 3 fat

Chicken Rostadoro	whole pizza	680	29	38	15	85	2040	66	4	35	4 1/2 starch, 3 medium-fat meat, 2 fat
Guinevere's Garden Delight	whole pizza	550	20	33	11	50	1440	66	5	23	4 starch, 1 veg, 1 high-fat meat, 2 fat
Italian Garlic Supreme	whole pizza	760	41	49	18	95	1780	63	3	30	4 starch, 2 high-fat meat, 5 fat
King Arthur's Supreme	whole pizza	750	39	47	16	105	2110	64	4	33	4 starch, 3 high-fat meat, 3 fat
Maui Zaui	whole pizza	590	22	34	12	70	1680	56	4	29	4 1/2 starch, 2 medium-fat meat, 2 fat
Montague's All Meat Marvel	whole pizza	780	44	51	17	110	2150	61	3	33	4 starch, 3 high-fat meat, 4 fat

(Continued)

✔ = Healthiest Bets; n/a = not available

THIN CRUST PIZZAS PERSONAL (*Continued*)	Amount	Cal.	Fat (g)	% Cal. Fat	Sat. Fat (g)	Chol. (mg)	Sod. (mg)	Carb. (g)	Fiber (g)	Pro. (g)	Servings/Exchanges
Pepperoni	whole pizza	620	30	44	11	80	830	58	2	28	4 starch, 2 medium-fat meat, 4 fat
Pepperoni Rostadoro	whole pizza	740	35	43	17	85	2130	70	4	33	4 1/2 starch, 3 high-fat meat, 2 fat
Roastin' Toastin' Chicken Club	whole pizza	710	33	42	15	90	1790	66	3	33	4 starch, 1 veg, 3 medium-fat meat, 3 fat
Western BBQ Chicken Supreme	whole pizza	590	20	31	12	90	1130	60	2	30	4 starch, 3 medium-fat meat, 1 fat
THIN CRUST PIZZAS, LARGE											
✔Cheese	1/12 pizza	210	8	34	5	25	530	23	1	9	1 1/2 starch, 1 high-fat meat
✔Chicken & Garlic Gourmet	1/12 pizza	230	9	35	4.5	30	590	24	1	11	1 1/2 starch, 1 medium-fat meat, 1 fat

✔ Chicken Rostadoro	1/12 pizza	250	10	36	5	30	750	25	2	12	1 1/2 starch, 1 medium-fat meat, 1 fat
✔ Gourmet Veggie	1/12 pizza	220	9	37	4.5	20	480	25	2	9	1 starch, 1 veg, 1 high-fat meat
✔ Guinevere's Garden Delight	1/12 pizza	210	7	30	4	20	550	25	2	9	1 starch, 1 veg, 1 medium-fat meat, 1/2 fat
King Arthur's Supreme	1/12 pizza	270	14	47	6	35	730	24	2	11	1 1/2 starch, 1 high-fat meat, 1 fat
✔ Maui Zaui	1/12 pizza	240	9	34	4.5	25	690	25	1	11	1 1/2 starch, 1 high-fat meat
Montague's All Meat Marvel	1/12 pizza	290	17	53	6	40	820	24	1	21	1 1/2 starch, 1 high-fat meat, 2 fat
✔ Pepperoni	1/12 pizza	240	11	41	5	30	660	23	1	10	1 1/2 starch, 1 high-fat meat

(Continued)

✔ = Healthiest Bets; n/a = not available

THIN CRUST PIZZAS, LARGE (*Continued*)	Amount	Cal.	Fat (g)	% Cal. Fat	Sat. Fat (g)	Chol. (mg)	Sod. (mg)	Carb. (g)	Fiber (g)	Pro. (g)	Servings/Exchanges
Pepperoni Rostadoro	1/12 pizza	270	12	40	6	30	770	26	1	12	1 1/2 starch, 1 high-fat meat, 1 fat
Roastin' Toastin' Chicken Club	1/12 pizza	260	12	42	6	30	650	25	1	12	1 1/2 starch, 1 medium-fat meat, 2 fat
✔ Western BBQ Chicken Supreme	1/12 pizza	240	9	34	4.5	35	710	23	1	11	1 1/2 starch, 1 medium-fat meat, 1 fat

✔ = Healthiest Bets; n/a = not available

Sbarro

❖Sbarro provided nutrition information for several of their menu items for this book.

Light 'n Lean Choice

Cheese pizza (*1 slice*)

Calories 485	Sodium (mg) 1,073
Fat (g) 18	Carbohydrate (g).........57
% calories from fat..33	Fiber (g) 2
Saturated fat (g)........9	Protein (g) 29
Cholesterol (mg) 61	

Exchanges: 4 starch, 2 medium fat meat, 1 fat

Healthy 'n Hearty Choice

Spinach & Broccoli Stuffed Pizza (*1 slice*)

Calories......................825	Sodium (mg) 1,536
Fat (g) 40	Carbohydrate (g).........85
% calories from fat..44	Fiber (g) 6
Saturated fat (g)......14	Protein (g) 33
Cholesterol (mg) 63	

Exchanges: 5 1/2 starch, 1 veg, 3 medium-fat meat, 5 fat

(*Continued*)

Sbarro

	Amount	Cal.	Fat (g)	% Cal. Fat	Sat. Fat (g)	Chol. (mg)	Sod. (mg)	Carb. (g)	Fiber (g)	Pro. (g)	Servings/Exchanges
OTHER ENTREES											
Baked Ziti	1 order	928	42	41	21.2	115	954	90	4	44	6 starch, 4 medium-fat meat, 4 fat
Chicken Parmigiana	1 order	364	21	52	4.7	73	743	13	0	31	1 starch, 4 medium-fat meat
Meat Lasagna	1 order	824	41	45	22.2	119	1431	68	34	42	4 1/2 starch, 4 medium-fat meat, 4 fat
Spaghetti with Sauce	1 order	911	23	23	3.2	3	848	144	7	27	10 starch, 4 1/2 fat

PIZZAS

	Amount	Cal.	Fat (g)	% Cal. Fat	Sat. Fat (g)	Chol. (mg)	Sod. (mg)	Carb. (g)	Fiber (g)	Pro. (g)	Exchanges
Cheese	1 slice	485	18	33	9.7	61	1073	56	2	25	3 1/2 starch, 2 medium-fat meat, 1 1/2 fat
Pepperoni	1 slice	591	27	41	13.4	73	1426	56	2	29	3 1/2 starch, 2 medium-fat meat, 2 1/2 fat
Sausage	1 slice	638	29	41	13.7	86	1559	57	2	33	3 1/2 starch, 2 medium-fat meat, 4 fat
Sausage & Pepper Stuffed Pizza	1 slice	961	47	44	19.3	120	2515	83	3	45	5 1/2 starch, 4 medium-fat meat, 5 fat
Spinach & Broccoli Stuffed Pizza	1 slice	825	40	44	14.2	63	1536	85	6	33	5 1/2 starch, 3 medium-fat meat, 5 fat
Supreme Pizza	1 slice	602	25	37	12.2	69	1583	60	3	29	4 starch, 2 medium-fat meat, 3 fat

✔ = Healthiest Bets; n/a = not available

Seafood Catches

RESTAURANTS

Captain D's

Long John Silver's

NUTRITION PROS

- Fish and seafood are naturally low in total and saturated fat and low in calories.
- During the years of nutrition and health consciousness, some fast-food restaurants began to bake, broil, or grill seafood.
- Some healthy sides are available: baked potatoes, rice, salad, and cooked vegetables.

NUTRITION CONS

- The nutritional virtues of fish and seafood are lost in most chain seafood restaurants because their favorite preparation method is frying.
- After fish and seafood have been battered and fried, you wonder what happened to the fish. When you read the nutrition numbers, there's not much fish to speak of.
- Fried fish is often surrounded by high-fat plate fillers—hush puppies, french fries, or creamy coleslaw. Thus, the once-healthy seafood is now part of a fat- and calorie-dense meal.
- Seafood restaurants load their starches—hush puppies, biscuits, cornbread, french fries, etc.—with fat.
- Fruit is nowhere to be found.

Healthy Tips

★ If you order a baked potato, have butter
  and sour cream held or served on the side.
★ Lemon is plentiful. Use it to add flavor
  without calories.
★ Use low-fat, low-calorie cocktail sauce to
  add flavor without extra calories.
  Substitute this for higher calorie tartar
  sauce.
★ Not all coleslaw is created equal. Some is
  high in fat, and some is relatively low.
  Check the nutrition numbers to know the
  score in the restaurant you choose.

Get It Your Way

★ Hold the tartar sauce and opt for lemon or
  vinegar.
★ Substitute a baked potato or rice for french
  fries or hush puppies.
★ Substitute a cooked vegetable, such as
  green beans or corn, for french fries.
★ Substitute breadsticks or a yeast roll for
  biscuits or corn bread if you have the
  option.

Captain D's

❖Captain D's provided nutrition information for only some of its menu items.

Light 'n Lean Choice

Broiled Fish & Chicken Lunch
(*with rice, vegetable medley, and breadstick*)

Calories	503	Sodium (mg)	n/a
Fat (g)	9	Carbohydrate (g)	n/a
% calories from fat	16	Fiber (g)	n/a
Saturated fat (g)	2	Protein (g)	39
Cholesterol (mg)	82		

Exchanges: insufficient information to calculate

Healthy 'n Hearty Choice

Broiled Shrimp Platter
(*with rice, vegetable medley, baked potato, salad with low-fat Italian dressing, and breadstick*)

Calories	720	Sodium (mg)	n/a
Fat (g)	8	Carbohydrate (g)	n/a
% calories from fat	10	Fiber (g)	n/a
Saturated fat (g)	1	Protein (g)	32
Cholesterol (mg)	155		

Exchanges: insufficient information to calculate

(*Continued*)

Captain D's

	Amount	Cal.	Fat (g)	% Cal. Fat	Sat. Fat (g)	Chol. (mg)	Sod. (mg)	Carb. (g)	Fiber (g)	Pro. (g)	Servings/Exchanges
BROILED MEALS											
Broiled Chicken Lunch	1	503	9	16	2	82	n/a	n/a	n/a	39	insufficient info. to calculate
Broiled Chicken Platter	1	802	10	11	2	82	n/a	n/a	n/a	46	insufficient info. to calculate
Broiled Fish & Chicken Lunch	1	478	8	15	1	66	n/a	n/a	n/a	34	insufficient info. to calculate
Broiled Fish & Chicken Platter	1	777	10	12	1	66	n/a	n/a	n/a	41	insufficient info. to calculate
Broiled Fish Lunch	1	435	7	14	1	49	n/a	n/a	n/a	28	insufficient info. to calculate
Broiled Fish Platter	1	734	7	9	1	49	n/a	n/a	n/a	36	insufficient info. to calculate
Broiled Shrimp Lunch	1	421	7	15	1	155	n/a	n/a	n/a	25	insufficient info. to calculate
Broiled Shrimp Platter	1	720	8	10	1	155	n/a	n/a	n/a	32	insufficient info. to calculate
CONDIMENTS											
✔Cocktail Sauce	1 oz/2 T	34	0	0	n/a	0	252	8	0	0	1/2 carb

Imitation Sour Cream	n/a	29	3	93	3	0	n/a	n/a	0	0	insufficient info. to calculate
✓Sweet & Sour Sauce	1.8 oz/4 T	52	0	0	n/a	0	5	13	0	0	1 carb
✓Tartar Sauce	1 oz/2 T	75	7	84	n/a	10	158	3	0	0	1 fat
DESSERTS											
Cheesecake	1 slice	420	31	66	n/a	141	480	30	0	7	2 carb, 6 fat
✓Chocolate Cake	1 slice	303	10	30	n/a	20	259	49	0	4	3 carb, 2 fat
Pecan Pie	1 slice	458	20	39	n/a	4	373	64	4	5	4 carb, 4 fat
SALAD DRESSINGS											
Blue Cheese	1 oz/2 T	105	12	103	n/a	14	101	0	0	0	2 fat
✓French	1 oz/2 T	111	11	89	n/a	7	187	4	0	0	2 fat
✓Light Italian Dressing	1 oz/2 T	16	1	56	0	0	n/a	n/a	n/a	0	insufficient info. to calculate
✓Ranch	1 oz/2 T	92	10	98	n/a	15	230	0	0	0	2 fat

✓ = Healthiest Bets; n/a = not available

(Continued)

	Amount	Cal.	Fat (g)	% Cal. Fat	Sat. Fat (g)	Chol. (mg)	Sod. (mg)	Carb. (g)	Fiber (g)	Pro. (g)	Servings/Exchanges
SANDWICHES											
✔Broiled Chicken Sandwich	1	451	19	38	n/a	105	858	29	0	40	2 starch, 7 lean meat
SIDES											
✔Baked Potato	1	278	0	0	0	0	n/a	n/a	n/a	0	insufficient info. to calculate
✔Breadstick	1	113	4	32	0	0	n/a	n/a	n/a	3	insufficient info. to calculate
Cole Slaw	4 oz	158	12	68	n/a	16	246	12	2	3	1 veg, 1/2 carb, 2 fat
✔Corn on the Cob	1	251	2	7	n/a	0	13	60	0	8	4 starch
✔Crackers	4	50	1	18	n/a	3	147	8	0	1	1/2 starch
Cracklins	1 oz	218	17	70	n/a	0	741	16	0	1	1 starch, 3 fat
✔French Fried Potatoes	1 order	302	10	30	n/a	0	152	50	0	3	3 starch, 2 fat
Fried Okra	4 oz	300	16	48	n/a	0	445	34	0	7	2 starch, 3 fat
✔Green Beans (seasoned)	4 oz	46	2	39	n/a	4	752	5	1	2	1 veg

Hushpuppies (6)	1 order	756	25	30	n/a	0	2790	119	1	13	8 starch, 5 fat
✔Rice	4 oz	124	0	0	n/a	0	9	28	1	3	2 starch
✔Rice (included w/ Broiler Platter)	n/a	184	0	0	0	0	n/a	n/a	n/a	1	insufficient info. to calculate
✔Salad	n/a	20	0	0	0	0	n/a	n/a	n/a	1	insufficient info. to calculate
✔Vegetable Medley (included w/ Broiler Platter)	n/a	36	1	25	0	0	n/a	n/a	n/a	1	insufficient info. to calculate

✔ = Healthiest Bets; n/a = not available

Long John Silver's

❖Long John Silver's provides nutrition information for most of its menu items on their website at www.longjohnsilvers.com.

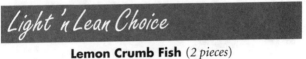

Light 'n Lean Choice

Lemon Crumb Fish (*2 pieces*)
Rice Pilaf
Corn Cobbette (*without butter*)
Coleslaw

Calories......................490	Sodium (mg)...........1,100
Fat (g) 20	Carbohydrate (g)..........52
% calories from fat..37	Fiber (g)..................n/a
Saturated fat (g)........4	Protein (g) 28
Cholesterol (mg).........55	

Exchanges: 3 starch, 1 veg, 3 lean meat, 1 fat

Healthy 'n Hearty Choice

Clam Chowder (*cup*)
Country Style Breaded Fish (*2 pieces*)
Corn Cobette (*without butter*)
Garden Salad w/Fat-Free French (*2 T*)

Calories......................825	Sodium (mg)...........1,885
Fat (g) 33	Carbohydrate (g)..........98
% calories from fat..36	Fiber (g)..................n/a
Saturated fat (g)........8	Protein (g) 38
Cholesterol (mg).........55	

Exchanges: 5 starch, 2 veg, 3 lean meat, 5 fat

Long John Silver's

	Amount	Cal.	Fat (g)	% Cal. Fat	Sat. Fat (g)	Chol. (mg)	Sod. (mg)	Carb. (g)	Fiber (g)	Pro. (g)	Servings/Exchanges
CONDIMENTS											
✓Honey Mustard Sauce	1 T	20	0	0	0	0	60	5	n/a	0	free
✓Shrimp Sauce	1 T	15	0	0	0	0	180	3	n/a	0	free
✓Sour Cream	1 oz/2 T	60	6	90	3.5	15	15	1	n/a	0	1 fat
✓Sweet 'N' Sour Sauce	1 T	20	0	0	0	0	45	5	n/a	0	free
✓Tartar Sauce	1 T	40	4	90	0.5	5	105	2	n/a	0	1 fat
DESSERTS											
Banana Split Sundae	1 order	300	17	51	9	15	130	34	n/a	4	2 carb, 3 fat
Chocolate Crème Pie	1 piece	280	17	55	8	15	125	29	n/a	4	2 carb, 3 fat

(Continued)

✓ = Healthiest Bets; n/a = not available

DESSERTS (*Continued*)	Amount	Cal.	Fat (g)	% Cal. Fat	Sat. Fat (g)	Chol. (mg)	Sod. (mg)	Carb. (g)	Fiber (g)	Pro. (g)	Servings/Exchanges
Double Lemon Pie	1 slice	350	18	46	10	40	180	41	n/a	6	2 1/2 carb, 3 1/2 fat
Dutch Apple Pie	1 piece	290	13	40	4	0	250	44	n/a	2	3 carb, 2 1/2 fat
Pecan Pie	1 piece	390	19	44	4	40	250	53	n/a	3	3 1/2 carb, 4 fat
Pineapple Crème	1 piece	310	17	49	9	5	105	36	n/a	4	2 1/2 carb, 3 fat
Cheesecake Pie											
Strawberries N' Crème Pie	1 piece	280	15	48	8	15	130	32	n/a	4	2 carb, 3 fat
FISH											
✓Lemon Crumb	1	240	12	45	4	55	790	10	n/a	23	1/2 starch, 3 very lean meat, 2 fat
FLAVORBAKED ITEMS											
✓Chicken	1 piece	140	8	51	2.5	20	400	9	n/a	8	1/2 starch, 1 very lean meat, 1 fat

	Amount	Calories	Fat (g)	% Fat Cal	Sat Fat (g)	Chol (mg)	Sod (mg)	Carb (g)	Fiber (g)	Pro (g)	Exchanges
✔ Country Style Breaded Fish	1 piece	200	10	45	1.5	10	300	17	n/a	10	1 starch, 1 very lean meat, 2 fat

FRIED ITEMS

	Amount	Calories	Fat (g)	% Fat Cal	Sat Fat (g)	Chol (mg)	Sod (mg)	Carb (g)	Fiber (g)	Pro (g)	Exchanges
✔ Batter-Dipped Chicken	1 piece	140	8	51	2.5	20	9	11	n/a	8	1 starch, 1 lean meat, 1/2 fat
Batter-Dipped Fish	1 piece	230	13	51	4	30	700	16	n/a	12	1 starch, 1 lean meat, 2 fat
Batter-Dipped Shrimp	1 piece	45	3	60	1	15	125	3	n/a	2	1/2 fat
Clams	1 order	250	14	50	3.5	35	560	26	n/a	9	2 starch, 1 lean meat, 2 fat
Popcorn Shrimp Munchers	1 order	320	15	42	2.5	85	1440	33	n/a	15	2 starch, 1 lean meat, 2 fat

GRAB N GO SANDWICHES

	Amount	Calories	Fat (g)	% Fat Cal	Sat Fat (g)	Chol (mg)	Sod (mg)	Carb (g)	Fiber (g)	Pro (g)	Exchanges
✔ Battered Chicken	1	340	14	37	3.5	25	840	40	n/a	13	2 1/2 starch, 1 lean meat, 2 fat
✔ Battered Chicken w/ Cheese	1	390	19	44	9	40	1090	40	n/a	16	2 1/2 starch, 1 lean meat, 3 fat

(Continued)

✔ = Healthiest Bets; n/a = not available

GRAB N GO SANDWICHES *(Continued)*	Amount	Cal.	Fat (g)	% Cal. Fat	Sat. Fat (g)	Chol. (mg)	Sod. (mg)	Carb. (g)	Fiber (g)	Pro. (g)	Servings/Exchanges
Battered Fish	1	430	20	42	5	35	1150	46	n/a	16	3 starch, 1 lean meat, 3 fat
Battered Fish w/ Cheese	1	480	25	47	10	50	1390	46	n/a	19	3 starch, 1 lean meat, 4 fat
OTHER ENTREES											
✔Crabcake	1	150	9	54	2	15	180	12	n/a	4	1 starch, 2 fat
Lemon Crumb Fish Meal	1	730	29	36	6	60	1720	89	n/a	31	6 starch, 2 lean meat, 5 fat
SALAD DRESSINGS											
✔Fat-Free French	1 oz/2 T	40	0	0	0	0	240	10	n/a	0	1/2 carb
✔Fat-Free Ranch	1 oz/2 T	40	0	0	0	0	290	9	n/a	0	1/2 carb
✔Italian	1 oz/2 T	90	9	90	1.5	0	290	2	n/a	0	2 fat
Ranch	1 oz/2 T	170	18	95	3	10	260	1	n/a	0	3 1/2 fat
Thousand Island	1 oz/2 T	120	10	75	1.5	15	290	5	n/a	0	2 fat

SALADS

	Amount	Cal	Fat	%Fat	Sat Fat	Chol	Sod	Carb	Fiber	Pro	Exchanges/Choices
✔Garden	1	45	0	0	0.0	0	25	9	n/a	3	2 veg
✔Grilled Chicken	1	140	3	19	0.5	45	260	10	n/a	20	2 veg, 2 very lean meat
✔Ocean Chef	1	130	2	14	0.0	60	540	15	n/a	14	3 veg, 2 very lean meat

SANDWICHES

	Amount	Cal	Fat	%Fat	Sat Fat	Chol	Sod	Carb	Fiber	Pro	Exchanges/Choices
Ultimate Fish	1	480	25	47	10	50	1400	46	n/a	19	3 starch, 1 very lean meat, 4 fat

SIDES

	Amount	Cal	Fat	%Fat	Sat Fat	Chol	Sod	Carb	Fiber	Pro	Exchanges/Choices
Cheese Sticks	1 order	160	9	51	4	10	360	12	n/a	6	1 starch, 2 fat
✔Coleslaw	4.0 oz	170	7	37	0	0	310	23	n/a	2	2 veg, 1 carb, 1 fat
Corn Cobbette	3.3 oz	140	8	51	1.5	0	0	19	n/a	3	1 starch, 1 1/2 fat
✔Corn Cobbette (w/o butter)	3.05 oz	80	1	11	0.5	0	0	19	n/a	3	1 starch
French Fries (large)	1 order	420	24	51	4	0	830	46	n/a	5	3 starch, 5 fat

(Continued)

✔ = Healthiest Bets; n/a = not available

SIDES (*Continued*)	Amount	Cal.	Fat (g)	% Cal. Fat	Sat. Fat (g)	Chol. (mg)	Sod. (mg)	Carb. (g)	Fiber (g)	Pro. (g)	Servings/Exchanges
French Fries (regular)	1 order	250	15	54	2.5	0	500	28	n/a	3	2 starch, 3 fat
✓ Hushpuppy	1 piece	60	3	45	0	0	25	9	n/a	1	1/2 starch, 1/2 fat
✓ Rice Pilaf	4 oz	180	4	20	0.5	0	560	34	n/a	3	2 starch, 1 fat
✓ Side Salad	1	20	0	0	0	0	10	3	n/a	1	free
SOUPS											
Broccoli Cheese	8 oz	180	12	60	4.5	15	1240	13	n/a	5	1 carb, 2 fat
Clam Chowder	8 oz	260	12	42	5	35	1020	26	n/a	12	1 1/2 starch, 1 lean meat, 2 fat
Clam Chowder	16 oz	520	24	42	10	70	2030	52	n/a	24	3 1/2 starch, 2 lean meat, 3 fat

✓ = Healthiest Bets; n/a = not available

Sit-Down Family Fare

RESTAURANTS

Big Boy Restaurant

Bob Evans Restaurants

Boston Market

Denny's

IHOP

Shoney's

Note: Nutrition information provided by most restaurants in this category is far from complete. You might not find a few large chains you expect to see in this chapter because they were unwilling to provide either a menu or nutrition information.

NUTRITION PROS

- Many sit-down American restaurants have added healthier options to their menus.
- You can pick and choose among the appetizers, salads, soups, and side dishes to put together healthy, portion-controlled meals.
- Healthier preparation methods are available— stir-frying, grilling, and blackening.
- Time and a desire to please is on your side. This makes special requests easier for you and possible for the kitchen.
- Portions are large, but take-home containers are at the ready.

- Some of these restaurants serve their breakfast-to-dinner menu 24 hours a day. This puts variety on your side.
- These restaurants hardly limit their menu to American specialties. They globe trot to bring you Mexican fajitas or salads, Italian pastas or pizzas, and Chinese pot stickers or stir-fry dishes. This helps to widen the variety of healthier choices.
- Raw and cooked vegetables are easier to find here than in fast-food restaurants. Just be careful they aren't drenched in fat or fried.
- Condiments to help you add taste without fat might be found in the kitchen—teriyaki or soy sauce, lemons, limes, a variety of vinegars, ketchup, barbecue sauce, and low-calorie salad dressings. Ask, and maybe you'll receive.

NUTRITION CONS

- Bread, rolls, crackers, or breadsticks and butter might greet you at the table.
- These restaurants love to fry—from fried mozzarella sticks to fried shrimp, chicken fingers, french fries, and onion rings.
- Sandwiches and other entrees may be accompanied by french fries, onion rings, potato chips, or creamy coleslaw.
- Some foods get a healthy start—vegetables, potatoes, or pasta. But then they are drenched in salad dressing or cheese sauce, or dropped a foot deep in oil and fried.
- Salads can start off healthy but end up with high-fat toppers—avocado, cheese, bacon, or croutons.

- Portions are frequently too big . . . many are *way* too big.
- Plain fruit is often not available. The apples buried between a double crust are not the healthiest way to count your fruits.
- Cheese is in, on, and around a startling number of menu items—melted cheese on a sandwich or cheese sauce on vegetables or pasta. This makes the calories, saturated fat, and cholesterol rise.

Healthy Tips

★ Combine a soup, salad, and side dish or combine one or two appetizers and a salad for a healthy, portion-controlled meal.

★ Share two complementary entrees—pasta topped with a tomato-based sauce or vegetables and a Mexican salad, for example.

★ Split everything with your dining partner, from appetizer to dessert.

★ Request a take-home container when you order your meal. Pack up the portion to take home when your food arrives.

Get It Your Way

★ Ask for your salad dressing on the side—
  all of the time.
★ Ask that high-fat salad toppers be used
  lightly or left in the kitchen.
★ Request to substitute high-fat, high-calorie
  sides with lower-fat, lower-calorie items.
  Substitute a baked potato for french fries
  or onion rings, request a sandwich on
  whole-wheat bread rather than on a croissant, opt for mustard rather than mayonnaise.
★ Ask the kitchen to hold the butter or
  cheese sauce on vegetables.
★ Forgo the fried tortilla shell in which big
  salads are served.
★ Request some lemon or lime slices, vinegar, or soy or teriyaki sauce on the side to
  flavor menu items with few calories.

Big Boy Restaurant

❖Big Boy provides nutrition information for their "Health Smart" items on the back of their menu. Their website is www.bigboy.com.

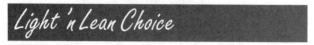

Light 'n Lean Choice

From Mini Breakfast:

Fresh Fruit
Hot Cakes 'n Bacon (*short stack of pancakes, substitute ham for bacon*)

Unable to calculate from limited nutrition information provided for these items.

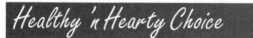

Healthy 'n Hearty Choice

Cabbage Soup (*bowl*)
Breast of Chicken w/ Mozzarella in Pita
(*with ranch dressing*)
Rice Pilaf
Fat-Free Frozen Yogurt (*4 oz/1/2 cup*)

Calories......................664	Sodium (mg)..........1,001
Fat (g) 15	Carbohydrate (g).........83
% calories from fat..20	Fiber (g).................n/a
Saturated fat (g) ....n/a	Protein (g) 48
Cholesterol (mg) 91	

Exchanges: 3 starch, 2 carb, 5 very lean meat, 2 1/2 fat

(*Continued*)

Big Boy Restaurant

	Amount	Cal.	Fat (g)	% Cal. Fat	Sat. Fat (g)	Chol. (mg)	Sod. (mg)	Carb. (g)	Fiber (g)	Pro. (g)	Servings/Exchanges
BREAKFAST											
✔ Plain Egg Beaters Omelet	1 order	305	10	30	n/a	0	603	36	n/a	19	2 1/2 starch, 2 lean meat
✔ Scrambled Egg Beaters	1 order	305	10	30	n/a	0	603	36	n/a	19	2 starch, 2 lean meat, 1 fat
✔ Vegetarian Egg Beaters Omelet	1 order	330	10	27	n/a	0	613	40	n/a	21	2 starch, 2 veg, 2 lean meat, 1 fat
DESSERTS											
✔ Frozen Yogurt (fat-free)	1 order	118	0	0	n/a	0	60	27	n/a	3	1 1/2 carb
✔ Frozen Yogurt Shake	1 order	158	0	0	n/a	2	120	33	n/a	7	2 carb
ENTREES											
✔ Baked Cod	1 order	744	21	25	n/a	76	655	82	n/a	57	5 1/2 starch, 6 very lean meat, 3 fat

	Amount									Exchanges/Choices
✔ Breast of Chicken w/ Mozzarella	1 order	697	20	26	n/a	76	613	80	n/a	50	5 starch, 5 very lean meat, 3 fat
Cajun Cod	1 order	736	21	26	n/a	76	745	80	n/a	56	5 starch, 6 very lean meat, 3 fat
✔ Chicken & Pasta Primavera	1 order	678	14	19	n/a	65	875	83	n/a	53	5 starch, 2 veg, 5 lean meat, 2 fat
✔ Chicken 'n Vegetable Stir Fry	1 order	795	18	20	n/a	65	845	109	n/a	51	6 starch, 3 veg, 4 lean meat, 1 fat
✔ Spaghetti Marinara	1 order	589	11	17	n/a	8	784	105	n/a	17	7 starch, 2 fat
✔ Vegetable Stir Fry	1 order	616	14	20	n/a	0	774	109	n/a	17	6 starch, 3 veg, 3 fat
PITAS											
✔ Breast of Chicken w/ Mozzarella (ranch dressing)	1 order	486	13	24	n/a	84	604	46	n/a	46	3 starch, 5 very lean meat, 1 fat

(Continued)

✔ = Healthiest Bets; n/a = not available

PITAS (*Continued*)	Amount	Cal.	Fat (g)	% Cal. Fat	Sat. Fat (g)	Chol. (mg)	Sod. (mg)	Carb. (g)	Fiber (g)	Pro. (g)	Servings/Exchanges
✔Turkey Pita (ranch dressing)	1 order	370	8	19	n/a	83	1173	46	n/a	30	3 starch, 3 very lean meat, 1 fat
SALAD DRESSINGS											
✔Fat-Free Oriental Dressing	1 oz/2 T	20	0	0	n/a	0	189	4	n/a	1	free
✔Italian Dressing (fat free)	1 oz/2 T	11	0	0	n/a	0	191	3	n/a	0	free
✔Reduced Calorie Ranch	1 oz/2 T	41	3	66	n/a	8	151	3	n/a	1	1/2 fat
SALADS											
✔Chicken Breast Salad (w/ roll, margarine)	1 order	523	16	28	n/a	73	654	50	n/a	44	2 starch, 3 veg, 5 lean meat

											Exchanges
✔Oriental Chicken Breast Salad (w/ roll, margarine)	1 order	660	20	27	n/a	65	855	73	n/a	48	4 starch, 3 veg, 5 lean meat, 1 fat
✔Tossed Salad	1 order	35	0	0	n/a	0	71	7	n/a	2	1 veg
SIDES											
✔Baked Potato (plain)	1	163	0	0	n/a	0	7	37	n/a	5	2 1/2 starch
✔Dinner Roll	1	210	5	21	n/a	0	340	36	n/a	6	2 starch, 1 fat
✔Promise Margarine	1 order	25	3	108	n/a	0	35	0	n/a	0	1/2 fat
✔Rice Pilaf	1 order	145	3	19	n/a	7	225	26	n/a	3	2 starch, 1/2 fat
SOUPS											
✔Cabbage Soup	1 bowl	40	1	23	n/a	0	347	7	n/a	1	1/2 starch

✔ = Healthiest Bets; n/a = not available

Bob Evans Restaurants

❖Bob Evans Restaurants provided nutrition information for several menu items. Their website is www.bobevans.com.

Light 'n Lean Choice

Bean Soup (*cup*)
Vegetable Stir Fry
1/2 Applesauce

Calories......................500	Sodium (mg)...............n/a
Fat (g) 8	Carbohydrate (g).........98
% calories from fat..12	Fiber (g) ....n/a
Saturated fat (g) ....n/a	Protein (g)...................n/a
Cholesterol (mg)........n/a	

Exchanges: insufficient information to calculate

Healthy 'n Hearty Choice

Grilled Chicken
Baked Potato
Green Beans
1/2 Blackberry Cobbler

Calories 658	Sodium (mg)...............n/a
Fat (g) 11	Carbohydrate (g).......100
% calories from fat...15	Fiber (g) ....n/a
Saturated fat (g) ....n/a	Protein (g)...................n/a
Cholesterol (mg)........n/a	

Exchanges: insufficient information to calculate

Bob Evans Restaurants

	Amount	Cal.	Fat (g)	% Cal. Fat	Sat. Fat (g)	Chol. (mg)	Sod. (mg)	Carb. (g)	Fiber (g)	Pro. (g)	Servings/Exchanges
BREADS											
✔Bagel (plain)	1	187	1	5	n/a	n/a	n/a	36	n/a	n/a	insufficient info. to calculate
✔English Muffin	1	120	1	8	n/a	n/a	n/a	27	n/a	n/a	insufficient info. to calculate
✔Toast (plain)	2 slices	180	2	10	n/a	n/a	n/a	36	n/a	n/a	insufficient info. to calculate
BREAKFAST											
✔French Toast	1 slice	161	3	17	n/a	n/a	n/a	27	n/a	n/a	insufficient info. to calculate
✔Hotcake	1	176	6	31	n/a	n/a	n/a	25	n/a	n/a	insufficient info. to calculate
✔Lite Sausage Link	1	104	6	52	n/a	n/a	n/a	0	n/a	n/a	insufficient info. to calculate
✔Oatmeal	1 order	252	4	14	n/a	n/a	n/a	44	n/a	n/a	insufficient info. to calculate

(Continued)

✔ = Healthiest Bets; n/a = not available

	Amount	Cal.	Fat (g)	% Cal. Fat	Sat. Fat (g)	Chol. (mg)	Sod. (mg)	Carb. (g)	Fiber (g)	Pro. (g)	Servings/Exchanges
CEREAL											
✔Grits	1	80	7	79	n/a	n/a	n/a	5	n/a	n/a	insufficient info. to calculate
DESSERTS											
Blackberry Cobbler	1	320	11	31	n/a	n/a	n/a	54	n/a	n/a	insufficient info. to calculate
ENTREES											
✔Spaghetti (w/o toast)	1	493	12	22	n/a	n/a	n/a	75	n/a	n/a	insufficient info. to calculate
✔Wildfire Chicken Breast	1	260	4	14	n/a	n/a	n/a	23	n/a	n/a	insufficient info. to calculate
✔Chicken Stir Fry	1 order	531	11	19	n/a	n/a	n/a	61	n/a	n/a	3 1/2 starch, 2 veg, 5 very lean meat, 1 fat
✔Grilled Chicken (1 piece)	1 order	165	4	22	n/a	n/a	n/a	0	n/a	n/a	insufficient info. to calculate
✔Vegetable Stir Fry	1 order	319	7	20	n/a	n/a	n/a	61	n/a	n/a	3 starch, 3 veg, 1 fat

PLATE

✔Fruit	1	245	1	4	n/a	n/a	62	n/a	n/a	insufficient info. to calculate

SALAD

✔Garden	1	50	1	18	n/a	n/a	10	n/a	n/a	insufficient info. to calculate
Cobb	1	480	24	45	n/a	n/a	15	n/a	n/a	insufficient info. to calculate

SIDES

✔Applesauce	1	155	0	0	n/a	n/a	40	n/a	n/a	insufficient info. to calculate
✔Baked Potato (plain)	1	278	0	0	n/a	n/a	64	n/a	n/a	insufficient info. to calculate
Bread & Celery Stuffing	1	174	8	41	n/a	n/a	22	n/a	n/a	insufficient info. to calculate
✔Cottage Cheese	1	112	5	40	n/a	n/a	4	n/a	n/a	insufficient info. to calculate
✔Dinner Rolls, plain	2	320	8	23	n/a	n/a	72	n/a	n/a	5 starch, 1 1/2 fat
✔Green Beans	1 order	55	1	16	n/a	n/a	9	n/a	n/a	2 veg
✔Long Grain & Wild Rice	1	133	4	27	n/a	n/a	23	n/a	n/a	insufficient info. to calculate

✔ = Healthiest Bets; n/a = not available

(Continued)

	Amount	Cal.	Fat (g)	% Cal. Fat	Sat. Fat (g)	Chol. (mg)	Sod. (mg)	Carb. (g)	Fiber (g)	Pro. (g)	Servings/Exchanges
SOUPS											
✔Bean Soup	1 bowl	146	1	6	n/a	n/a	n/a	23	n/a	n/a	1 1/2 starch, 1 very lean meat
✔Bean Soup	1 cup	104	1	9	n/a	n/a	n/a	17	n/a	n/a	1 starch, 1 very lean meat
✔Vegetable	1 bowl	213	10	42	n/a	n/a	n/a	22	n/a	n/a	insufficient info. to calculate
✔Vegetable	1 cup	123	6	44	n/a	n/a	n/a	13	n/a	n/a	insufficient info. to calculate
TOPPINGS											
Appleberry	n/a	80	0	0	n/a	n/a	n/a	20	n/a	n/a	insufficient info. to calculate
Cream Cheese light	n/a	60	5	75	n/a	n/a	n/a	1	n/a	n/a	insufficient info. to calculate
Oregon Berry	n/a	110	0	0	n/a	n/a	n/a	28	n/a	n/a	insufficient info. to calculate
Syrup	n/a	243	0	0	n/a	n/a	n/a	61	n/a	n/a	insufficient info. to calculate

✔ = Healthiest Bets; n/a = not available

Boston Market

❖Boston Market provides nutrition information
for all its menu items on their website at
www.bostonmarket.com.

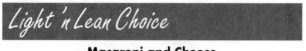

Light 'n Lean Choice

Macaroni and Cheese
Whole Kernel Corn
Zucchini Marinara
Fruit Salad

Calories.......................590 Sodium (mg) 1,340
Fat (g) ....19 Carbohydrate (g).........84
  % calories from fat..29   Fiber (g) 6
  Saturated fat (g)........7 Protein (g) 20
Cholesterol (mg) 30

Exchanges: 4 starch, 1 veg, 1 fruit, 2 medium-fat
meat, 1 fat

Healthy 'n Hearty Choice

1/4 White Meat Chicken (*no skin or wing*)
Chicken Gravy (*4 T*)
Homestyle Mashed Potatoes (*2/3 cup*)
Green Beans (*3/4 cup*)
1/2 Toll House Cookie

Calories.......................865 Sodium (mg) 2,155
Fat (g) ....37 Carbohydrate (g)........ 93
  % calories from fat..38   Fiber (g) 6
  Saturated fat (g)......13 Protein (g) 42
Cholesterol (mg) 142

Exchanges: 4 1/2 starch, 1 veg, 1 carb, 4 lean meat,
4 fat

(*Continued*)

Boston Market

	Amount	Cal.	Fat (g)	% Cal. Fat	Sat. Fat (g)	Chol. (mg)	Sod. (mg)	Carb. (g)	Fiber (g)	Pro. (g)	Servings/Exchanges
BREADS											
✔Corn Bread	1 piece	200	6	27	1.5	25	390	33	1	3	2 starch, 1 fat
✔Honey Wheat Roll	1/2 roll	150	2	12	0	0	280	29	2	5	2 starch
COLD SIDES											
Cole Slaw	3/4 cup	280	16	51	2.5	0	520	32	3	2	1 veg, 1 1/2 carb, 2 fat
✔Cranberry Relish	3/4 cup	370	5	12	0.5	0	5	84	5	2	1 fruit, 4 carb, 1 fat
✔Fruit Salad	3/4 cup	70	1	13	0	0	10	17	2	1	1 fruit
Mediterranean Pasta Salad	3/4 cup	170	10	53	2.5	10	490	16	2	4	1 starch, 2 fat
Tortellini Salad	3/4 cup	380	24	57	4.5	25	530	29	2	14	2 starch, 1 medium-fat meat, 4 fat

DESSERTS

Brownie	1	450	27	54	7	80	190	47	3	6	3 carb, 5 fat
Chocolate Chip Cookie	1	340	17	45	6	25	240	48	1	4	3 carb, 3 fat
Oatmeal Raisin Cookie	1	320	13	37	2.5	25	260	48	1	4	3 carb, 2 fat

ENTREES

1/2 Chicken with Skin	1	590	33	50	10	290	1010	4	0	70	10 lean meat, 1/2 fat
✔1/4 Dark Meat Chicken w/o Skin	1	190	10	47	3	115	440	1	0	22	3 lean meat
1/4 Dark Meat Chicken with Skin	1	320	21	59	6	155	500	2	0	30	4 lean meat, 2 fat
✔1/4 White Meat Chicken w/o Skin or Wing	1	170	4	21	1	85	480	2	0	33	5 very lean meat
1/4 White Meat Chicken with Skin	1	280	12	39	3.5	135	510	2	0	40	6 very lean meat, 1 fat
✔Ham with Cinnamon Apples	1	320	11	31	4.0	75	1510	35	2	25	1 fruit, 1 carb, 4 lean meat

(Continued)

✔ = Healthiest Bets; n/a = not available

ENTREES (*Continued*)	Amount	Cal.	Fat (g)	% Cal. Fat	Sat. Fat (g)	Chol. (mg)	Sod. (mg)	Carb. (g)	Fiber (g)	Pro. (g)	Servings/Exchanges
Meat Loaf & Brown Gravy	1 order	390	22	51	8	120	1040	19	1	30	1 starch, 4 medium-fat meat
✔Meat Loaf & Chunky Tomato Sauce	1 order	370	18	44	8	120	1170	22	2	30	1 1/2 carb, 4 medium-fat meat
Original Chicken Pot Pie	1	750	34	41	9	115	2380	78	6	34	5 starch, 3 lean meat, 5 fat
✔Skinless Rotisserie Turkey Breast	1 order	170	1	5	0.5	100	850	1	0	36	5 very lean meat
HOT SIDES											
✔BBQ Baked Beans	3/4 cup	270	5	17	2	0	540	48	12	8	3 starch, 1 fat
✔Butternut Squash	3/4 cup	160	6	34	4	15	580	25	3	2	1 1/2 starch, 1 fat
✔Chicken Gravy	1 oz/2 T	15	1	60	0	0	170	2	0	0	free
✔Cinnamon Apples	3/4 cup	250	5	18	0.5	0	45	56	3	0	1 fruit, 2 1/2 carb, 1 fat
Creamed Spinach	3/4 cup	260	20	69	13	55	740	11	2	9	2 veg, 4 fat

Homestyle Mashed Potatoes & Gravy	3/4 cup	210	10	43	6	25	740	26	1	4	2 starch, 2 fat
Macaroni & Cheese	3/4 cup	280	11	35	6	30	830	32	1	13	2 starch, 1 high-fat meat
Mashed Potatoes	2/3 cup	190	9	43	6	25	570	24	1	3	1 1/2 starch, 2 fat
✔New Potatoes	3/4 cup	130	3	21	0	0	150	25	2	3	1 1/2 starch, 1/2 fat
Penne Marinara	1	190	9	43	3.5	5	460	20	2	7	1 starch, 1 veg, 2 fat
✔Rice Pilaf	2/3 cup	180	5	25	1	0	600	32	2	5	2 starch, 1 fat
✔Steamed Vegetables	2/3 cup	35	1	26	0	0	35	7	3	2	1 veg
Stuffing	3/4 cup	310	12	35	2	0	1140	44	3	6	3 starch, 2 fat
✔Whole Kernel Corn	3/4 cup	180	4	20	0.5	0	170	30	2	5	2 starch, 1 fat

✔ = Healthiest Bets; n/a = not available

(Continued)

SALADS

	Amount	Cal.	Fat (g)	% Cal. Fat	Sat. Fat (g)	Chol. (mg)	Sod. (mg)	Carb. (g)	Fiber (g)	Pro. (g)	Servings/Exchanges
Caesar Salad Entree	1	510	42	74	11	35	1130	17	3	17	3 veg, 2 medium-fat meat, 6 fat
✓Caesar Salad without Dressing	1	230	12	47	6	20	500	14	3	16	3 veg, 1 medium-fat meat, 1 fat
✓Caesar Side Salad	1	200	17	77	4.5	15	450	7	1	7	1 veg, 3 fat
Chicken Caesar Salad	1	650	45	62	12	105	1580	17	3	43	3 veg, 2 medium-fat meat, 7 fat

SANDWICHES

	Amount	Cal.	Fat (g)	% Cal. Fat	Sat. Fat (g)	Chol. (mg)	Sod. (mg)	Carb. (g)	Fiber (g)	Pro. (g)	Servings/Exchanges
Chicken w/o Sauce or Cheese	1	420	6	13	2	50	1260	64	4	29	4 starch, 3 very lean meat
Chicken w/ Cheese & Sauce	1	750	33	40	12	135	1860	72	5	41	5 starch, 4 lean meat, 4 fat

Item	Amount	Cal	Fat	%	Sat	Chol	Sod	Carb	Fib	Pro	Exchanges/Choices
Ham and Turkey Club w/o Cheese or Sauce	1	430	6	13	2	55	1330	64	4	29	4 starch, 3 lean meat
Ham and Turkey Club w/ Cheese & Sauce	1	890	43	43	20	150	2280	76	4	48	5 starch, 5 lean meat, 5 1/2 fat
Ham w/o Cheese or Sauce	1	440	8	16	2.5	45	1450	66	4	25	4 1/2 starch, 2 lean-fat meat
Ham w/ Cheese & Sauce	1	750	34	41	12	100	1730	72	5	38	4 1/2 starch, 4 medium-fat meat, 3 fat
Meat Loaf w/o Cheese	1	690	21	27	7	120	1610	86	6	40	5 1/2 starch, 4 medium-fat meat
Meat Loaf w/ Cheese	1	860	33	35	16	165	2270	95	6	46	6 starch, 4 medium-fat meat, 2 1/2 fat
✔ Turkey w/o Cheese or Sauce	1	400	4	9	1	60	1070	61	4	32	4 starch, 4 very lean meat

(Continued)

✔ = Healthiest Bets; n/a = not available

SANDWICHES (Continued)	Amount	Cal.	Fat (g)	% Cal. Fat	Sat. Fat (g)	Chol. (mg)	Sod. (mg)	Carb. (g)	Fiber (g)	Pro. (g)	Servings/Exchanges
Turkey w/ Cheese & Sauce	1	710	28	35	10	110	1390	68	4	45	4 1/2 starch, 5 lean meat, 2 1/2 fat
SOUPS											
✔Chicken Noodle Soup	3/4 cup	100	3	27	1	30	990	9	1	9	1/2 carb, 1 lean meat
Chicken Tortilla Soup	1 cup	220	11	45	4	35	1410	19	2	10	1 carb, 2 fat

✔ = Healthiest Bets; n/a = not available

Denny's

❖Denny's provides nutrition information for all of its menu items on their website at www.dennys.com.

Light 'n Lean Choice

Waffle
Grilled Ham
Syrup (*2 T*)
Banana/Strawberry Medley

Calories......................529	Sodium (mg)..........1,038
Fat (g) 25	Carbohydrate (g).........61
% calories from fat..42	Fiber (g) 2
Saturated fat (g)........4	Protein (g) 23
Cholesterol (mg) 169	

Exchanges: 2 starch, 2 fruit, 2 lean meat, 3 fat

Healthy 'n Hearty Choice

Grilled Chicken Sandwich
Carrots in Honey Glaze
Side Garden Salad with
Fat-Free Honey Mustard Dressing (*2 T*)
Applesauce

Calories......................725	Sodium (mg)..........2,206
Fat (g) 16	Carbohydrate (g).......108
% calories from fat..20	Fiber (g) 11
Saturated fat (g)........5	Protein (g) 39
Cholesterol (mg) 82	

Exchanges: 4 starch, 3 veg, 1 fruit, 3 lean meat, 1 fat

(*Continued*)

Denny's

	Amount	Cal.	Fat (g)	% Cal. Fat	Sat. Fat (g)	Chol. (mg)	Sod. (mg)	Carb. (g)	Fiber (g)	Pro. (g)	Servings/Exchanges
APPETIZER											
Smothered Cheese Fries	1	767	48	56	17	78	875	69	0	27	4 1/2 starch, 2 high-fat meat, 4 fat
Buffalo Chicken Strips	1 order	734	42	51	4	96	1673	43	0	48	3 starch, 6 lean meat, 5 fat
Buffalo Wings (12)	1 order	856	54	57	17	500	5552	1	1	92	12 medium-fat meat
Chicken Strips, fried (5)	1 order	720	33	41	4	95	1666	56	0	47	4 starch, 5 lean meat, 3 fat
Mozzarella Sticks (8)	1 order	710	41	52	24	48	5220	49	6	36	3 starch, 4 high-fat meat, 4 1/2 fat
Sampler	1 order	1405	80	51	24	75	5305	124	4	47	8 starch, 3 high-fat meat, 10 fat

BEVERAGES

	Serving	Cal	Fat (g)	% Fat Cal	Sat Fat (g)	Chol (mg)	Sod (mg)	Carb (g)	Fiber (g)	Prot (g)	Exchanges
✔Apple Juice	10 oz	126	0	0	0	0	24	33	0	0	2 fruit
✔Cappuccino French Vanilla	8 oz	100	2	18	2	0	220	28	1	3	2 carb
✔Cappuccino Original Flavor	8 oz	100	3	27	3	0	100	17	0	2	1 1/2 carb
Chocolate Milk	10 oz	235	9	34	6	37	189	30	0	9	1 whole milk, 1 carb
✔French Vanilla Coffee	8 oz	76	1	12	1	2	4	16	0	0	1 carb
✔Grapefruit Juice	10 oz	115	0	0	0	0	0	29	0	1	2 fruit
✔Hazelnut Coffee	8 oz	66	1	14	1	2	4	14	0	0	1 carb
✔Hot Chocolate	8 oz	90	2	20	0	0	155	18	0	4	1 carb
✔Irish Cream Coffee	8 oz	73	1	12	1	2	4	16	0	0	1 carb
Lemonade	16 oz	150	0	0	0	0	38	35	0	0	2 carb
✔Raspberry Iced Tea	16 oz	78	0	0	0	0	0	21	0	0	1 1/2 carb
✔Tomato Juice	10 oz	56	0	0	0	0	921	11	2	2	2 veg

✔ = Healthiest Bets; n/a = not available

(Continued)

	Amount	Cal.	Fat (g)	% Cal. Fat	Sat. Fat (g)	Chol. (mg)	Sod. (mg)	Carb. (g)	Fiber (g)	Pro. (g)	Servings/Exchanges
BREAKFAST											
All American Slam	13 oz	712	62	78	20	686	1281	9	1	38	1/2 starch, 5 medium-fat meat, 7 fat
Bacon (4 slices)	1 order	162	18	100	5	36	640	1	0	12	2 high-fat meat
✓Bagel, dry, whole	1	235	1	4	0	0	495	46	0	9	3 starch
Big Texas Chicken Fajita Skillet	1	1217	70	52	19	518	1817	25	8	49	1 starch, 1 veg, 6 high-fat meat, 11 fat
Biscuit & Sausage Gravy	1	398	21	47	6	12	1267	45	0	8	3 starch, 4 fat
✓Biscuit, buttered	1	272	11	36	4	0	790	39	0	5	2 1/2 starch, 2 fat
✓Blueberry Flav. Syrup	1.5 oz/3 T	102	0	0	0	0	15	26	0	0	1 1/2 carb
Breakfast Dagwood	1	1251	90	65	38	802	3597	35	1	75	2 starch, 10 high-fat meat, 2 fat

✔Cereal, dry	1	100	0	0	0	0	276	23	1	2	1 1/2 starch
Chicken Fried Steak & Eggs	1	723	36	45	12	440	861	9	4	22	2 starch, 3 medium-fat meat, 8 fat
Chili Cheese Fries	1	815	44	49	17	74	917	77	3	29	5 starch, 2 high-fat meat, 5 fat
Corned Beef Hash Skillet	1	733	40	49	15	523	2116	29	11	38	2 starch, 5 high-fat meat, 2 fat
Country Scramble	1	1231	61	45	10	497	8059	139	3	32	9 starch, 2 medium-fat meat, 8 fat
✔Eggbeaters	1 order	71	5	63	0	1	138	1	0	5	1 medium-fat meat
Eggs Benedict	1	695	46	60	11	515	1718	34	1	34	2 starch, 4 medium-fat meat, 5 fat

✔ = Healthiest Bets; n/a = not available

(*Continued*)

BREAKFAST (*Continued*)	Amount	Cal.	Fat (g)	% Cal. Fat	Sat. Fat (g)	Chol. (mg)	Sod. (mg)	Carb. (g)	Fiber (g)	Pro. (g)	Servings/Exchanges
✔English Muffin, dry, whole	1	125	1	7	0	0	198	24	1	5	1 1/2 starch
Farmer's Slam	1	1200	80	60	24	704	3204	82	3	51	5 1/2 starch, 5 medium-fat meat, 9 fat
French Slam	1	1029	71	62	20	777	1428	58	2	44	4 starch, 5 medium-fat meat, 9 fat
French Toast, plain (2 slices)	1 order	507	24	43	6	219	594	54	3	16	3 1/2 starch, 1 medium-fat meat, 4 fat
Grand Slam Slugger	1	789	46	52	14	487	1438	58	2	32	4 starch, 3 medium-fat meat, 5 fat
✔Grits	1	80	0	0	0	0	520	18	0	2	1 starch
✔Ham	1	94	3	29	1	23	761	2	0	15	2 very lean meat
Ham 'n' Cheddar Omelet	1	581	45	70	8	672	1180	4	2	37	5 medium-fat meat, 5 fat

	Amount										Exchanges/Choices
Hashed Browns	1 order	218	14	58	2	0	424	20	2	2	1 starch, 3 fat
Hashed Browns, Covered	1 order	318	23	65	7	30	604	21	2	9	1 1/2 starch, 4 1/2 fat
Hashed Browns, Covered & Smothered	1 order	359	26	65	7	30	790	26	2	9	1 1/2 starch, 5 fat
✔ Hotcakes, plain (3)	1 order	491	7	13	1	0	1818	95	3	12	6 starch, 1 fat
Lumberjack Slam 2	1	1259	70	50	18	481	4028	118	5	54	8 starch, 5 medium-fat meat, 5 fat
Meat Lover's Sampler	1	503	36	64	13	548	1138	3	0	41	6 medium-fat meat, 1 fat
Meat Lover's Skillet	1	1147	93	73	25	460	2507	24	7	41	1 1/2 starch, 6 high-fat meat, 13 fat
Moons Over My Hammy	1	922	59	58	24	581	2810	42	2	54	3 starch, 6 medium-fat meat, 5 fat

✔ = Healthiest Bets; n/a = not available

(Continued)

BREAKFAST (Continued)	Amount	Cal.	Fat (g)	% Cal. Fat	Sat. Fat (g)	Chol. (mg)	Sod. (mg)	Carb. (g)	Fiber (g)	Pro. (g)	Servings/Exchanges
✓ Oatmeal	1	100	2	18	0	0	175	18	3	5	1 starch
✓ One Egg	1	120	10	75	3	210	120	1	0	6	1 medium-fat meat, 1 fat
Original Grand Slam	1	795	50	57	14	460	2237	65	2	34	4 starch, 3 medium-fat meat, 5 fat
Rollover Fruit Slam	1	787	47	54	15	530	116	65	1	30	4 starch, 3 medium-fat meat, 5 fat
Sausage (4 links)	1 order	354	32	81	2	64	944	0	0	16	2 high-fat meat, 3 fat
Scram Slam	1	740	62	75	20	686	1293	14	3	39	2 1/2 starch, 4 medium-fat meat, 5 fat
Sirloin Steak & Eggs	1	622	49	71	18	572	632	1	1	43	6 medium-fat meat, 4 fat

	Amount	Calories	Fat (g)	% Cal. Fat	Sat. Fat (g)	Chol. (mg)	Sodium (mg)	Carb. (g)	Fiber (g)	Prot. (g)	Servings/Exchanges
Slim Slam w/out syrup	1	495	12	22	3	34	1746	98	1	34	6 1/2 starch, 2 medium-fat meat
Slim Slam with syrup	1	638	12	17	3	34	1772	98	1	34	6 1/2 starch, 3 lean meat, 1/2 fat
Smoked Ham Steak & Eggs	1	991	75	68	18	599	3382	26	2	53	1 1/2 starch, 7 medium-fat meat, 8 fat
Strawberry Flav. Syrup	1.5 oz/3 T	91	0	0	0	0	36	23	0	0	1 1/2 carb
✔ Sugar Free Maple Flav. Syrup	1.5 oz/3 T	23	0	0	0	0	71	9	0	0	1/2 carb
✔ Sunshine Slam w/Fruit	1	339	13	35	4	426	750	45	2	18	3 carb, 1 medium-fat meat, 1 fat
Sunshine Slam w/Hashed Browns	1	536	28	47	6	426	1207	55	3	19	3 1/2 starch, 1 medium-fat meat, 4 fat

✔ = Healthiest Bets; n/a = not available

(Continued)

BREAKFAST (*Continued*)	Amount	Cal.	Fat (g)	% Cal. Fat	Sat. Fat (g)	Chol. (mg)	Sod. (mg)	Carb. (g)	Fiber (g)	Pro. (g)	Servings/Exchanges
✔Sunshine Slam w/Tomatoes	1	305	13	38	4	426	734	36	2	18	2 1/2 carb, 1 medium-fat meat, 2 fat
✔Syrup	1.5 oz/3 T	143	0	0	0	0	26	36	0	0	2 1/2 carb
T-bone Steak & Eggs	1	991	77	70	31	657	1003	1	2	73	10 medium-fat meat, 5 fat
✔Toast, dry	1 slice	92	1	10	0	0	166	17	1	3	1 starch
Two Egg Breakfast	1	825	67	73	17	538	1765	24	2	21	1 1/2 starch, 2 medium-fat meat, 12 fat
Ultimate Omelet	1	564	47	75	12	639	939	9	2	30	1 veg, 4 medium-fat meat, 5 fat
Veggie-Cheese Omelet	1	480	39	73	13	644	535	9	2	26	1 veg, 3 medium-fat meat, 5 fat
✔Waffle, plain	1	304	21	62	3	146	200	23	0	7	1 1/2 starch, 4 fat

CONDIMENTS

	Amount	Cal	Fat (g)	% Fat Cal	Sat Fat (g)	Chol (mg)	Sod (mg)	Carb (g)	Fiber (g)	Pro (g)	Choices/Exch
✔ BBQ Sauce	1.5 oz/3 T	47	1	19	0	0	595	11	0	0	1 starch
✔ Brown Gravy	1 oz/2 T	13	0	0	0	0	184	2	0	0	free
✔ Chicken Gravy	1 oz/2 T	14	1	64	0	2	139	2	0	0	free
✔ Country Gravy	1 oz/2 T	17	1	53	0	0	93	2	0	0	free
✔ Cream Cheese	1 oz/2 T	100	10	90	6	31	90	1	0	2	2 fat
Horseradish Sauce	1.5 oz/3 T	170	20	106	3	43	227	3	0	1	4 fat
✔ Marinara Sauce	1.5 oz/3 T	48	2	38	1	0	206	7	1	1	1/2 carb
✔ Salsa	2 oz/4 T	10	0	0	0	0	221	3	1	0	free
✔ Sour Cream	1.5 oz/3 T	91	9	89	6	19	23	2	0	1	2 fat
Tartar Sauce	1.5 oz/3 T	230	24	94	3	17	185	5	0	0	4 fat
✔ Whipped Margarine	0.5 oz/1 T	87	10	103	2	0	117	0	0	0	2 fat

✔ = Healthiest Bets; n/a = not available

(Continued)

DESSERTS

	Amount	Cal.	Fat (g)	% Cal. Fat	Sat. Fat (g)	Chol. (mg)	Sod. (mg)	Carb. (g)	Fiber (g)	Pro. (g)	Servings/Exchanges
Apple Pie	1 slice	470	24	46	6	0	470	64	1	3	3 carb, 1 fruit, 4 fat
Banana Split Sundae	1	894	43	43	19	78	177	121	6	15	7 carb, 8 1/2 fat
Blueberry Topping	2 oz/4 T	71	0	0	0	0	10	17	0	0	1 carb
Cheesecake Pie	1 slice	470	27	52	13	90	290	48	0	6	3 carb, 5 fat
Cherry Pie	1 slice	630	25	36	6	0	550	101	2	3	6 1/2 carb, 5 fat
Chocolate Cake	1 slice	275	12	39	3	26	62	42	0	4	3 carb, 2 fat
Chocolate Peanut Butter Pie	1 slice	653	39	54	19	27	319	64	3	15	4 carb, 7 fat
Chocolate Topping	2 oz/4 T	317	25	71	0	0	83	27	0	2	1 1/2 carb, 5 fat
Double Scoop/Sundae	1	375	27	65	12	74	86	29	0	6	2 carb, 5 fat
Dutch Apple Pie	1 slice	440	19	39	5	0	290	65	1	10	3 carb, 1 fruit, 4 fat
Fudge Topping	2 oz/4 T	201	10	45	7	3	96	30	1	1	2 carb, 2 fat

Grasshopper Blender Blaster	1	735	37	45	23	140	299	92	0	13	6 carb, 7 fat
Grasshopper Sundae	1	734	34	42	21	118	290	97	1	13	6 1/2 carb, 7 fat
Hershey's Chocolate Chunks N' Chips Pie	1 piece	600	36	54	25	10	270	58	3	6	4 carb, 7 fat
Hot Fudge Cake Sundae	1	620	35	51	17	60	170	73	1	7	5 carb, 7 1/2 fat
Ice Cream Float	12 oz	280	10	32	6	0	109	47	0	3	3 carb, 2 fat
✔Low Fat Choc/Chip Yogurt	4 oz	110	2	16	0.5	5	60	19	1	4	1 carb
Oreo Cookies & Cream Pie	1 piece	651	40	55	26	20	401	67	2	6	4 carb, 8 fat
Peaches & Cream Parfait	1	568	22	35	15	81	227	91	1	5	6 carb, 4 fat
Peachy Cheesecake	1 piece	590	30	46	16	105	306	74	1	8	5 carb, 6 fat
✔Rainbow Sherbet	4 oz	120	2	15	1	5	30	25	0	1	1 1/2 carb
Single Scoop Sundae	1	188	14	67	6	37	43	14	0	3	1 carb, 3 fat

✔ = Healthiest Bets; n/a = not available

(Continued)

	Amount	Cal.	Fat (g)	% Cal. Fat	Sat. Fat (g)	Chol. (mg)	Sod. (mg)	Carb. (g)	Fiber (g)	Pro. (g)	Servings/Exchanges
DESSERTS (*Continued*)											
Strawberry Topping	2 oz/4 T	77	1	12	0	0	8	17	1	1	1 carb
Whipped Cream	2 T	23	2	78	0	7	3	2	0	0	free
DINNERS, PLATES, ETC.											
✔Chicken Strip & Fried Shrimp	1	395	14	32	1	90	1587	43	1	26	3 starch, 2 lean meat, 1 fat
✔Shrimp Scampi Combo	1	346	20	52	4	241	1104	15	1	27	1 starch, 3 lean meat, 2 fat
✔Shrimp Scampi Skillet Dinner	1	289	19	59	4	192	766	3	0	25	3 lean meat, 2 fat
✔Grilled Chicken Stir-Fry	1	864	10	10	1	67	3635	149	10	43	9 starch, 2 veg, 2 lean meat
✔Charleston Chicken	1	327	18	50	4	65	993	16	1	25	1 starch, 3 lean meat, 2 fat
✔Chicken Fried Steak	1	265	17	58	8	27	668	14	1	15	1 starch, 2 medium-fat meat, 1 fat
Chicken Strips (5)	1 order	635	25	35	1	95	1510	55	0	47	3 1/2 starch, 5 lean meat, 2 fat

✔ Grilled Alaskan Salmon	1	210	4	17	1	101	103	1	0	43	6 very lean meat
✔ Grilled Chicken Breast	1	130	4	28	1	67	566	0	0	24	3 very lean meat
✔ Grilled Chicken Dinner (fit fare)	1	130	4	28	1	67	560	0	0	24	3 very lean meat
✔ Pot Roast Dinner w/Gravy	1	292	11	34	5	87	927	5	0	42	6 lean meat
✔ Roast Turkey & Stuffing w/Gravy	1	388	3	7	1	116	2467	38	2	46	2 1/2 starch, 6 very lean meat
✔ Shrimp Dinner (fried)	1	219	10	41	2	133	774	18	1	17	1 starch, 2 lean meat, 1 fat
Sirloin Steak Dinner	1	337	28	75	8	687	344	1	1	18	3 medium-fat meat, 2 fat
Steak and Shrimp Dinner	1	645	42	59	14	150	1143	31	2	36	2 starch, 4 medium-fat meat, 4 fat
T-bone Steak Dinner	1	860	65	68	29	196	867	0	0	65	9 medium-fat meat, 4 fat
Sirloin Steak & Shrimp Combo	1	816	48	53	14	349	813	4	1	87	12 lean meat, 3 fat
FRUIT											
✔ Banana	1	110	0	0	0	0	0	29	4	1	2 fruit

✔ = Healthiest Bets; n/a = not available

(Continued)

FRUIT (*Continued*)	Amount	Cal.	Fat (g)	% Cal. Fat	Sat. Fat (g)	Chol. (mg)	Sod. (mg)	Carb. (g)	Fiber (g)	Pro. (g)	Servings/Exchanges
✔ Banana/Strawberry Medley	4 oz	108	1	8	0	0	6	27	2	1	2 fruit
✔ Cantaloupe	3 oz	32	0	0	0	0	16	8	1	1	1/2 fruit
✔ Fresh Fruit Mix	3 oz	36	0	0	0	0	16	9	1	1	1/2 fruit
✔ Grapefruit	1/2	60	0	0	0	0	0	16	6	1	1 fruit
✔ Grapes	3 oz	55	1	16	0	0	0	15	1	1	1 fruit
✔ Honeydew	3 oz	31	0	0	0	0	22	8	1	1	1/2 fruit
KID'S MEALS											
✔ BURGERlicious	1	296	17	52	6	28	368	24	1	13	1 1/2 starch, 2 medium-fat meat, 1 fat
✔ BURGERlicious w/ cheese	1	341	20	53	6	40	580	24	1	15	1 1/2 starch, 2 medium-fat meat, 2 fat
✔ DENNYSAUR Chicken Nuggets	1	260	9	31	0	35	1088	27	0	18	2 starch, 2 medium-fat meat, 1/2 fat

FRENCHtastic Slam	1	452	33	66	9	311	664	22	19	1 1/2 starch, 2 high-fat meat, 2 1/2 fat
Junior GRAND SLAM	1	397	25	57	7	230	1118	33	17	2 starch, 2 high-fat meat, 1 fat
PIGS in a Blanket	1	479	21	39	7	32	1684	63	16	4 starch, 1 high-fat meat, 2 fat
✔PIZZA PARTY	1	400	15	34	3	10	1090	47	18	3 starch, 1 high-fat meat, 1 fat
✔SHRIMPsational Basket	1	291	16	49	3	68	774	27	10	2 starch, 1 lean meat, 2 1/2 fat
✔SMILEY-FACE hot cakes w/out meat	1	344	9	24	3	13	1014	62	7	4 starch, 2 fat

(Continued)

✔ = Healthiest Bets; n/a = not available

KID'S MEALS (*Continued*)	Amount	Cal.	Fat (g)	% Cal. Fat	Sat. Fat (g)	Chol. (mg)	Sod. (mg)	Carb. (g)	Fiber (g)	Pro. (g)	Servings/Exchanges
✔SMILEY-FACE hot cakes with meat	1	463	22	43	7	38	1410	63	2	14	4 starch, 1 high-fat meat, 2 fat
✔THE BIG Cheese	1	334	20	54	2	24	828	28	2	9	2 starch, 2 high-fat meat
✔WACKY WAFFLES	1	215	12	50	3	78	102	23	0	4	1 1/2 starch, 2 fat
SALAD DRESSINGS											
Blue Cheese	1 oz/2 T	163	18	99	3	20	205	1	0	1	4 fat
Caesar	1 oz/2 T	133	14	95	2	2	380	1	0	1	3 fat
✔Fat Free Honey Mustard	1 oz/2 T	38	0	0	0	0	121	9	0	0	1/2 carb
✔French	1 oz/2 T	106	10	85	2	7	274	3	0	0	2 fat
Ranch	1 oz/2 T	129	14	98	2	8	189	1	0	0	3 fat
✔Reduced Calorie Italian	1 oz/2 T	15	1	60	0	0	390	3	0	0	free
Thousand Island	1 oz/2 T	118	11	84	2	15	170	5	0	0	2 fat

SALADS

Garden Deluxe Salad w/Buffalo Chicken	1	516	35	61	8	79	1197	26	4	33	1 starch, 2 veg, 4 lean meat, 3 fat
✔ Garden Deluxe Salad w/Chicken Breast	1	264	11	38	5	89	714	10	4	32	2 veg, 4 lean meat
✔ Garden Deluxe Salad w/Fried Chicken Strips	1	438	26	53	6	78	1030	26	4	33	1 starch, 2 veg, 4 lean meat, 2 fat
✔ Garden Deluxe Salad w/Salmon Fillet	1	389	9	21	5	124	349	10	4	67	2 veg, 9 very lean meat
Garden Salad Deluxe w/Turkey & Ham	1	322	11	31	6	100	1706	12	4	43	2 veg, 8 very lean meat
Grilled Chicken Caesar w/dressing	1	600	41	62	10	101	1792	19	4	37	2 veg, 1/2 starch, 4 lean meat, 7 fat

✔ = Healthiest Bets; n/a = not available

(Continued)

SALADS *(Continued)*	Amount	Cal.	Fat (g)	% Cal. Fat	Sat. Fat (g)	Chol. (mg)	Sod. (mg)	Carb. (g)	Fiber (g)	Pro. (g)	Servings/Exchanges
Side Caesar w/dressing	1	362	26	65	7	23	913	20	3	11	1 starch, 2 veg, 5 fat
✓ Side Garden Salad	1	113	4	32	1	0	147	16	3	3	3 veg, 1 fat
SANDWICHES AND BURGERS											
Albacore Tuna Melt	1	668	41	55	14	121	1351	44	3	31	3 starch, 3 lean meat, 7 fat
Bacon Cheddar Burger	1	875	52	53	19	163	1672	58	5	53	4 starch, 6 lean meat, 5 fat
Bacon, Lettuce & Tomato	1	610	38	56	9	35	862	50	2	15	3 starch, 1 veg, 2 high-fat meat, 3 fat
Big Texas BBQ Burger	1	929	58	56	24	163	2271	53	3	53	3 1/2 starch, 6 medium-fat meat, 5 1/2 fat
Boca Burger	1	616	28	41	5	14	861	66	10	29	4 1/2 starch, 2 lean meat, 3 fat
Buffalo Chicken Burger	1	803	45	50	9	77	2143	67	5	37	4 1/2 starch, 3 lean meat, 6 fat

											Exchanges/Choices
Charleston Chicken Ranch Melt	1	858	47	49	10	83	2294	62	4	41	4 starch, 4 lean meat, 7 fat
Chicken Burger	1	632	32	46	7	81	1967	53	4	35	3 1/2 starch, 3 lean meat, 4 fat
Chicken Parmesan Sandwich	1	792	44	50	15	106	2424	47	4	45	3 starch, 5 lean meat, 6 fat
Classic Burger	1	673	40	53	15	106	1142	42	3	37	3 starch, 4 medium-fat meat, 4 fat
Classic Burger w/ Cheese	1	836	53	57	19	137	1595	43	3	47	3 starch, 5 medium-fat meat, 5 1/2 fat
Classic Double Decker Burger	1	1377	92	60	34	210	2209	81	7	62	5 1/2 starch, 6 medium-fat meat, 6 fat
Club	1	718	38	48	7	75	1666	62	3	32	4 starch, 3 medium-fat meat, 4 1/2 fat

✔ = Healthiest Bets; n/a = not available

(Continued)

SANDWICHES AND BURGERS (*Continued*)	Amount	Cal.	Fat (g)	% Cal. Fat	Sat. Fat (g)	Chol. (mg)	Sod. (mg)	Carb. (g)	Fiber (g)	Pro. (g)	Servings/Exchanges
Delidinger	1	852	45	48	6	80	3142	62	3	56	4 starch, 6 medium-fat meat, 3 fat
Deluxe Grilled Cheese	1	506	30	53	14	54	1347	40	3	19	2 1/2 starch, 2 high-fat meat, 2 fat
Gardenburger	1	665	33	45	8	36	1051	75	8	18	5 starch, 1 lean meat, 6 fat
✓Gardenburger (patty only)	1	172	4	21	2	20	424	25	5	8	1 1/2 starch, 1 lean meat
Garlic Mushroom Swiss Burger	1	872	51	53	14	116	1529	58	5	48	4 starch, 5 medium-fat meat, 4 fat
Grilled Chicken	1	520	14	24	3	77	1613	64	3	35	4 starch, 4 lean meat
Grilled Chicken, Fit Fare	1	434	9	19	3	82	1705	56	4	35	3 1/2 starch, 4 lean meat
Ham & Swiss on Rye	1	533	31	52	4	36	1638	40	5	23	2 1/2 starch, 2 medium-fat meat, 4 fat

Item	Amount									Exchanges
Patty Melt	1	788	50	57	21	127	1285	37	4	45	2 1/2 starch, 4 medium-fat meat, 5 fat
Reuben	1	586	32	49	15	67	1933	38	4	35	2 1/2 starch, 4 medium-fat meat, 2 fat
Super Bird	1	620	32	46	5	60	1880	48	2	35	3 starch, 4 lean meat, 4 fat
Turkey Breast, on multigrain	1	476	26	49	5	57	1107	39	5	23	2 1/2 starch, 2 lean meat, 4 fat

SHAKES

Item	Amount									Exchanges
Chocolate	12 oz	583	26	40	16	100	278	82	0	12	1 whole milk, 5 carb, 1 fat
Vanilla	12 oz	583	26	40	16	100	278	82	1	12	1 whole milk, 5 carb, 1 fat

SIDES

Item	Amount									Exchanges
✓Applesauce	3 oz	60	0	0	0	0	13	15	1	0	1 fruit
✓Baked Potato, plain	1	220	0	0	0	0	16	51	5	5	3 starch

✓ = Healthiest Bets; n/a = not available

(Continued)

SIDES (*Continued*)	Amount	Cal.	Fat (g)	% Cal. Fat	Sat. Fat (g)	Chol. (mg)	Sod. (mg)	Carb. (g)	Fiber (g)	Pro. (g)	Servings/Exchanges
Biscuit, plain	1	375	22	53	5	0	750	40	0	5	2 1/2 starch, 4 fat
✓Bread Stuffing, plain	3 oz	100	1	9	0	0	405	19	1	3	1 starch
✓Carrots in honey glaze	4 oz	80	3	34	1	0	220	12	3	1	1 veg, 1/2 carb, 1/2 fat
✓Corn in butter sauce	4 oz	120	4	30	2	5	260	19	5	3	1 starch, 1 fat
✓Cottage Cheese	3 oz/6 T	72	3	38	2	10	281	2	0	9	1 lean meat
French Fries, unsalted	1 order	323	14	39	3	0	130	44	0	5	3 starch, 3 fat
✓Green Beans with bacon	4 oz	60	4	60	2	5	390	6	3	1	1 veg, 1 fat
✓Green Peas in butter sauce	4 oz	100	2	18	2	5	360	14	4	5	1 starch
✓Grilled Mushrooms	2 oz	14	0	0	0	0	0	2	1	2	free
Herb Toast	1 order	170	11	58	2	0	325	15	1	2	1 1/2 starch, 2 fat
✓Mashed Potato w/Cheddar	6 oz	117	2	15	0.6	2	405	22	2	3	2 1/2 starch
✓Mashed Potatoes, plain	6 oz	105	1	9	0	0	378	21	2	3	1 1/2 starch

Onion Rings	1 order	381	23	54	6	6	1003	38	1	5	2 1/2 starch, 4 fat
Seasoned French Fries	1 order	261	12	41	3	0	556	35	0	5	2 starch, 2 fat
✔ Sliced Tomatoes	3 slices	13	0	0	0	0	6	3	1	1	free
✔ Vegetable Rice Pilaf	3 oz	85	1	11	0	0	325	16	1	3	1 1/2 starch

SOUPS

✔ Chicken Noodle	8 oz	60	2	30	0	10	640	8	0	2	1/2 starch
Chili w/cheese	8 oz	401	19	43	8	57	1039	21	7	26	1 starch, 4 fat
✔ Clam Chowder	8 oz	214	11	46	9	5	903	22	1	5	1 1/2 carb, 2 fat
Cream of Broccoli	8 oz	193	12	56	9	0	818	15	2	4	1 carb, 2 fat
Cream of Potato	8 oz	222	12	49	9	0	761	23	2	4	1 1/2 starch, 2 fat
✔ Split Pea	8 oz	146	6	37	2	5	819	18	2	8	1 carb, 1 fat
✔ Vegetable Beef	8 oz	79	1	11	1	5	820	11	2	6	1 starch

✔ = Healthiest Bets; n/a = not available

IHOP

❖IHOP provided nutrition information for several items for this book. Their website is www.ihop.com.

Light 'n Lean Choice

Note: Too little information provided to put together meals.

Healthy 'n Hearty Choice

Note: Too little information provided to put together meals.

IHOP

BREAKFAST

	Amount	Cal.	Fat (g)	% Cal. Fat	Sat. Fat (g)	Chol. (mg)	Sod. (mg)	Carb. (g)	Fiber (g)	Pro. (g)	Servings/Exchanges
✔Buckwheat	1 pancake	110	3	25	1	50	280	15	1	3	1 starch, 1/2 fat
✔Buttermilk	1 pancake	110	3	25	1	30	450	17	1	3	1 starch, 1/2 fat
✔Country Griddle	1 pancake	120	4	30	1	35	440	19	1	3	1 starch, 1 fat
✔Egg Crepe	1	120	6	45	1.5	80	230	14	0	3	1 starch, 1 fat
✔Harvest Grain 'N Nut	1 pancake	180	9	45	1.5	40	410	20	2	5	1 starch, 2 fat
Old Fashion Syrup	2 oz/4 T	230	0	0	0	0	230	58	1	0	4 starch
Regular Belgian Waffle	1	390	19	44	12	140	850	48	1	8	3 starch, 4 fat
✔Regular Waffle	1	310	15	44	4	70	380	37	1	6	2 1/2 starch, 3 fat

✔ = Healthiest Bets; n/a = not available

Shoney's

❖Shoney's provided nutrition information for all of
its menu items for use in this book. Their website is
www.shoneysrestaurants.com.

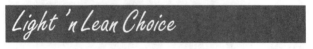

From Breakfast Bar
Eggs *(1/2 c)*; **French Toast** *(4 pieces)*
Low Calorie Syrup *(2 T)*
Strawberries *(3/4 cup)*

Calories 591	Sodium (mg) 947
Fat (g) 23	Carbohydrate (g)..........78
% calories from fat..35	Fiber (g) 5
Saturated fat (g) ....n/a	Protein (g) 18
Cholesterol (mg) 342	

Exchanges: 4 starch, 1 fruit, 2 medium-fat meat,
1 1/2 fat

Raymond's French Dip Sandwich
Corn *(1/2 cup)*; **Collard Greens** *(1/2 cup)*
Watermelon *(1 cup)*

Calories......................807	Sodium (mg) 3,774
Fat (g) 32	Carbohydrate (g)..........96
% calories from fat..36	Fiber (g) 5
Saturated fat (g) ....n/a	Protein (g) 46
Cholesterol (mg) 76	

Exchanges: 4 1/2 starch, 1 veg, 1 fruit, 4 medium-fat
meat, 1 1/2 fat

Shoney's

	Amount	Cal.	Fat (g)	% Cal. Fat	Sat. Fat (g)	Chol. (mg)	Sod. (mg)	Carb. (g)	Fiber (g)	Pro. (g)	Servings/Exchanges
BLUE PLATE SPECIALS											
✔Baked Whitefish	1	507	8	14	n/a	94	2231	58	0	48	4 starch, 5 very lean meat
✔Cajun Whitefish	1	480	10	19	n/a	73	883	56	0	40	3 1/2 starch, 4 very lean meat, 1 fat
Grandma's Meatloaf w/ Glaze	1	1092	47	39	n/a	188	2276	93	1	72	6 starch, 7 medium-fat meat, 2 fat
Grandma's Meatloaf w/ Gravy	1	1089	49	40	n/a	189	2451	87	1	72	6 starch, 7 medium-fat meat, 2 fat
Grilled Liver 'n' Onions	1	711	22	28	n/a	683	1115	79	2	49	5 starch, 5 lean meat, 1 fat
Ham Steak Dinner	1	667	76	103	n/a	100	3210	60	1	48	4 starch, 5 lean meat, 2 fat

(Continued)

✔ = Healthiest Bets; n/a = not available

BLUE PLATE SPECIALS (Continued)	Amount	Cal.	Fat (g)	% Cal. Fat	Sat. Fat (g)	Chol. (mg)	Sod. (mg)	Carb. (g)	Fiber (g)	Pro. (g)	Servings/Exchanges
Original Country Fried Steak	1	1151	62	48	n/a	107	4073	103	1	47	7 starch, 4 medium-fat meat, 6 fat
Roast Beef Platter	1	880	30	31	n/a	136	3253	96	5	59	6 1/2 starch, 6 lean meat, 1 fat
BREAKFAST											
✓All Star Breakfast	1	190	15	71	n/a	850	180	1	0	13	2 medium-fat meat, 1 fat
Big Eater Steak Breakfast	1	629	41	59	n/a	1003	511	1	0	60	8 medium-fat meat, 1 fat
Country Fried Steak Breakfast	1	994	66	60	n/a	957	3594	49	0	50	3 starch, 6 medium-fat meat, 7 fat
Deluxe Pancake Platter	1	1609	32	18	n/a	850	4988	299	0	29	20 starch, 6 fat
Half Stack Pancake Platter	1	932	14	14	n/a	147	2592	167	0	15	11 starch, 3 fat
✓Peach Topping	1/4 cup	54	0	0	n/a	0	2	13	1	0	1 carb
Sausage/Biscuit	1	539	34	57	n/a	48	1655	42	1	16	3 starch, 1 high-fat meat, 4 1/2 fat

	Amount	Cal	Fat (g)	% Cal. Fat	Sat. Fat (g)	Chol. (mg)	Sod. (mg)	Carb. (g)	Fiber (g)	Pro. (g)	Choices/Exchanges
Sunrise Breakfast	1	973	59	55	n/a	852	4001	88	2	22	6 starch, 1 medium-fat meat, 9 fat

BREAKFAST BAR

	Amount	Cal	Fat (g)	% Cal. Fat	Sat. Fat (g)	Chol. (mg)	Sod. (mg)	Carb. (g)	Fiber (g)	Pro. (g)	Choices/Exchanges
Apple Crisp Topping	1/4 cup	87	0	0	n/a	0	9	22	0	0	1 1/2 carb
Apple Topping	1/4 cup	96	0	0	n/a	0	6	24	0	0	1 1/2 carb
✓ Banana	8 long	109	0	0	n/a	0	1	28	3	1	2 fruit
✓ Blackberries	1/4 cup	19	0	0	n/a	0	0	5	2	0	free
✓ Blueberries	1/4 cup	20	0	0	n/a	0	2	5	1	0	free
✓ Breakfast Bar Gravy	2 oz/4 T	54	4	67	n/a	0	324	1	0	2	1 fat
✓ Breakfast Potato Casserole	4 oz	90	4	40	n/a	7	69	12	1	2	1 carb, 1 fat
Bundt Cake—Apple Spice	1 piece	120	13	98	n/a	10	115	13	0	1	1 carb, 2 1/2 fat
✓ Bundt Cake—Banana Bash	1 piece	130	9	62	n/a	10	120	13	0	2	1 carb, 2 fat

(Continued)

✓ = Healthiest Bets; n/a = not available

BREAKFAST BAR (*Continued*)	Amount	Cal.	Fat (g)	% Cal. Fat	Sat. Fat (g)	Chol. (mg)	Sod. (mg)	Carb. (g)	Fiber (g)	Pro. (g)	Servings/Exchanges
✔Bundt Cake—Buttercreme	1 piece	130	8	55	n/a	10	125	15	0	1	1 carb, 1 fat
✔Bundt Cake—Double Chocolate	1 piece	130	8	55	n/a	10	150	15	1	1	1 carb, 1 1/2 fat
✔Bundt Cake—Luscious Lemon	1 piece	130	7	48	n/a	15	115	15	0	1	1 carb, 1 fat
✔Bundt Cake—Orange Cranberry	1 piece	120	0	0	n/a	0	5	19	0	1	1 carb
Cake, Brunch Berry	1 piece	120	13	98	n/a	n/a	270	41	1	4	2 1/2 carb, 2 1/2 fat
✔Cake, Shortcake	1 piece	50	3	54	n/a	70	70	11	0	1	1/2 carb, 1/2 fat
✔Cantaloupe	1/4 cup	14	0	0	0	0	4	3	0	0	free
✔Cheese Sauce	1 T	27	2	67	n/a	7	42	1	0	2	free

✔Chicken Wings, Mild	1 piece	64	3	42	n/a	28	191	3	0	5	1 lean meat
✔Cottage Cheese	1 T	15	0	0	n/a	1	67	0	0	2	free
✔Diced Ham	1 T	16	1	56	n/a	5	137	0	0	2	free
✔Eggs	1/2 cup	120	7	53	n/a	285	320	3	0	11	2 lean meat
✔Fancy Cheddar Cheese	1 T	27	2	67	n/a	7	42	1	0	2	free
French Toast Sticks	4 pieces	380	16	38	n/a	0	570	53	2	7	3 1/2 starch, 3 fat
✔Grapefruit	1/4 cup	19	0	0	n/a	0	0	5	0	0	free
Honey	1 packet	45	0	0	n/a	0	0	11	0	0	1/2 carb
✔Honeydew Melon	1/4 cup	15	0	0	n/a	0	4	4	0	0	free
✔Pancakes	1 piece	318	7	20	n/a	73	1168	56	n/a	7	3 1/2 starch, 1 fat
✔Peppers, Jalapeno	1 T	2	0	0	n/a	0	109	0	0	0	free
✔Pineapple	1/4 cup	30	0	0	n/a	0	5	8	1	0	1/2 carb
✔Powdered Donut	1	175	9	46	n/a	11	200	23	0	0	1 1/2 carb

(Continued)

✔ = Healthiest Bets; n/a = not available

BREAKFAST BAR (*Continued*)	Amount	Cal.	Fat (g)	% Cal. Fat	Sat. Fat (g)	Chol. (mg)	Sod. (mg)	Carb. (g)	Fiber (g)	Pro. (g)	Servings/Exchanges
✔Prunes, pitted	1/4 cup	61	0	0	n/a	0	2	16	2	0	1 fruit
✔Sauce, Hot Louisiana	1 t	0	0	0	n/a	0	240	0	0	0	free
✔Sauce, Salsa	1 T	5	0	0	n/a	0	69	1	0	0	free
✔Seedless Grapes	1/4 cup	15	0	0	n/a	0	0	4	0	0	free
✔Strawberries	1/4 cup	11	0	0	n/a	0	0	3	1	0	free
✔Strawberry Banana Topping	4 oz	84	0	0	n/a	0	1	20	2	1	1 1/2 fruit
Strawberry Topping	1/2 cup	158	0	0	n/a	0	13	41	0	0	2 1/2 carb
✔Syrup	2 T	80	0	0	n/a	0	5	21	0	0	1 1/2 carb
✔Syrup, Diet Smuckers	1 oz/2 T	46	0	0	n/a	0	57	13	0	0	1 carb
✔Tangerine	1 medium	37	0	0	n/a	0	1	9	2	0	1/2 fruit
✔Tortillas, flour	1	133	3	20	n/a	0	338	21	1	4	1 1/2 starch, 1/2 fat
✔Tropical Fruit Salad	1/4 cup	48	0	0	n/a	0	3	17	1	0	1 fruit

(Continued)

	Amount	Cal.	Fat (g)	% Cal. Fat	Sat. Fat (g)	Chol. (mg)	Sod. (mg)	Carb. (g)	Fiber (g)	Prot. (g)	Servings/Exchanges
✓Watermelon	1/4 cup	12	0	0	n/a	0	0	3	0	0	free
Whipped Topping	1 scoop	9	1	100	n/a	1	3	1	0	0	free
BREAKFAST SIDES											
✓Apple Cinnamon Jelly	1 packet	35	0	0	n/a	0	0	9	0	0	1/2 carb
Bacon	3 strips	120	11	83	n/a	23	405	0	0	6	1 high-fat meat
Biscuit	1 piece	309	14	41	n/a	1	894	41	1	5	2 1/2 starch, 3 fat
Biscuits & Gravy	1 order	683	32	42	n/a	2	2113	88	2	11	6 starch, 5 fat
✓Grape Jelly	1 packet	35	0	0	n/a	0	0	9	0	0	1/2 carb
✓Grits	4 oz	105	6	51	n/a	0	158	11	0	1	1/2 carb
Hash Browns	4 oz	238	15	57	n/a	15	457	25	0	3	1 1/2 starch, 3 fat
✓Margarine	1 packet	36	4	100	n/a	0	47	0	0	0	1 fat
Sausage Patty	1 piece	209	18	78	n/a	47	74	0	0	11	1 high-fat meat, 2 fat
✓Sourdough Toast w/marg	2 slices	206	5	22	n/a	0	527	50	1	9	3 starch, 1 fat

✓ = Healthiest Bets; n/a = not available

BREAKFAST SIDES (*Continued*)	Amount	Cal.	Fat (g)	% Cal. Fat	Sat. Fat (g)	Chol. (mg)	Sod. (mg)	Carb. (g)	Fiber (g)	Pro. (g)	Servings/Exchanges
✓Strawberry Jam	1 packet	35	0	0	0	0	0	9	0	0	1/2 carb
✓Wheat Toast w/marg	2 slices	188	9	43	n/a	0	352	24	4	5	1 1/2 starch, 2 fat
✓White Toast w/marg	2 slices	202	9	40	n/a	1	356	26	1	4	1 1/2 starch, 2 fat
BURGERS											
All-American Burger	1	688	32	42	n/a	150	932	44	2	54	3 starch, 6 medium-fat meat
Bacon Cheeseburger	1	891	49	49	n/a	195	1490	44	3	66	3 starch, 7 medium-fat meat, 3 fat
Famous Patty Melt	1	946	60	57	n/a	190	1276	40	5	59	2 1/2 starch, 7 medium-fat meat, 5 fat
Half-O-Pound Burger	1	1351	53	35	n/a	224	1884	130	1	89	8 1/2 starch, 9 medium-fat meat
Mushroom Swiss Burger	1	969	58	54	n/a	176	1122	49	4	64	3 starch, 8 medium-fat meat, 3 fat

CHICKEN

Item											Servings/Exchanges
Charbroiled Blackened Chicken	1	831	26	28	n/a	97	2017	99	1	47	6 1/2 starch, 4 lean meat, 2 fat
Charbroiled Chicken Breast	1	796	23	26	n/a	37	1831	99	1	47	6 1/2 starch, 4 lean meat, 1 fat
Chicken Stir Fry	1	1200	35	26	n/a	103	4317	172	5	48	10 starch, 2 veg, 2 lean meat, 5 fat
Fried Chicken Tenderloins	1	1157	61	47	n/a	45	2514	121	6	30	8 starch, 2 lean meat, 9 fat
Monterey Chicken	1	909	39	39	n/a	126	2067	84	3	53	5 1/2 starch, 5 lean meat, 4 fat
Smothered Chicken	1	891	34	34	n/a	125	2199	90	2	56	6 starch, 6 lean meat, 2 fat

DESSERTS

Item											Servings/Exchanges
Apple Nutrasweet Pie	1 piece	454	18	36	n/a	0	415	64	3	4	4 carb, 3 fat

✔ = Healthiest Bets; n/a = not available

(Continued)

DESSERTS *(Continued)*	Amount	Cal.	Fat (g)	% Cal. Fat	Sat. Fat (g)	Chol. (mg)	Sod. (mg)	Carb. (g)	Fiber (g)	Pro. (g)	Servings/Exchanges
Apple Pie a la Mode	1 piece	1203	53	40	n/a	49	1116	174	8	12	11 1/2 carb, 5 fat
Caramel Sundae	1	621	27	39	n/a	88	332	83	0	10	5 1/2 carb, 5 fat
Cheesecake	1 piece	364	26	64	n/a	62	188	23	0	5	1 1/2 carb, 5 fat
Cherry Nutrasweet Pie	1 piece	467	18	35	n/a	0	441	66	4	6	4 1/2 carb, 3 fat
Chocolate Milk Shake	1	1082	51	42	n/a	190	531	141	4	25	9 carb, 10 fat
Hot Fudge Sundae	1	599	30	45	n/a	80	228	75	0	10	5 carb, 6 fat
Original Strawberry Pie	1 piece	332	16	43	n/a	0	247	45	2	2	3 carb, 3 fat
Peach Nutrasweet Pie	1 piece	479	21	39	n/a	0	467	68	4	4	4 1/2 carb, 4 fat
Strawberry Milk Shake	1	1115	50	40	n/a	190	447	151	1	23	10 carb, 10 fat
Strawberry Sundae	1	609	27	40	n/a	88	189	85	0	9	5 1/2 carb, 5 fat
Ultimate Hot Fudge Cake	1	875	32	33	n/a	99	784	126	1	14	8 1/2 carb, 6 fat
Vanilla Milk Shake	1	1076	50	42	n/a	190	432	140	0	23	9 carb, 10 fat

Walnut Brownie a la Mode	1	576	34	53	n/a	35	435	61	0	10	4 carb, 7 fat

FOOD BAR

✔Beets & Onions Salad	1/2 cup	16	0	0	n/a	0	56	4	1	1	free
✔Beets, sliced	1/4 cup	13	0	0	n/a	0	83	3	1	0	free
✔Black Olives, sliced	1 T	25	3	108	n/a	0	130	0	0	0	free
✔Black-eyed Peas	4 oz	141	6	38	n/a	5	992	16	4	6	1 starch, 1 fat
✔Bleu Cheese Dressing	2 T	186	20	97	n/a	18	267	1	0	1	4 fat
✔Broccoli Florets	1/4 cup	5	0	0	0	0	4	1	0	1	free
✔Broccoli Rice Casserole	4 oz	106	4	34	n/a	11	700	14	1	5	1 starch, 1 fat
Cabbage	4 oz	130	12	83	n/a	0	641	6	2	1	1 veg, 2 fat
✔Carrots, shredded	4 oz	10	0	0	n/a	0	8	2	1	0	free
✔Cauliflower	1/4 cup	6	0	0	n/a	0	8	1	1	1	free
✔Chow Mein Noodles	1/2 cup	130	5	35	n/a	0	110	16	0	0	1 starch, 1 fat

✔ = Healthiest Bets; n/a = not available

(Continued)

FOOD BAR (Continued)	Amount	Cal.	Fat (g)	% Cal. Fat	Sat. Fat (g)	Chol. (mg)	Sod. (mg)	Carb. (g)	Fiber (g)	Pro. (g)	Servings/Exchanges
✓Club Crackers	1 package	30	2	60	n/a	0	75	4	0	0	free
Cole Slaw	1/4 cup	127	8	57	n/a	7	224	11	2	1	2 veg, 1 1/2 fat
✓Collard Greens	4 oz	44	4	82	n/a	4	346	4	2	1	1 veg, 1 fat
Corn, seasoned	4 oz	173	9	47	n/a	0	267	23	1	2	1 1/2 starch, 2 fat
✓Dave's Pasta Salad	2/3 cup	170	6	32	n/a	5	450	25	2	4	1 1/2 starch, 1 fat
✓Green Beans	4 oz	71	6	76	n/a	6	859	4	2	1	1 veg, 1 fat
Honey French Dressing	2 T	130	10	69	n/a	0	170	10	0	0	1/2 carb, 2 fat
Honey Mustard Dressing	2 T	173	17	88	n/a	14	134	5	0	0	3 fat
Italian Dressing	2 T	137	15	99	n/a	0	305	1	0	0	3 fat
✓Italian Dressing, fat free	2 T	20	0	0	n/a	0	430	4	0	0	free
✓Lettuce	1 cup	7	0	0		0	5	1	1	1	free
✓Lima Beans	4 oz	83	3	33	n/a	3	451	11	2	4	1 starch

Macaroni & Cheese	1/2 cup	241	14	52	n/a	n/a	588	18	1	11	1 starch, 1 high-fat meat, 1 fat
Macaroni Salad	1/2 cup	310	22	64	n/a	15	580	26	1	4	1 1/2 starch, 4 fat
✔Mushrooms	1/4 cup	4	0	0	n/a	0	1	1	0	1	free
✔Pickled Okra	6 pieces	23	0	0	n/a	0	822	5	0	0	free
✔Pinto Beans	4 oz	137	6	39	n/a	5	1000	17	6	5	1 starch, 1 fat
Potato Salad	1/2 cup	190	8	38	n/a	10	550	29	2	2	2 starch, 1 1/2 fat
Ranch Dressing	2 T	114	12	95	n/a	13	276	1	0	1	2 fat
✔Ranch Dressing, fat free	2 T	50	0	0	n/a	0	350	11	0	0	1 carb
Red Potato Salad	1/2 cup	280	20	64	n/a	15	180	26	2	2	1 1/2 starch, 4 fat
✔Spinach, cooked	4 oz	105	6	51	n/a	0	589	11	4	3	2 veg
✔Spring Salad	1/2 cup	29	0	0	n/a	0	422	7	1	0	1 veg
Sunflower Seeds, salted	1/4 cup	186	16	77	n/a	0	250	8	3	6	1/2 starch, 3 fat

(Continued)

✔ = Healthiest Bets; n/a = not available

FOOD BAR (*Continued*)	Amount	Cal.	Fat (g)	% Cal. Fat	Sat. Fat (g)	Chol. (mg)	Sod. (mg)	Carb. (g)	Fiber (g)	Pro. (g)	Servings/Exchanges
✔Sweet Potato Casserole	4 oz	244	6	22	n/a	56	260	44	0	5	3 starch, 1 fat
Thousand Island Dressing	2 T	179	18	91	n/a	12	268	4	0	0	4 fat
✔Thousand Island Dressing, fat free	2 T	40	0	0	n/a	0	270	9	0	0	1/2 carb
✔Turnip Greens	4 oz	43	4	84	n/a	4	354	4	1	1	1 veg, 1 fat
✔Vegetable Oil	1 T	130	4	28	n/a	0	0	0	0	0	1 fat
PASTA											
Chicken Alfredo	1	1705	78	41	n/a	427	3144	170	6	85	11 starch, 8 lean meat, 9 fat
Italian Feast	1	1435	45	28	n/a	262	4630	204	8	64	13 1/2 starch, 4 lean meat, 3 fat
Pasta Ya Ya	1	1847	81	39	n/a	467	4738	176	7	110	11 1/2 starch, 11 medium-fat meat, 2 fat

	Amount	Calories	Fat (g)	% Fat Cal.	Sat. Fat (g)	Chol. (mg)	Sodium (mg)	Carb. (g)	Fiber (g)	Prot. (g)	Servings/Exchanges
Shrimp Alfredo	1	1781	85	43	n/a	545	3243	172	6	87	11 1/2 starch, 8 medium-fat meat, 6 fat
RIB COMBOS W/ FRIES											
1/4 Rack & BBQ Chicken	1	1228	54	40	n/a	95	3258	104	4	80	7 starch, 8 medium-fat meat, 2 fat
1/4 Rack & Fried Shrimp	1	1144	51	40	n/a	88	2862	113	4	58	7 1/2 starch, 5 medium-fat meat, 5 fat
1/4 Rack & Grilled Shrimp	1	1125	53	42	n/a	96	2808	103	4	59	7 starch, 5 medium-fat meat, 5 fat
1/4 Rack & Tenderloins	1	1372	70	46	n/a	47	3486	121	4	65	8 starch, 6 medium-fat meat, 6 fat
SANDWICHES											
Blackened Chicken Sandwich	1	885	21	21	n/a	95	2130	122	0	54	8 starch, 5 lean meat

✔ = Healthiest Bets; n/a = not available

(Continued)

SANDWICHES (*Continued*)	Amount	Cal.	Fat (g)	% Cal. Fat	Sat. Fat (g)	Chol. (mg)	Sod. (mg)	Carb. (g)	Fiber (g)	Pro. (g)	Servings/Exchanges
Charbroiled Chicken Sandwich	1	893	22	22	n/a	95	1914	122	1	55	8 starch, 5 lean meat
Chicken Parm Sandwich	1	751	30	36	n/a	99	2520	80	4	42	5 starch, 4 lean meat, 3 fat
Corned Beef Reuben	1	793	53	60	n/a	179	4144	37	5	40	2 1/2 starch, 5 medium-fat meat, 5 fat
Fish Sandwich	1	827	17	19	n/a	67	2598	127	0	44	8 1/2 starch, 3 very lean meat, 1 fat
Fried Chicken Sandwich	1	561	15	24	n/a	66	3307	77	4	32	5 starch, 3 lean meat
Hot Roast Beef w/Mashed Potatoes	1	771	24	28	n/a	97	2897	95	5	44	6 starch, 3 lean meat, 3 fat
Hot Turkey w/Mashed Potatoes	1	842	30	32	n/a	95	1914	94	5	45	6 starch, 3 lean meat, 4 1/2 fat
Original Slim Jim	1	1004	34	30	n/a	98	4392	123	0	54	8 1/2 starch, 4 medium-fat meat, 3 fat

Item	Amount	Cal	Fat		Chol	Sod	Carb	Fiber		Exchanges
✓ Raymond's French Dip	1	498	15	27	n/a	76	2802	53	2	41	3 1/2 starch, 4 lean meat
Turkey Club	1	952	53	50	n/a	178	2691	47	3	71	3 starch, 8 lean meat, 6 fat
Ultimate Grilled Cheese	1	896	46	46	n/a	102	2097	77	4	42	5 starch, 4 high-fat meat, 2 fat

SEAFOOD PLATTERS

Item	Amount	Cal	Fat		Chol	Sod	Carb	Fiber		Exchanges
Fish 'n' Shrimp	1	1098	39	32	n/a	162	2155	129	6	53	8 1/2 starch, 4 lean meat, 4 fat
Fried Fish	1	1049	39	33	n/a	97	2047	123	6	49	8 starch, 3 lean meat, 5 fat
Grilled Salmon	1	749	19	23	n/a	62	1623	95	1	50	6 starch, 4 lean meat, 1 fat
Grilled Shrimp	1	720	19	24	n/a	194	1401	96	1	39	6 1/2 starch, 3 lean meat, 1 fat
Shrimp Stir-Fry	1	873	19	20	n/a	200	3975	131	5	41	8 1/2 starch, 3 lean meat, 1 fat

✓ = Healthiest Bets; n/a = not available

(*Continued*)

SEAFOOD (*Continued*)	Amount	Cal.	Fat (g)	% Cal. Fat	Sat. Fat (g)	Chol. (mg)	Sod. (mg)	Carb. (g)	Fiber (g)	Pro. (g)	Servings/Exchanges
Shrimper's Feast	1	1032	39	34	n/a	182	2131	123	6	39	8 starch, 2 very lean meat, 7 fat
SIDES / CONDIMENTS											
✓A1 Steak Sauce	1 T	12	0	0	n/a	0	230	3	0	0	free
American Cheese	1 slice	107	9	76	n/a	27	228	1	0	6	1 high-fat meat
✓BBQ Sauce	1.5 oz/3 T	71	1	13	n/a	0	327	11	0	0	1/2 carb
✓Cheese, Parmesan	1 T	23	2	78	n/a	4	15	0	0	2	free
✓Cocktail Sauce	1.5 oz/3 T	55	0	0	n/a	0	499	12	1	1	1 carb
Corn	1 order	173	9	47	n/a	0	267	23	1	2	1 1/2 starch, 2 fat
✓Cranberry Sauce	1.5 oz/3 T	64	0	0	n/a	0	12	17	0	0	1 carb
✓French Fries	4 oz	213	11	46	n/a	0	896	83	4	12	5 1/2 starch, 2 fat
✓Green Beans	1 order	70	6	77	n/a	6	859	4	2	1	1 veg, 1 fat

	Serving	Cal	Fat (g)	% Fat Cal	Sat Fat	Chol	Sodium	Carb	Fiber	Protein	Exchanges
✔ Grilled Onions	1.5 oz	67	6	81	n/a	0	68	4	1	1	1 veg, 1 fat
✔ Heinz 57 Steak Sauce	1 T	14	0	0	n/a	0	247	3	0	0	free
Macaroni & Cheese	1 order	241	14	52	n/a	n/a	588	18	1	10	1 starch, 1 high-fat meat, 1 fat
Mashed Potatoes/Gravy	1 order	223	10	40	n/a	7	575	30	1	4	2 starch, 2 fat
Monterey Jack Cheese	1 slice	159	13	74	n/a	38	228	0	0	10	1 high-fat meat, 1 fat
Onion Rings	1 order	500	15	27	n/a	25	896	4	0	0	1 veg, 3 fat
Sautéed Mushrooms	3 oz	107	10	84	n/a	0	356	5	1	2	1 veg, 2 fat
Secret Sauce	1.5 oz/3 T	168	16	86	n/a	14	258	4	0	0	3 fat
✔ Sweet & Sour Sauce	1.5 oz/3 T	67	0	0	n/a	0	149	14	0	0	1 carb
Swiss Cheese	1 slice	160	12	68	n/a	39	111	1	0	12	2 high-fat meat
Tartar Sauce	1.5 oz/3 T	225	25	100	n/a	22	301	2	0	1	5 fat

(Continued)

✔ = Healthiest Bets; n/a = not available

STEAKS

	Amount	Cal.	Fat (g)	% Cal. Fat	Sat. Fat (g)	Chol. (mg)	Sod. (mg)	Carb. (g)	Fiber (g)	Pro. (g)	Servings/Exchanges
Choice Sirloin	8 oz	1224	51	38	n/a	154	2073	128	5	63	8 1/2 starch, 5 medium-fat meat, 4 fat
Half 0 Pound w/ Grilled Onions	1	1337	52	35	n/a	224	1872	133	7	84	8 1/2 starch, 8 medium-fat meat, 1 fat
Half 0 Pound w/Grilled Mushrooms	1	1317	52	36	n/a	225	3038	127	6	84	8 1/2 starch, 8 medium-fat meat, 1 fat
Ribeye	8 oz	1481	75	46	n/a	189	2111	128	5	73	8 1/2 starch, 7 medium-fat meat, 6 fat
Ribeye & 5 Fried Shrimp	1	1639	82	45	n/a	284	2287	139	5	85	9 starch, 8 medium-fat meat, 7 fat

Item	Serving									Exchanges
Ribeye & 6 Grilled Shrimp	1	1589	81	46	n/a	286	2258	128	5	85	8 1/2 starch, 8 medium-fat meat, 7 fat
Sirloin & 5 Fried Shrimp	1	1382	58	38	n/a	248	2249	139	5	76	9 starch, 7 medium-fat meat, 3 fat
Sirloin & 6 Grilled Shrimp	1	1332	57	39	n/a	250	2220	128	5	76	8 1/2 starch, 7 medium-fat meat, 3 fat
Southwest Half O Pound	1	1304	69	48	n/a	244	2943	83	3	85	5 1/2 starch, 10 medium-fat meat, 2 fat
T-Bone	12 oz	1809	100	50	n/a	219	2187	128	5	96	8 1/2 starch, 9 medium-fat meat, 11 fat
T-Bone & 5 Fried Shrimp	1	1967	107	49	n/a	313	2363	139	5	109	9 starch, 10 medium-fat meat, 11 fat

(Continued)

✔ = Healthiest Bets; n/a = not available

Soups, Sandwiches, Salads, and Subs

RESTAURANTS

Arby's

Au Bon Pain

Blimpie Subs and Salads

Jamba Juice

Panera Bread

Schlotsky's Deli

Subway

Togo's Eatery

NUTRITION PROS

- Healthier condiments, such as mustard and vinegar, are available. They keep your sub or sandwich moist without adding a lot of calories and fat.
- Subs and sandwiches are often made to order. That's good because you can specify what you want and don't want.
- Healthy breads, even whole wheat with extra fiber, are usually available.
- Healthy sub and sandwich fillers are available— turkey, smoked turkey, ham, chicken breast, or roast beef.
- Healthy broth-based vegetable and grain soups are warm and ready in some sandwich shops.
- Sub shops offer smaller-sized sandwiches. No need to order the foot-long size.

- Salads with light or fat-free salad dressings are an option in most sub and sandwich shops.

NUTRITION CONS

- Large sandwiches and long subs can be stuffed with enough protein for the whole day.
- Common sub and sandwich condiments, such as mayonnaise and oil, are high in fat.

Healthy Tips

★ To keep your sodium meter on low, go light on or hold the pickles and olives.
★ Complement a sub or sandwich with a healthier side than a fried snack food (potato chips, tortilla chips, and the like). For some crunch, try a side salad, popcorn, baked chips, or pretzels.
★ Ask to have large subs cut into two. Pack half for another day.
★ In sandwich shops, order a cup of broth-based vegetable or bean soup. They'll fill you up and not out.
★ A Greek salad and piece of pita bread makes a high-carbohydrate and light-on-protein meal. Ask for dressing on the side.
★ Pack a piece of fruit from home to bring to the sub or sandwich shop.

Get It Your Way

★ Hold the mayonnaise and oil. Substitute mustard or vinegar.
★ Ask the sub maker to go light on the meat and heavy on the lettuce, onions, tomatoes, and peppers.
★ Hold the cheese.
★ Ask for the salad dressing on the side.

■ Tuna fish, chicken, and seafood salads sound healthy, but they are chock full of fat and calories.
■ Cheese is a frequent sub or sandwich addition. Some restaurants give their nutrition information minus the cheese. Make sure you read the numbers for the way you eat yours.
■ Fruit and cooked vegetables are rarely available.

Arby's

❖Arby's provides nutrition information for all of its menu items on their website at www.arbys.com.

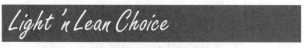

Light 'n Lean Choice

Jr. Roast Beef Sandwich
Garden Salad
Reduced Calorie Buttermilk Ranch Dressing (*2 T*)
1/2 Curly Fries

Calories......................565	Sodium (mg) 1,640
Fat (g) 22	Carbohydrate (g).........75
% calories from fat..35	Fiber (g) 10
Saturated fat (g)........7	Protein (g) 22
Cholesterol (mg) 70	

Exchanges: 4 starch, 2 veg, 1 medium-fat meat, 3 fat

Healthy 'n Hearty Choice

Broccoli 'n Cheddar Baked Potato
Garden Salad
Honey French Salad Dressing (*2 T*)

Calories......................683	Sodium (mg) 830
Fat (g) 31	Carbohydrate (g).........90
% calories from fat..40	Fiber (g) 13
Saturated fat (g)......13	Protein (g) 16
Cholesterol (mg) 50	

Exchanges: 5 1/2 starch, 2 veg, 4 fat

Arby's

	Amount	Cal.	Fat (g)	% Cal. Fat	Sat. Fat (g)	Chol. (mg)	Sod. (mg)	Carb. (g)	Fiber (g)	Pro. (g)	Servings/Exchanges
ARBY'S SUPER-STUFFED BAKED POTATOES											
Chicken Broccoli	1	841	56	60	6	49	850	56	n/a	29	3 1/2 starch, 3 lean meat, 9 fat
Cool Ranch	1	480	25	47	7	25	190	56	n/a	8	3 1/2 starch, 5 fat
Jalapeno	1	640	38	53	13	48	970	61	n/a	15	4 starch, 7 1/2 fat
Philly Chicken	1	860	54	57	10	69	1060	64	n/a	32	4 starch, 3 lean meat, 9 fat
BEVERAGES											
✔Hot Chocolate	8 oz	110	1	8	0.7	0	120	23	3	2	1 1/2 carb

(Continued)

✔ = Healthiest Bets; n/a = not available

BREAKFAST

	Amount	Cal.	Fat (g)	% Cal. Fat	Sat. Fat (g)	Chol. (mg)	Sod. (mg)	Carb. (g)	Fiber (g)	Pro. (g)	Servings/Exchanges
Bacon	1 order	90	7	70	3	15	220	0	0	5	1 medium-fat meat
Biscuit w/bacon	1	360	24	60	7	10	220	27	1	9	2 starch, 1 high-fat meat, 3 fat
Biscuit w/butter	1	280	17	55	4	0	780	27	1	5	2 starch, 1 high-fat meat, 1 fat
Biscuit w/ham	1	330	20	55	5	30	830	28	1	12	2 starch, 1 high-fat meat, 4 fat
Biscuit w/sausage	1	460	33	65	9	25	300	28	1	12	2 starch, 1 high-fat meat, 4 1/2 fat
Biscuit, plain	1	280	15	48	3	0	730	34	1	6	2 starch, 3 fat
Croissant w/bacon	1	340	23	61	13	30	520	28	1	10	2 starch, 1 high-fat meat, 2 1/2 fat

	Amount	Cal.	Fat (g)	% Cal. Fat	Sat. Fat (g)	Chol. (mg)	Sod. (mg)	Carb. (g)	Fiber (g)	Pro. (g)	Exchanges/Choices
Croissant w/ham	1	310	19	55	11	50	1130	29	0	13	2 starch, 1 high-fat meat, 2 fat
Croissant w/sausage	1	440	32	65	15	45	600	29	0	13	2 starch, 1 high-fat meat, 4 fat
Croissant, plain	1	220	12	49	7	25	230	25	0	4	1 1/2 starch, 2 fat
✔ Egg Portion	1	110	9	74	2	175	170	2	0	5	1 medium-fat meat, 1/2 fat
French-Toastix	1 order	370	17	41	4	0	440	48	4	7	3 starch, 3 1/2 fat
✔ Ham	1	45	1	20	0.5	20	405	0	0	7	1 very lean meat
Sausage	1 order	163	15	83	6	25	321	0	0	7	1 high-fat meat, 1 fat
Sourdough w/bacon	1	420	10	21	2.5	10	960	66	3	16	4 1/2 starch, 1 medium-fat meat, 1 fat
✔ Sourdough w/ham	1	390	6	14	1	30	1570	67	2	19	4 1/2 starch, 1 medium-fat meat

(Continued)

✔ = Healthiest Bets; n/a = not available

BREAKFAST (Continued)	Amount	Cal.	Fat (g)	% Cal. Fat	Sat. Fat (g)	Chol. (mg)	Sod. (mg)	Carb. (g)	Fiber (g)	Pro. (g)	Servings/Exchanges
Sourdough w/sausage	1	520	19	33	5	25	1040	67	2	19	4 1/2 starch, 1 medium-fat meat, 3 fat

CONDIMENTS

	Amount	Cal.	Fat (g)	% Cal. Fat	Sat. Fat (g)	Chol. (mg)	Sod. (mg)	Carb. (g)	Fiber (g)	Pro. (g)	Servings/Exchanges
✔ Arby's Sauce	0.5 oz/1 T	15	0	0	0	0	180	4	0	0	free
✔ Au Jus Sauce	3 oz/6 T	85	5	53	0	0	386	0	0	0	1 fat
✔ Barbeque Sauce	1 oz/2 T	40	0	0	0	0	350	10	0	0	1/2 carb
✔ Bronco Berry Sauce	1.5 oz/3 T	90	0	0	0	0	35	23	0	0	1 1/2 carb
Honey Mustard	1 oz/2 T	130	12	83	1.5	10	160	5	0	0	2 fat
✔ Horsey Sauce	0.5 oz/1 T	60	5	75	0.5	5	150	3	0	0	1 fat
✔ Marinara Sauce	1.5 oz/3 T	35	1	26	0	0	260	5	0	1	free
✔ Table Syrup	0.5 oz/1 T	130	0	0	0	0	45	32	0	0	2 carb
Tangy Southwest Sauce	1.5 oz/3 T	250	26	94	4.5	30	290	3	0	0	5 fat

DESSERTS

Apple Turnover	1	420	16	34	4.5	0	230	65	2	4	4 carb, 3 fat
Cherry Turnover	1	410	16	35	4.5	0	250	63	1	4	4 carb, 3 fat

MARKET FRESH SALADS

✔Caesar Salad	1	90	4	40	2.5	10	170	8	3	7	2 veg, 1 lean meat
✔Caesar Side Salad	1	45	2	40	1	5	95	4	2	4	1 veg, 1 very lean meat
Chicken Finger Salad	1	570	34	54	9	65	1300	39	3	30	2 starch, 2 veg, 3 lean meat, 5 fat
✔Grilled Chicken Caesar	1	230	8	31	3.5	80	920	8	3	33	2 veg, 4 very lean meat, 1 fat
✔Turkey Club Salad	1	350	21	54	10	90	920	9	3	33	2 veg, 4 lean meat, 1 fat

MARKET FRESH SANDWICHES

Roast Beef & Swiss	1	810	42	47	13	130	1780	73	5	37	5 starch, 3 lean meat, 7 fat

(Continued)

✔ = Healthiest Bets; n/a = not available

MARKET FRESH SANDWICHES (Continued)	Amount	Cal.	Fat (g)	% Cal. Fat	Sat. Fat (g)	Chol. (mg)	Sod. (mg)	Carb. (g)	Fiber (g)	Pro. (g)	Servings/Exchanges
Roast Chicken Caesar	1	820	38	42	9	140	2160	75	5	43	5 starch, 3 lean meat, 6 fat
Roast Ham & Swiss	1	730	34	42	8	125	2180	74	5	36	5 starch, 3 lean meat, 5 fat
Roast Turkey & Swiss	1	760	33	39	6	130	1920	75	5	43	5 starch, 3 lean meat, 4 fat
MISCELLANEOUS											
Chicken Finger Snack (2 pieces with Curly Fries)	1 order	580	32	50	7	35	1450	55	3	19	3 1/2 starch, 1 lean meat, 6 fat
SALAD DRESSINGS											
✔BBQ Vinaigrette	2 oz/4 T	140	11	71	1.5	0	660	9	0	0	1/2 carb
Blue Cheese	2 oz/4 T	300	31	93	6	45	580	3	0	2	6 fat
Buttermilk Ranch	2 oz/4 T	360	39	98	6	5	490	2	0	1	8 fat
Caesar	2 oz/4 T	310	34	99	5	60	470	0	1	1	5 fat
Honey French	2 oz/4 T	290	24	74	4	0	410	18	0	0	1 carb, 5 fat

Italian Parmesan	2 oz/4 T	240	24	90	4	0	950	4	0	1	free
✔ Reduced Calorie Buttermilk Ranch	2 oz/4 T	60	0	0	0	0	750	13	1	1	1 carb
✔ Reduced Calorie Italian	2 oz/4 T	25	1	36	1	0	1030	3	0	0	free
Thousand Island	2 oz/4 T	290	28	87	4.5	35	480	9	0	1	1/2 carb, 5 1/2 fat

SALADS

✔ Garden	1	70	1	13	0	0	45	14	6	4	2 veg
✔ Roast Chicken	1	160	3	17	0.5	40	700	15	6	20	2 veg, 3 very lean meat
✔ Side	1	25	0	0	0	0	20	5	2	2	1 veg

SANDWICHES

Fish Fillet (seasonal for Lent)	1	529	27	46	7	43	864	50	2	23	3 starch, 2 medium-fat meat, 3 fat

(Continued)

✔ = Healthiest Bets; n/a = not available

SANDWICHES (*Continued*)	Amount	Cal.	Fat (g)	% Cal. Fat	Sat. Fat (g)	Chol. (mg)	Sod. (mg)	Carb. (g)	Fiber (g)	Pro. (g)	Servings/Exchanges
Hot Ham N' Swiss	1	340	13	34	4.5	90	1450	35	1	23	2 starch, 2 medium-fat meat, 1/2 fat
SANDWICHES, CHICKEN											
Breaded Chicken Fillet	1	540	30	50	5	90	1160	47	2	24	3 starch, 2 medium-fat meat, 4 fat
Chicken Bacon and Swiss	1	610	33	49	8	110	1550	49	2	31	3 starch, 3 lean meat, 5 fat
Chicken Cordon Bleu	1	630	35	50	8	120	1820	47	2	34	3 starch, 4 lean meat, 4 fat
Grilled Chicken Deluxe	1	450	22	44	4	110	1050	37	2	29	3 starch, 2 medium-fat meat, 2 fat
Roast Chicken Club	1	520	28	48	7	115	1440	38	2	29	2 1/2 starch, 3 medium-fat meat, 3 fat

SANDWICHES, LIGHT MENU

Grilled Chicken	1	280	5	16	1.5	55	1170	30	3	29	2 starch, 3 lean meat
✔ Roast Chicken Deluxe	1	260	5	17	1	40	1010	33	3	23	2 starch, 2 lean meat
✔ Roast Turkey Deluxe	1	260	5	17	0.5	40	980	33	3	23	2 starch, 2 lean meat

SANDWICHES, ROAST BEEF

Arby Q	1	360	14	35	4	70	1530	40	2	16	2 1/2 starch, 2 medium-fat meat, 1 fat
✔ Arby's Melt	1	340	15	40	5	70	890	36	2	16	2 1/2 starch, 1 medium-fat meat, 2 fat
Beef 'n Cheddar	1	480	24	45	8	90	1240	43	2	23	3 starch, 2 medium-fat meat, 3 fat
Big Montana	1	630	32	46	15	155	2080	41	3	47	2 1/2 starch, 4 medium-fat meat, 2 fat

(Continued)

✔ = Healthiest Bets; n/a = not available

SANDWICHES, ROAST BEEF (*Continued*)	Amount	Cal.	Fat (g)	% Cal. Fat	Sat. Fat (g)	Chol. (mg)	Sod. (mg)	Carb. (g)	Fiber (g)	Pro. (g)	Servings/Exchanges
Giant Roast Beef	1	480	23	43	10	110	1440	41	3	32	2 1/2 starch, 4 medium-fat meat, 1/2 fat
✔ Junior Roast Beef	1	310	13	38	4.5	70	740	34	2	16	2 starch, 2 medium-fat meat, 1/2 fat
✔ Regular Roast Beef	1	350	16	41	6	85	950	34	2	21	2 starch, 3 medium-fat meat
Super Roast Beef	1	470	23	44	7	85	1130	47	3	22	3 starch, 2 medium-fat meat, 1 1/2 fat
S H A K E S											
Chocolate	14 oz	480	16	30	8	45	370	84	0	10	5 carb, 3 fat
Jamocha	14 oz	470	15	29	7	45	390	82	0	10	4 carb, 3 fat
Vanilla	14 oz	470	15	29	7	45	360	45	0	10	3 carb, 2 fat

SIDES

Baked Potato, with butter & sour cream	1	500	24	43	15	55	170	65	6	8	4 starch, 5 fat
Broccoli 'n Cheddar Baked Potato	1	540	24	40	12	50	680	71	7	12	6 starch, 5 fat
Cheddar Curly Fries	1 order	460	24	47	6	5	1290	54	4	6	3 1/2 starch, 4 fat
Chicken Finger 4 Pack	1 order	640	38	53	8	70	1590	42	0	31	3 starch, 3 lean meat, 6 fat
Curly Fries (large)	1 order	620	30	44	7	0	1540	78	7	8	5 starch, 6 fat
Curly Fries (medium)	1 order	400	20	45	5	0	990	50	4	5	3 starch, 4 fat
Curly Fries (small)	1 order	310	15	44	3.5	0	770	39	3	4	2 1/2 starch, 3 fat
Deluxe Baked Potato	1	650	34	47	20	90	750	67	6	20	4 1/2 starch, 7 fat
✔Homestyle French Fries (kids)	1 order	220	10	41	2.5	0	430	32	3	3	2 starch, 2 fat

✔ = Healthiest Bets; n/a = not available

(Continued)

SIDES (*Continued*)	Amount	Cal.	Fat (g)	% Cal. Fat	Sat. Fat (g)	Chol. (mg)	Sod. (mg)	Carb. (g)	Fiber (g)	Pro. (g)	Servings/Exchanges
Homestyle Fries (large)	1 order	560	24	39	6	0	1070	79	6	6	5 starch, 5 fat
Homestyle Fries (medium)	1 order	370	16	39	4	0	710	53	4	4	3 1/2 starch, 3 fat
Homestyle Fries (small)	1 order	300	13	39	3.5	0	570	42	3	3	3 starch, 2 1/2 fat
Jalapeno Bites	1 order	330	21	57	9	40	670	30	2	7	2 starch, 4 fat
Mozzarella Sticks	1 order	470	29	56	14	60	1330	34	2	18	2 starch, 2 high-fat meat, 2 fat
Onion Petals	1 order	410	24	53	3.5	0	300	43	2	4	3 starch, 5 fat
Potato Cakes	1 order	250	16	58	4	0	490	26	3	2	1 1/2 starch, 3 fat
SUB ROLL SANDWICHES											
Roast Beef Sub	1	760	48	57	16	130	2230	47	3	35	3 starch, 3 medium-fat meat, 5 fat

	Amount	Calories	Fat (g)	% Cal. Fat	Sat. Fat (g)	Chol. (mg)	Sodium (mg)	Carb. (g)	Fiber (g)	Protein (g)	Exchanges/Choices
French Dip	1	440	18	37	8	100	1680	42	2	28	2 1/2 starch, 3 medium-fat meat, 1 fat
Hot Ham 'n Swiss	1	530	27	46	8	110	1860	45	3	29	3 starch, 3 medium-fat meat, 1 1/2 fat
Italian Sub	1	780	53	61	15	120	2440	49	3	29	3 starch, 2 medium-fat meat, 5 fat
Philly Beef 'n Swiss	1	700	42	54	15	130	1940	46	4	36	3 starch, 4 medium-fat meat, 5 fat
Turkey Sub	1	630	37	53	9	100	2170	51	2	26	3 starch, 2 lean meat, 4 fat

✔ = Healthiest Bets; n/a = not available

Au Bon Pain

❖Au Bon Pain provides some nutrition information
for its menu items on their website at
www.aubonpain.com. They provided complete
nutrition information for this book.

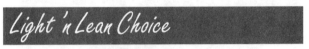

Light 'n Lean Choice

Thai Chicken Sandwich
Garden Salad (*small*)
Lite Honey Mustard Dressing (*2 T*)

Calories	613	Sodium (mg)	1,657
Fat (g)	13	Carbohydrate (g)	102
% calories from fat	19	Fiber (g)	7
Saturated fat (g)	2	Protein (g)	26
Cholesterol (mg)	33		

Exchanges: 5 1/2 starch, 2 veg, 1/2 carb, 2 lean meat,
1 fat

Healthy 'n Hearty Choice

Vegetarian Chili (*medium, 12 oz*)
Hearth Roll
Garden Salad (*large*)
Fat Free Tomato Basil Dressing (*4 T*)

Calories	627	Sodium (mg)	2,520
Fat (g)	13	Carbohydrate (g)	114
% calories from fat	19	Fiber (g)	11
Saturated fat (g)	2	Protein (g)	25
Cholesterol (mg)	0		

Exchanges: 6 starch, 3 veg, 1 very lean meat, 1 fat

Au Bon Pain

	Amount	Cal.	Fat (g)	% Cal. Fat	Sat. Fat (g)	Chol. (mg)	Sod. (mg)	Carb. (g)	Fiber (g)	Pro. (g)	Servings/Exchanges
BAGEL SANDWICHES											
✔ Egg	1	500	12	9	1	120	880	83	3	29	5 1/2 starch, 2 very lean meat
Egg with Bacon	1	580	12	19	3.5	130	1100	83	3	33	5 1/2 starch, 2 lean meat, 1 fat
Egg with Bacon and Cheese	1	660	19	26	7	155	1240	83	3	39	5 1/2 starch, 2 lean meat, 1 fat
Egg with Cheese	1	580	12	19	4.5	140	1010	83	3	34	5 1/2 starch, 3 medium-fat meat

(Continued)

✔ = Healthiest Bets; n/a = not available

	Amount	Cal.	Fat (g)	% Cal. Fat	Sat. Fat (g)	Chol. (mg)	Sod. (mg)	Carb. (g)	Fiber (g)	Pro. (g)	Servings/Exchan
BAGELS											
✔Asiago Cheese	1	380	6	14	3.5	15	690	66	3	17	4 1/2 starch, 1 medium-fat meat
✔Cheddar & Scallion	1	310	5	15	3	10	600	50	2	16	3 1/2 starch, 1 fat
✔Cinnamon Raisin	1	390	1	2	0	0	550	83	4	14	5 1/2 starch
✔Cranberry Walnut	1	460	4	8	0.5	0	590	93	7	15	6 starch, 1 fat
✔Dutch Apple with Walnut Streusel	1	350	5	13	0	0	480	77	4	11	5 starch, 1 fat
✔Everything	1	360	3	8	0	0	710	72	3	14	5 starch, 1/2 fat
✔Focaccia	1	330	5	14	1	0	990	61	4	12	4 starch, 1 fat
✔Honey 9 Grain	1	360	2	5	0	0	580	72	6	14	5 starch
✔Jalapeno Double Cheddar	1	390	8	18	5	20	710	62	3	17	4 starch, 1 1/2 fat

✓Onion	1	360	1	3	0	0	540	75	4	14	5 starch
✓Plain	1	350	1	3	0	0	540	71	3	13	5 starch
✓Sesame	1	380	4	9	0.5	0	540	71	3	15	4 1/2 starch, 1 fat
✓Wild Blueberry	1	380	2	5	0	0	570	80	4	14	5 starch
BEVERAGES											
Apple Cider	24 oz	350	1	3	0	0	22	87	0	0	6 fruit
Apple Cider	20 oz	290	1	3	0	0	19	72	0	0	5 fruit
Apple Cider	16 oz	230	1	4	0	0	15	58	0	0	4 fruit
Apple Cider	12 oz	175	0	0	0	0	11	43	0	0	3 fruit
Frozen Mocha Blast (large)	24 oz	480	4	8	3	15	230	96	3	13	1 1/2 low-fat milk, 5 carb
Frozen Mocha Blast	16 oz	320	3	8	2	10	150	64	2	9	1 low-fat milk, 3 carb
Iced Cappuccino	20 oz	270	10	33	6	40	270	26	0	18	2 low-fat milk, 1 fat
✓Iced Cappuccino	12 oz	150	6	36	3.5	25	150	15	0	10	1 low-fat milk, 1 fat

(Continued)

✓ = Healthiest Bets; n/a = not available

BEVERAGES (Continued)	Amount	Cal.	Fat (g)	% Cal. Fat	Sat. Fat (g)	Chol. (mg)	Sod. (mg)	Carb. (g)	Fiber (g)	Pro. (g)	Servings/Exchanges
✓Iced Cappuccino	9 oz	110	4	33	2.5	15	110	10	0	7	1 low-fat milk
Iced Strawberry Banana Blast	16 oz	280	5	16	3.5	25	190	45	0	13	1 1/2 low-fat milk, 1 1/2 carb, 1 fat
Malt Shoppe Blast	16 oz	460	9	18	6	35	350	74	1	19	2 low-fat milk, 3 carb, 1 fat
Peach Iced Tea (large)	16 oz	170	0	0	0	0	30	44	0	0	3 carb
Peach Iced Tea (medium)	12 oz	130	0	0	0	0	20	33	0	0	2 carb
✓Peach Iced Tea (small)	8 oz	90	0	0	0	0	15	22	0	0	1 1/2 carb
BREAD											
Bowl	1	680	3	4	0	0	1930	134	6	29	9 starch
✓Pita	1/2 wrap	130	0	0	0	0	150	29	2	5	2 starch
✓Stick—Rosemary Garlic	1	180	3	15	0	0	550	34	2	7	2 starch, 1/2 fat
✓Tomato Herb	1 slice	130	1	7	0	0	340	25	1	6	1 1/2 starch

COOKIES

Item											
Chocolate Chip	1	280	13	42	8	40	85	40	2	3	2 1/2 carb, 2 1/2 fat
Chocolate-Dipped Shortbread	1	410	27	59	19	55	160	41	2	4	3 carb, 5 fat
✔ Cranberry Almond Macaroon	1	160	8	45	5	0	115	22	2	2	2 carb, 1 1/2 fat
Ginger Pecan	1	260	15	52	6	40	115	30	1	5	2 carb, 3 fat
✔ Gingerbread Man	1	300	8	24	1.5	35	280	54	1	4	3 1/2 carb, 1 fat
✔ Holiday Tree with Icing	1	200	4	18	1	10	75	42	6	2	3 carb
Red Sugar Shortbread Heart	1	350	22	57	14	6	170	37	1	3	2 1/2 carb, 3 fat
Shortbread	1	390	25	58	15	65	190	39	1	3	2 1/2 carb, 5 fat

CROISSANTS

Item											
Almond	1	570	38	60	16	110	330	50	3	11	3 starch, 7 fat
✔ Apple	1	280	10	32	6	25	180	46	1	4	3 starch, 2 fat
Chocolate	1	440	23	47	15	30	230	53	4	7	4 1/2 starch

(Continued)

✔ = Healthiest Bets; n/a = not available

CROISSANTS (*Continued*)	Amount	Cal.	Fat (g)	% Cal. Fat	Sat. Fat (g)	Chol. (mg)	Sod. (mg)	Carb. (g)	Fiber (g)	Pro. (g)	Servings/Exchanges
Cinnamon Raisin	1	340	5	13	2.5	10	350	69	3	9	4 starch, 2 1/2 fat
✓Ham and Cheese	1	330	10	27	6	35	740	46	2	18	2 1/2 starch, 1 high-fat meat
✓Plain	1	250	6	22	3.5	15	340	43	2	8	2 starch, 3 fat
Raspberry Cheese	1	340	11	29	6	40	360	55	2	8	3 starch, 1/2 carb, 2 fat
✓Spinach and Cheese	1	240	9	34	6	25	390	32	2	10	2 starch, 1 high-fat meat
Sweet Cheese	1	350	14	36	8	50	390	50	1	9	3 starch, 2 fat
DANISHES											
Cinnamon Roll	1	340	15	40	9	35	320	48	2	7	3 carb, 3 fat
Lemon Swirl	1	360	11	28	4	40	370	60	6	9	4 carb, 1 fat
Sweet Cheese	1	420	18	39	8	70	450	46	2	10	3 starch, 4 fat
DESSERTS											
7 Layer Bar	1	300	10	30	5	10	250	51	2	5	3 1/2 starch, 1 fat

	Amount	Cal.	Fat (g)	% Fat Cal.	Sat. Fat (g)	Chol. (mg)	Sod. (mg)	Carb. (g)	Fiber (g)	Prot. (g)	Exchanges
Mochaccino Bar	1	404	24	53	10	37	294	44	1	5	3 carb, 5 fat
Oreo Cookie Bar	1	550	29	47	5	75	190	58	1	5	4 starch, 5 fat
Pecan Roll	1	770	30	35	7	15	580	116	4	14	7 1/2 starch, 4 fat
Walnut Fudge Brownie	1	380	18	43	11	100	150	56	4	5	3 1/2 carb, 3 1/2 fat
FRUIT											
✔Fresh Fruit Cup	8 oz	90	1	10	0	0	15	21	2	0	1 1/2 fruits
✔Fresh Fruit Cup	10 oz	110	1	8	0	0	15	27	2	0	2 fruits
LOAF BREADS											
✔Baguette	1 slice	130	1	7	0	0	300	26	1	5	1 1/2 starch
✔Parisienne	1 slice	130	0	0	0	0	330	25	1	5	1 1/2 starch
MUFFINS											
Blueberry	1	420	18	39	4.5	50	420	60	2	7	4 starch, 3 fat
Carrot Walnut	1	580	30	47	3.5	65	880	71	5	9	4 1/2 starch, 5 fat

(Continued)

✔ = Healthiest Bets; n/a = not available

MUFFINS (*Continued*)	Amount	Cal.	Fat (g)	% Cal. Fat	Sat. Fat (g)	Chol. (mg)	Sod. (mg)	Carb. (g)	Fiber (g)	Pro. (g)	Servings/Exchanges
✓Chocolate Cake (low fat)	1	290	3	9	0.5	20	630	68	3	4	4 starch, 1/2 fat
Chocolate Chip	1	600	26	39	6	50	720	92	2	10	6 starch, 5 fat
Corn	1	520	23	40	4	85	660	81	1	9	5 carb, 3 fat
Cranberry Walnut	1	480	26	49	5	45	400	55	3	8	3 1/2 starch, 4 fat
Pumpkin with Streusel Topping	1	570	20	32	3.5	70	600	81	3	10	4 starch, 1 carb, 3 fat
Raisin Bran	1	450	14	28	4.5	45	1020	81	9	10	4 1/2 starch, 1 carb, 1 fat
ROLLS											
✓3 Seed—Pecan Raisin	1	250	6	22	1	0	240	43	3	9	3 starch, 1 fat
✓Hearth	1	200	2	9	0.5	0	410	38	2	9	2 1/2 starch
✓Petit Pain	1	210	1	4	0	0	560	42	2	9	3 starch
SALAD DRESSINGS											
Bleu Cheese	3 oz/6 T	410	41	90	8	40	910	8	0	4	1/2 carb, 8 fat

✓Buttermilk Ranch	3 oz/6 T	310	32	93	4	35	270	4	0	3	6 fat
Caesar	3 oz/6 T	380	39	92	5	25	410	3	0	5	8 fat
✓Fat Free Tomato Basil	3 oz/6 T	70	0	0	0	0	650	17	1	1	1 carb
Greek	3 oz/6 T	440	50	102	7	0	820	2	0	0	10 fat
Lemon Basil Vinaigrette	3 oz/6 T	330	32	87	2	0	460	15	0	0	1 carb, 6 fat
✓Lite Honey Mustard	3 oz/6 T	280	17	55	2.5	40	560	30	1	2	2 carb, 3 fat
✓Lite Italian	3 oz/6 T	230	20	78	1.5	0	570	15	0	0	1 carb, 4 fat
Mandarin Orange	3 oz/6 T	380	33	78	3	0	310	23	0	0	1 1/2 carb, 6 fat
Sesame French	3 oz/6 T	370	30	73	4.5	0	1010	26	1	1	2 carb, 6 fat
✓Thai Peanut	2 oz/4 T	130	6	42	0	0	1000	16	0	2	1 carb, 1 fat
SALADS											
✓Caesar Salad	1	270	10	33	6	20	800	27	5	19	2 veg, 1 carb, 1 medium-fat meat, 1 fat

(Continued)

✓ = Healthiest Bets; n/a = not available

SALADS (*Continued*)	Amount	Cal.	Fat (g)	% Cal. Fat	Sat. Fat (g)	Chol. (mg)	Sod. (mg)	Carb. (g)	Fiber (g)	Pro. (g)	Servings/Exchanges
Chef	1	390	26	60	11	70	1460	12	4	30	1 carb, 4 medium-fat meat, 1 fat
✔Chicken Caesar Salad	1	360	11	28	6	65	910	28	5	36	2 veg, 1 carb, 4 lean meat
Chicken Tarragon with Almonds	1	470	23	44	4	80	500	38	6	32	2 veg, 2 carb, 3 lean meat, 2 fat
Field Greens, Gorgonzola & Roasted Walnut Salad	1	400	34	77	13	50	800	9	3	20	2 veg, 2 high-fat meat, 3 fat
✔Garden Salad (large)	1	160	2	11	0	0	290	34	6	7	3 veg, 1 carb
✔Garden Salad (small)	1	100	1	9	0	0	150	20	4	5	2 veg, 1/2 carb
✔Mozzarella & Roasted Red Pepper Salad	1	340	18	48	10	60	135	26	10	22	2 veg, 1 carb, 2 high-fat meat
✔Oriental Chicken	1	270	4	13	0.5	70	700	17	5	40	2 veg, 7 very lean meat

✔Pesto Chicken Salad	1	230	11	43	2	45	250	11	4	20	2 veg, 2 lean meat, 1 fat
✔Thai Chicken	1	330	8	22	1	70	980	23	6	41	2 veg, 1 carb, 7 very lean meat
Tuna Salad (w/mayonnaise on greens)	1	490	27	50	4.5	45	750	40	7	26	2 veg, 2 carb, 3 lean meat, 3 fat

SANDWICH BREADS

✔Braided Roll	1 roll	370	11	27	2.5	30	670	57	3	12	4 starch, 2 fat
✔Country White	1 slice	130	1	7	0	0	190	27	1	5	2 starch
✔Four Grain	1 slice	170	2	11	0	0	470	32	1	7	2 starch
✔French Roll	1 roll	300	1	3	0	0	810	60	3	12	4 starch
✔Hearth	1 roll	290	3	9	1	0	580	53	2	13	3 1/2 starch
✔Multigrain Loaf	1 slice	140	2	13	0	0	210	26	1	6	2 starch

(Continued)

✔ = Healthiest Bets; n/a = not available

	Amount	Cal.	Fat (g)	% Cal. Fat	Sat. Fat (g)	Chol. (mg)	Sod. (mg)	Carb. (g)	Fiber (g)	Pro. (g)	Servings/Exchanges
SANDWICH FILLINGS											
Cheddar Cheese	43 g	170	14	74	9	45	260	1	0	11	2 medium-fat meat, 1 fat
Chicken Tarragon	113 g	240	17	64	3	65	170	1	0	20	3 lean meat, 2 fat
✓Country Ham	106 g	150	7	42	2.5	55	1370	1	0	21	3 lean meat
✓Grilled Chicken	112 g	140	2	13	0	72	184	2	0	27	4 very lean meat
Provolone Cheese	43 g	150	11	66	7	30	370	1	0	11	2 medium-fat meat
✓Roast Beef	106 g	140	4	26	0	50	550	1	0	22	3 very lean meat
Swiss Cheese	43 g	160	12	68	8	40	110	1	0	12	2 medium-fat meat
Tuna Salad	128 g	360	29	73	4.5	50	520	3	1	21	3 lean meat, 4 fat
✓Turkey Breast	106 g	120	1	8	0	20	1110	1	0	24	3 very lean meat
SANDWICHES											
Arizona Chicken	1	720	33	41	12	125	1190	57	4	49	4 starch, 5 lean meat, 3 1/2 fat

	Amount	Cal.	Fat (g)	% Cal. Fat	Sat. Fat (g)	Chol. (mg)	Sod. (mg)	Carb. (g)	Fiber (g)	Prot. (g)	Exchanges/Choices
Chicken of Ca-cha-cha	1	870	29	30	5.0	130	2280	80	10	74	1 veg, 5 starch, 8 lean meat, 1 fat
Fresh Mozzarella, Tomato & Pesto	1	650	30	42	12	55	1090	69	4	30	4 1/2 starch, 3 medium-fat meat, 3 fat
Grilled Chicken & Mozzarella Focaccia	1	910	20	20	1.5	130	2670	83	7	96	5 1/2 starch, 11 very lean meat, 2 fat
Honey Dijon Chicken	1	730	18	22	6	135	1990	85	4	57	5 1/2 starch, 7 very lean meat, 2 fat
Hot Roasted Turkey Club	1	950	50	47	16	135	2240	80	4	50	5 starch, 5 lean meat, 7 fat
✔Thai Chicken	1	420	6	13	1	20	1320	72	3	20	5 starch, 2 lean meat
SCONES											
Cinnamon	1	440	17	35	7	82	310	82	2	10	5 1/2 starch, 3 fat
Cranberry Almond Orange	1	500	18	32	8	65	220	75	3	9	5 starch, 2 fat

(Continued)

✔ = Healthiest Bets; n/a = not available

	Amount	Cal.	Fat (g)	% Cal. Fat	Sat. Fat (g)	Chol. (mg)	Sod. (mg)	Carb. (g)	Fiber (g)	Pro. (g)	Servings/Exchanges
SCONES (*Continued*)											
Orange with icing	1	430	15	31	8	130	350	64	2	12	4 starch, 3 fat
✓Sour Cream Lemon	1	390	8	18	4	55	320	74	2	8	5 starch, 1 fat
SOUP IN A BREAD BOWL											
Beef Barley w/bowl	1	760	7	8	2	20	2940	147	8	36	9 starch, 1 medium-fat meat
Caribbean Black Bean w/bowl	1	830	5	5	1	10	3100	163	17	36	10 starch, 1 lean meat
Chicken Chili w/bowl	1	990	22	20	11	65	3970	162	12	48	10 starch, 3 lean meat, 2 fat
Chicken Noodle w/bowl	1	760	6	7	1	20	2950	146	7	39	9 starch, 2 lean meat
Clam Chowder w/bowl	1	1050	32	27	15	100	3040	155	5	43	10 starch, 2 lean meat, 5 fat
Cream of Broccoli w/bowl	1	970	31	29	15	60	3100	152	7	34	10 starch, 6 fat
French Onion w/bowl	1	760	8	9	2	0	3860	148	8	30	9 starch, 1 1/2 fat
New England Potato & Cheese with Ham w/bowl	1	860	15	16	9	40	3170	152	9	34	9 starch, 1 lean meat, 2 fat

Tomato Florentine w/bowl	1	760	5	6	2	10	3490	150	8	33	9 starch, 1 lean meat
Vegetarian Chili w/bowl	1	870	7	7	1	0	3550	171	8	36	11 starch, 1 fat

SOUPS

Artichoke Portabella with Chicken	12 oz	270	18	60	11	75	1600	21	3	11	1 1/2 starch, 1 lean meat, 2 fat
Artichoke Portabella with Chicken	16 oz	370	25	61	15	105	2220	30	4	15	2 starch, 2 lean meat, 2 fat
Asiago Cheese Bisque	8 oz	230	16	63	8	35	660	16	1	5	1 starch, 3 fat
Asiago Cheese Bisque	12 oz	370	25	61	13	60	1050	26	2	8	1 1/2 starch, 1 high-fat meat, 3 fat
Asiago Cheese Bisque	16 oz	460	32	63	16	75	1310	33	3	10	2 starch, 1 high-fat meat, 4 fat

(Continued)

✔ = Healthiest Bets; n/a = not available

SOUPS *(Continued)*	Amount	Cal.	Fat (g)	% Cal. Fat	Sat. Fat (g)	Chol. (mg)	Sod. (mg)	Carb. (g)	Fiber (g)	Pro. (g)	Servings/Exchanges
Asiago Tomato Lentil	16 oz	240	4	15	0.5	5	1740	37	12	14	2 1/2 starch, 1 very lean meat, 1/2 fat
Asiago Tomato Lentil	12 oz	180	3	15	0.5	5	1310	27	9	10	2 starch, 1 very lean meat
✔Asiago Tomato Lentil	8 oz	120	2	15	0	0	870	18	6	7	1 starch, 1 very lean meat
Autumn Pumpkin	16 oz	330	18	49	9	45	1540	35	9	7	2 starch, 3 fat
Autumn Pumpkin	12 oz	270	14	47	7	35	1230	29	8	7	2 starch 2 fat
✔Autumn Pumpkin	8 oz	170	9	48	4.5	20	770	18	5	6	1 starch, 2 fat
Beef Barley (large)	16 oz	150	4	24	2	25	1310	22	5	12	1 starch, 1 lean meat
✔Beef Barley (medium)	12 oz	112	3	24	1.5	18	980	16	3	9	1 starch, 1 lean meat
✔Beef Barley (small)	8 oz	75	2	24	.5	15	660	14	2	6	1 starch
Chicken Noodle (large)	16 oz	170	2	11	0.5	35	1340	19	2	16	1 starch, 2 lean meat
Chicken Noodle (medium)	12 oz	120	2	15	0.5	25	1000	14	2	12	1 starch, 1 very lean meat

✓Chicken Noodle (small)	8 oz	80	2	23	0	15	670	10	1	8	1/2 starch, 1 very lean meat
Clam Chowder (large)	16 oz	540	39	65	18	125	1460	32	0	22	2 starch, 2 lean meat, 6 fat
Clam Chowder (medium)	12 oz	400	29	65	14	95	1090	24	0	16	1 1/2 starch, 2 lean meat, 4 fat
Clam Chowder (small)	8 oz	270	19	63	19	65	730	16	0	11	1 starch, 1 lean meat, 3 fat
Corn & Green Chile Bisque (large)	16 oz	380	20	47	12	60	2290	41	5	8	3 starch, 4 fat
Corn Chowder	16 oz	530	33	56	19	95	1530	58	3	11	4 starch, 4 fat
Corn Chowder	12 oz	390	24	55	14	70	1150	43	2	8	3 starch, 3 fat
Corn Chowder	8 oz	260	16	55	10	50	760	29	1	5	2 starch, 2 fat
Corn Green & Chile Bisque (medium)	12 oz	300	16	48	9	45	1830	33	4	7	2 starch, 3 fat

(Continued)

✔ = Healthiest Bets; n/a = not available

SOUPS (*Continued*)	Amount	Cal.	Fat (g)	% Cal. Fat	Sat. Fat (g)	Chol. (mg)	Sod. (mg)	Carb. (g)	Fiber (g)	Pro. (g)	Servings/Exchanges
Corn Green & Chile Bisque (small)	8 oz	190	10	47	6	30	1140	21	3	4	1 1/2 starch, 2 fat
Cream of Broccoli (large)	16 oz	440	37	76	17	80	1550	28	3	10	2 starch, 7 fat
Cream of Broccoli (medium)	12 oz	330	28	76	13	60	1160	21	2	8	1 1/2 starch, 5 1/2 fat
Cream of Broccoli (small)	8 oz	220	18	74	9	40	770	14	1	5	1 starch, 3 1/2 fat
Forest Mushroom Bisque	16 oz	250	12	43	6	40	1940	25	3	12	1 1/2 starch, 1 high-fat meat, 1 fat
Forest Mushroom Bisque	12 oz	200	9	41	5	35	1550	20	2	9	1 starch, 1 high-fat meat
✓Forest Mushroom Bisque	8 oz	130	6	42	3	20	970	12	1	6	1 starch, 1 fat
✓Garden Vegetable	8 oz	29	0	0	0	0	820	8	2	2	1 veg
Garden Vegetable	12 oz	45	0	0	0	0	1240	12	3	2	2 veg
Garden Vegetable	16 oz	58	0	0	0	0	1650	16	4	3	2 veg

	Serving	Cal	Fat (g)	% Cal from Fat	Sat Fat (g)	Chol (mg)	Sod (mg)	Carb (g)	Fiber (g)	Prot (g)	Exchanges
Lobster Bisque	12 oz	460	30	59	13	120	1830	32	3	16	2 starch, 1 lean meat, 6 fat
Lobster Bisque	16 oz	580	37	57	17	150	2280	40	4	20	2 1/2 starch, 2 lean meat, 6 fat
✔ Maryland Crab & Red Lentil	8 oz	180	4	20	0.5	5	980	28	8	9	2 starch, 1 fat
Maryland Crab & Red Lentil	12 oz	300	7	21	1	10	1570	44	13	15	3 starch, 1 fat
Maryland Crab & Red Lentil	16 oz	370	8	19	1.5	10	1960	55	16	19	3 1/2 starch, 1 lean meat, 1 fat
✔ Mushroom Orzo	8 oz	60	2	30	0	0	870	11	1	2	1/2 starch
Mushroom Orzo	12 oz	90	3	30	0	0	1300	17	2	4	1 starch
Mushroom Orzo	16 oz	130	4	28	0.5	0	1730	22	3	5	1 1/2 starch, 1 fat
✔ Roasted Vegetable Bisque	8 oz	210	11	47	6	35	840	22	3	5	1 1/2 starch, 2 fat
Roasted Vegetable Bisque	12 oz	340	18	48	10	55	1350	36	5	9	2 1/2 starch, 3 fat
Roasted Vegetable Bisque	16 oz	430	23	48	13	65	1690	45	6	11	3 starch, 4 fat

✔ = Healthiest Bets; n/a = not available

(Continued)

SOUPS *(Continued)*	Amount	Cal.	Fat (g)	% Cal. Fat	Sat. Fat (g)	Chol. (mg)	Sod. (mg)	Carb. (g)	Fiber (g)	Pro. (g)	Servings/Exchanges
Tomato Florentine (large)	16 oz	122	2	15	1	5	2070	27	3	8	2 starch
Tomato Florentine (medium)	12 oz	90	2	20	1	5	1550	20	2	6	1 starch
Tomato Florentine (small)	8 oz	61	1	15	0.5	5	1030	13	2	4	1 starch
Vegetarian Chili (large)	16 oz	278	5	16	0.5	0	2150	53	4	13	3 1/2 starch, 1 lean meat
Vegetarian Chili (medium)	12 oz	210	4	17	0	0	1610	40	3	9	2 1/2 starch, 1 fat
✔Vegetarian Chili (small)	8 oz	139	2	13	0	0	1070	27	2	6	2 starch
SPREADS											
✔Lite Cream Cheese	2 oz/4 T	100	8	72	5	20	280	4	0	6	1 high-fat meat
✔Lite Honey Walnut Cream Cheese	2 oz/4 T	150	11	66	7	30	190	9	1	4	1/2 carb, 1 high-fat meat
✔Lite Raspberry Cream Cheese	2 oz/4 T	130	10	69	7	30	200	7	1	6	1/2 carb, 1 high-fat meat

✔ Lite Sun-Dried Tomato Cream Cheese	2 oz/4 T	120	8	60	5	20	320	6	0	6	1/2 carb, 1 high-fat meat
✔ Lite Vanilla Hazelnut Spread	2 oz/4 T	140	11	71	7	35	210	6	1	5	1/2 carb, 1 high-fat meat
✔ Plain Cream Cheese	2 oz/4 T	180	18	90	11	50	150	2	0	4	1 high-fat meat, 1 1/2 fat
✔ Veggie Lite Cream Cheese	2 oz/4 T	130	11	76	7	35	230	4	1	5	1 high-fat meat

STRUDEL DESSERTS

Apple	1	490	26	48	0	0	130	60	1	5	4 starch, 4 fat
Cherry	1	490	26	48	0	0	130	60	1	5	4 starch, 4 fat

WRAP SANDWICHES

Chicken Caesar	1	630	31	44	8	80	1140	46	2	38	3 starch, 3 lean meat, 4 fat
Fields & Feta	1	560	17	27	4	10	850	89	13	20	5 starch, 2 veg, 3 fat

(Continued)

✔ = Healthiest Bets; n/a = not available

WRAP SANDWICHES (*Continued*)	Amount	Cal.	Fat (g)	% Cal. Fat	Sat. Fat (g)	Chol. (mg)	Sod. (mg)	Carb. (g)	Fiber (g)	Pro. (g)	Servings/Exchanges
Honey Smoked Turkey	1	540	7	12	1.5	35	1520	89	12	38	6 starch, 3 very lean meat
Roast Beef & Brie	1	770	34	40	13	135	1270	63	6	48	4 starch, 5 lean meat, 4 fat
Southwestern Tuna	1	950	64	61	17	110	1230	53	4	41	3 1/2 starch, 4 lean meat, 10 fat

YOGURTS

	Amount	Cal.	Fat (g)	% Cal. Fat	Sat. Fat (g)	Chol. (mg)	Sod. (mg)	Carb. (g)	Fiber (g)	Pro. (g)	Servings/Exchanges
✓ Blueberry with Fresh Berries	8.5 oz	210	3	13	1	10	100	42	1	7	2 carb, 1 fruit
✓ Blueberry with Granola	8 oz	230	4	16	1.5	10	100	45	1	8	2 carb, 1 fruit, 1/2 fat
✓ Plain with Fresh Berries	8.5 oz	210	3	13	1	10	115	38	1	7	1 1/2 carb, 1 fruit
✓ Plain with Granola	8 oz	230	4	16	1.5	10	120	41	1	8	1 1/2 carb, 1 fruit, 1 fat
✓ Strawberry with Fresh Berries	8.5 oz	210	3	13	1	10	100	42	1	7	1 1/2 carb, 1 fruit
✓ Strawberry with Granola	8 oz	230	4	16	1.5	10	100	45	1	8	2 carb, 1 fruit

✓ = Healthiest Bets; n/a = not available

Blimpie Subs and Salads

❖Blimpie provides nutrition information for all of its menu items on their website at www.blimpie.com.

Light 'n Lean Choice

6″ Roast Beef Sub on Wheat

Calories......................390	Sodium (mg)..........1,380
Fat (g) 8	Carbohydrate (g).........45
% calories from fat..18	Fiber (g) 5
Saturated fat (g)........3	Protein (g) 37
Cholesterol (mg) 65	

Exchanges: 3 starch, 4 very lean meat

Healthy 'n Hearty Choice

6″ Ham & Swiss Sub on Wheat

Calories......................400	Sodium (mg)..........1,040
Fat (g) 14	Carbohydrate (g).........46
% calories from fat..31	Fiber (g) 5
Saturated fat (g)........7	Protein (g) 26
Cholesterol (mg) 50	

Exchanges: 3 starch, 2 medium-fat meat

(Continued)

Blimpie Subs and Salads

	Amount	Cal.	Fat (g)	% Cal. Fat	Sat. Fat (g)	Chol. (mg)	Sod. (mg)	Carb. (g)	Fiber (g)	Pro. (g)	Servings/Exchanges
BAKED GOODS											
✓Fudge Brownies	1	243	11	41	n/a	34	169	34	n/a	3	3 carb, 2 fat
White Roll Icing	1 oz	97	1	9	n/a	0	6	23	n/a	0	1 1/2 carb
COOKIES											
✓Chocolate Chunk Cookie	1	201	10	45	6	15	201	26	1	2	1 1/2 carb, 2 fat
✓Macadamia White Chunk	1	210	10	43	5	20	140	26	1	2	1 1/2 carb, 2 fat
✓Oatmeal Raisin	1	191	8	38	2	15	201	27	1	3	2 carb, 1 1/2 fat
Peanut Butter	1	221	12	49	5	15	201	27	1	4	2 carb, 2 fat
Sugar	1	330	17	46	4.5	30	290	24	0	3	1 1/2 carb, 3 fat
DESSERTS											
Chocolate Roll Icing	1 oz	97	1	9	n/a	0	27	22	n/a	0	1 1/2 carb

	Amount	Calories	Fat (g)	% Cal. Fat	Sat. Fat (g)	Chol. (mg)	Sod. (mg)	Carb. (g)	Fiber (g)	Prot. (g)	Servings/Exchanges
Cinnamon Roll	1	631	25	36	n/a	0	692	90	n/a	9	6 starch, 5 fat
✔ Donut	1	131	9	62	n/a	0	131	11	n/a	2	1/2 carb, 2 fat
DRESSINGS & SAUCES											
BLIMPIE Dressing	3/4 oz/1.5 T	120	8	60	1	0	570	16	1	1	1 carb, 1 1/2 fat
✔ BLIMPIE Special Sub Dressing	3/4 oz/1.5 T	70	7	90	1	0	0	0	0	0	1 fat
Blue Cheese	1 oz/2 T	220	24	98	4	40	440	2	0	2	5 fat
Buttermilk Ranch	1 oz/2 T	270	29	97	4	5	360	1	0	0	6 fat
✔ Fat Free Italian	1 oz/2 T	20	0	0	0	0	670	5	0	0	free
Guacamole	1 oz/2 T	194	18	84	2.7	1	468	7	1	2	1/2 carb, 3 1/2 fat
Honey French	1 oz/2 T	240	20	75	3	0	350	16	0	0	1 carb, 4 fat
✔ Light Buttermilk Ranch	1.5 oz/3 T	90	5	50	1	0	350	10	0	1	1/2 carb, 1 fat
✔ Light Italian	1.5 oz/3 T	20	1	45	0	0	810	3	0	0	free

✔ = Healthiest Bets; n/a = not available

(Continued)

DRESSINGS & SAUCES (*Continued*)	Amount	Cal.	Fat (g)	% Cal. Fat	Sat. Fat (g)	Chol. (mg)	Sod. (mg)	Carb. (g)	Fiber (g)	Pro. (g)	Servings/Exchanges
Mayonnaise	1 T	100	11	99	1.5	10	60	1	0	0	2 fat
Thousand Island	1 oz/2 T	210	21	90	3	25	360	7	0	0	4 fat
MUFFIN											
Banana Nut	1	472	23	44	n/a	55	442	55	n/a	8	3 1/2 starch, 4 1/2 fat
Blueberry	1	412	18	39	n/a	55	452	55	n/a	7	3 1/2 starch, 3 1/2 fat
Bran & Raisin	1	442	18	37	n/a	20	502	64	n/a	7	4 starch, 3 1/2 fat
POTATO CHIPS											
✓Blimpie Jalapeno	1	210	11	47	2	5	250	25	1	2	1 1/2 starch, 2 fat
✓Blimpie Lea & Perrins	1	210	10	43	2	0	270	25	2	3	1 1/2 starch, 2 fat
✓Blimpie Regular Flavored	1	210	11	47	2	0	190	25	2	3	1 1/2 starch, 2 fat
✓Blimpie Zesty	1	210	11	47	2	5	220	25	2	3	1 1/2 starch, 2 fat
✓Blimpie Cheddar & Sour Cream	1	210	11	47	2	5	220	25	1	3	1 1/2 starch, 2 fat

SALADS

	Amount	Cal.	Fat (g)	% Cal. Fat	Sat. Fat (g)	Chol. (mg)	Sod. (mg)	Carb. (g)	Fiber (g)	Prot. (g)	Exchanges/Choices
✔Club	1	130	6	42	3	30	450	7	3	14	1 veg, 2 lean meat
Grilled Chicken Salad	1	350	12	31	0	140	1190	13	0	47	2 veg, 6 very lean meat, 2 fat
✔Ham & Swiss Cheese	1	170	8	42	6	40	500	7	3	16	1/2 carb, 2 lean meat
✔Italian Pasta Supreme	1	180	7	35	1	0	840	20	1	3	1 starch, 1 fat
Macaroni	2/3 cup	360	25	63	4	10	660	25	1	4	1 1/2 starch, 5 fat
✔Mustard Potato	2/3 cup	160	5	28	1	5	660	21	1	2	1 1/2 starch, 1 fat
Potato	2/3 cup	270	19	63	3	10	560	19	1	2	1 starch, 4 fat
✔Roast Beef	1	120	3	23	1.5	25	480	8	3	19	1/2 carb, 3 very lean meat
✔Tossed Green	1	35	1	26	0	0	20	7	3	2	1 veg
✔Tuna	1	130	2	14	0	45	400	7	3	22	1/2 carb, 3 very lean meat
✔Turkey	1	90	1	10	0	25	580	8	3	15	1/2 carb, 2 very lean meat

✔ = Healthiest Bets; n/a = not available

(Continued)

	Amount	Cal.	Fat (g)	% Cal. Fat	Sat. Fat (g)	Chol. (mg)	Sod. (mg)	Carb. (g)	Fiber (g)	Pro. (g)	Servings/Exchanges
SIDES											
Antipasto Salad	1	200	11	50	5	50	950	9	3	19	2 veg, 2 medium-fat meat
✔Chef Salad	1	150	6	36	3	40	600	8	3	17	2 veg, 2 lean meat
Cole Slaw	1/2 cup	180	13	65	2	5	280	13	1	1	1 veg, 2 1/2 fat
SOUPS											
Chicken Noodle	1 cup	140	3	19	1	30	1190	20	2	8	1 starch, 1 lean meat
Chicken w/White & Wild Rice	1 cup	230	12	47	2	30	1210	21	2	10	1 1/2 starch, 1 lean meat, 2 fat
✔Classic Chili w/Beans & Beef	1 cup	240	8	30	3.5	40	1060	27	10	14	2 starch, 1 lean meat, 1 fat
✔Cream of Potato	1 cup	190	9	43	2.5	5	860	24	3	5	1 1/2 starch, 2 fat
6" SUBS											
Blimpie Best on White	1	410	13	29	5	50	1480	47	4	39	3 starch, 4 lean meat

Blimpie's Best on Wheat	1	410	13	29	5	50	1480	47	4	39	3 starch, 4 lean meat
Cheese Trio on Wheat	1	490	23	42	12	55	1110	55	5	26	3 1/2 starch, 2 lean meat
Cheese Trio on White	1	490	23	42	12	55	1130	48	3	25	3 starch, 2 high-fat meat, 1/2 fat
Chik Max on Wheat	1	495	13	24	1	0	1370	69	4	26	4 1/2 starch, 2 medium-fat meat, 1/2 fat
Chik Max on White	1	483	12	22	1	0	1293	70	4	34	4 1/2 starch, 3 lean meat, 1/2 fat
Club on Wheat	1	370	11	27	4.5	30	1180	48	5	23	3 starch, 2 medium-fat meat
Club on White	1	370	10	24	4.5	30	1200	48	3	23	3 starch, 3 medium-fat meat
✓ Grille Max on Wheat	1	425	7	15	1	5	900	71	5	18	4 1/2 starch, 1 medium-fat meat

(Continued)

✓ = Healthiest Bets; n/a = not available

6" SUBS (*Continued*)	Amount	Cal.	Fat (g)	% Cal. Fat	Sat. Fat (g)	Chol. (mg)	Sod. (mg)	Carb. (g)	Fiber (g)	Pro. (g)	Servings/Exchanges
✔Grille Max on White	1	413	6	13	1	5	823	72	5	18	4 1/2 starch, 1 medium-fat meat
✔Grilled Chicken	1	400	9	20	11	30	950	52	2	28	3 1/2 starch, 3 lean meat
✔Ham & Swiss on Wheat	1	400	14	32	7	50	1040	46	5	26	3 starch, 2 medium-fat meat, 1 fat
✔Ham & Swiss on White	1	410	14	31	7	48	1050	48	3	25	3 starch, 2 medium-fat meat, 1 fat
Ham, Salami & Provolone on Wheat	1	450	20	40	8	55	1350	47	5	24	3 starch, 2 medium-fat meat, 2 fat
Ham, Salami, Provolone on White	1	480	20	38	8	55	1370	49	3	24	3 starch, 3 medium-fat meat, 1 fat
Italian Meatball	1	500	22	40	8	25	970	52	2	23	3 1/2 starch, 2 medium-fat meat, 2 fat

✔ Mexi Max on Wheat	1	405	6	13	1	0	1080	65	5	25	4 starch, 2 lean meat
✔ Mexi Max on White	1	393	5	11	1	0	1003	66	5	25	4 starch, 2 lean meat
Roast Beef	1	390	7	16	3	65	1370	47	3	27	3 starch, 3 very lean meat
Roast Beef on Wheat	1	390	8	18	3	65	1380	45	5	37	3 starch, 4 very lean meat
Roast Turkey Cordon Bleu	1	430	7	15	1	0	1293	43	1	29	3 starch, 2 lean meat
Smokey Cheddar Roast Beef Melt	1	380	12	28	6	50	1200	42	1	23	3 starch, 2 lean meat, 1 fat
Steak & Cheese	1	550	26	43	4	70	1080	51	2	27	3 1/2 starch, 3 medium-fat meat, 3 fat
Tuna on Wheat	1	650	45	62	6	55	860	49	5	18	3 starch, 2 lean meat, 8 fat
Tuna on White	1	660	44	60	8	55	880	51	3	18	3 starch, 2 lean meat, 8 fat
Turkey on Wheat	1	330	7	19	1.5	0	1190	48	5	19	4 starch, 2 lean meat
Turkey on White	1	330	6	16	1.5	0	1200	48	3	19	3 starch, 2 lean meat

(Continued)

✔ = Healthiest Bets; n/a = not available

6" SUBS (Continued)	Amount	Cal.	Fat (g)	% Cal. Fat	Sat. Fat (g)	Chol. (mg)	Sod. (mg)	Carb. (g)	Fiber (g)	Pro. (g)	Servings/Exchanges
✔Vegi Max on Wheat	1	415	8	17	0.5	0	1050	60	5	24	4 starch, 2 lean meat
✔Vegi Max on White	1	403	7	16	0.5	0	980	61	5	24	4 starch, 2 lean meat
WRAPS											
Chicken Caesar	1	610	31	46	6	35	1770	56	3	26	3 1/2 starch, 2 lean meat, 5 fat
Southwestern	1	590	28	43	7	75	1990	56	3	28	3 1/2 starch, 2 lean meat, 4 fat
Zesty Italian Wrap	1	530	22	37	7	45	1850	59	3	24	3 1/2 starch, 2 lean meat, 3 fat

✔ = Healthiest Bets; n/a = not available

Jamba Juice

❖Jamba Juice provides nutrition information for their drinks on their website at www.jambajuice.com. They provided additional information for this book.

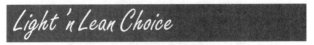

Light 'n Lean Choice

Mama's Minestrone Soup (*16 oz*)
Sunny Tomato & Herb Bread (*1 serving*)

Calories 460	Sodium (mg) 1,920
Fat (g) 11	Carbohydrate (g).........71
% calories from fat..22	Fiber (g) 7
Saturated fat (g)........2	Protein (g) 16
Cholesterol (mg) 5	

Exchanges: 4 1/2 starch, 2 fat

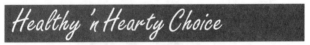

Healthy 'n Hearty Choice

Bistro Lentil Soup (*16 oz*)
Pizza Protein Bread (*1 serving*)
1/2 Orange Berry Blitz

Calories......................605	Sodium (mg) 1,640
Fat (g) 7	Carbohydrate (g).......119
% calories from fat..10	Fiber (g) 16
Saturated fat (g)........2	Protein (g) 24
Cholesterol (mg) 5	

Exchanges: 4 1/2 starch, 3 carb, 1 very lean meat

(*Continued*)

Jamba Juice

	Amount	Cal.	Fat (g)	% Cal. Fat	Sat. Fat (g)	Chol. (mg)	Sod. (mg)	Carb. (g)	Fiber (g)	Pro. (g)	Servings/Exchanges
BREADS											
✓Lively Lemon Poppyseed	1 slice	230	6	23	2	0	190	40	1	5	2 1/2 starch, 1 fat
✓Mind Over Blueberry	1 slice	250	5	18	1	5	310	45	3	6	3 starch, 1 fat
✓Pizza Protein	1 slice	230	6	23	1.5	5	450	33	2	9	2 starch, 1 fat
✓Sunny Tomato & Herb	1 slice	230	6	23	1.5	5	580	32	2	8	2 starch, 1 fat
FLAVORFUL FRUIT SMOOTHIES											
Aloha Pineapple	24 oz	470	2	4	n/a	n/a	n/a	89	5	7	6 carb
Banana Berry	24 oz	470	2	4	n/a	n/a	n/a	102	6	21	6 1/2 carb
Berry Lime Sublime	24 oz	450	2	4	n/a	n/a	n/a	104	6	3	6 1/2 carb
Caribbean Passion	24 oz	440	2	4	n/a	n/a	n/a	102	4	4	6 1/2 carb
Citrus Squeeze	24 oz	450	2	4	n/a	n/a	n/a	93	5	4	6 carb

Cranberry Craze	24 oz	420	2	4	n/a	n/a	97	4	6	6 1/2 carb
Mango-A-Go-Go	24 oz	500	2	4	n/a	n/a	117	4	4	7 1/2 carb
Orange Berry Blitz	24 oz	410	3	7	n/a	n/a	94	5	5	5 carb
Orange-A-Peel	24 oz	440	1	2	n/a	n/a	102	5	9	6 1/2 carb
Peach Pleasure	24 oz	460	2	4	n/a	n/a	108	5	4	6 1/2 carb
Peenya Kowlada	24 oz	650	5	7	n/a	n/a	118	3	8	8 carb
Razzmatazz	24 oz	480	2	4	n/a	n/a	112	4	3	7 1/2 carb
Strawberries Wild	24 oz	450	0	0	n/a	n/a	105	4	6	7 carb

MOO'D SMOOTHIES

Chocolate Moo'd	24 oz	690	8	10	n/a	n/a	141	2	16	9 1/2 carb
Peanut Butter Moo'd	24 oz	840	22	24	n/a	n/a	139	5	23	9 1/2 carb, 1 high-fat meat

POWER SMOOTHIES

Kiwi Berry Burner	24 oz	470	0	0	n/a	n/a	112	5	4	7 1/2 carb

✔ = Healthiest Bets; n/a = not available

(Continued)

POWER SMOOTHIES (*Continued*)	Amount	Cal.	Fat (g)	% Cal. Fat	Sat. Fat (g)	Chol. (mg)	Sod. (mg)	Carb. (g)	Fiber (g)	Pro. (g)	Servings/Exchanges
Protein Berry Pizzazz	24 oz	490	2	4	n/a	n/a	n/a	102	6	21	7 carb, 1 very lean meat
The Coldbuster	24 oz	430	2.5	5	n/a	n/a	n/a	100	5	5	6 1/2 carb
The Jamba Powerboost	24 oz	440	1.5	3	n/a	n/a	n/a	103	7	6	6 1/2 carb
SOUPS											
Beyond Broccoli	16 oz	220	8	33	2.5	10	1590	27	6	8	1 starch, 2 veg, 1 1/2 fat
Bistro Lentil	16 oz	170	1	5	0	0	1190	39	12	12	2 starch, 1 very lean meat
Chicken Noodle	16 oz	140	4	26	3	25	1280	16	4	7	2 starch, 1 lean meat
Dill-icious Creamy Potato	16 oz	190	7	33	4	20	1450	26	2	8	1 1/2 starch, 1 fat
Mama's Minestrone	16 oz	230	5	20	0	0	1340	39	5	8	2 starch, 1 veg, 1 fat
Santa Fe Corn	16 oz	270	9	30	5	5	1220	46	6	8	3 starch, 1 fat

✔ = Healthiest Bets; n/a = not available

Panera Bread

❖Panera Bread provided complete nutrition
information for use in this book. Their website is
www.panerabread.com.

Light 'n Lean Choice

Strawberry Poppyseed Salad with Fat Free Poppyseed Dressing *(2 T)*
Santa Fe Roasted Corn Soup

Calories 420	Sodium (mg) 965
Fat (g) 11	Carbohydrate (g).........79
% calories from fat..24	Fiber (g) 11
Saturated fat (g)........1	Protein (g) 7
Cholesterol (mg) 0	

Exchanges: 1 1/2 starch, 1 carb, 2 veg, 2 fruit, 1 fat

Healthy 'n Hearty Choice

Savory Vegetable Bean Soup
1/2 Festiago Chicken Sandwich
1/2 Nutty Oatmeal Raisin Cookie

Calories......................655	Sodium (mg) 1,430
Fat (g) 22	Carbohydrate (g).........70
% calories from fat..30	Fiber (g) 7
Saturated fat (g)........8	Protein (g) 41
Cholesterol (mg) 87	

Exchanges: 3 starch, 1 1/2 carb, 4 lean meat, 2 fat

(Continued)

Panera Bread

BAGELS

	Amount	Cal.	Fat (g)	% Cal. Fat	Sat. Fat (g)	Chol. (mg)	Sod. (mg)	Carb. (g)	Fiber (g)	Pro. (g)	Servings/Exchanges
✔ Asiago Cheese	1	330	5	14	3	15	470	57	2	15	3 1/2 starch, 1 fat
✔ Blueberry	1	330	1	3	0	0	490	69	3	12	4 starch
Choc-o-Nut	1	310	13	38	1.5	0	1040	41	4	7	2 1/2 starch, 2 fat
✔ Cinnamon Crunch	1	510	9	16	5	0	520	95	3	12	6 starch, 1 fat
✔ Cranberry Walnut	1	350	5	13	0	0	540	65	4	12	4 starch, 1 fat
✔ Dutch Apple	1	350	3	8	0	0	430	73	3	10	5 starch
✔ Everything	1	300	2	6	0	0	550	60	3	12	4 starch
✔ French Toast	1	380	5	12	1	5	850	73	3	11	4 1/2 starch, 1/2 fat
Morning Glory	1	380	7	17	2.5	10	1640	71	3	11	4 1/2 starch, 1 fat

✔Multigrain	1	290	2	6	0	0	400	60	3	12	4 starch
✔Peanut Butter Banana Crunch	1	390	6	14	3	0	460	76	3	11	5 starch
✔Plain	1	290	1	3	0	0	460	59	2	11	4 starch
✔Sesame Seed	1	300	2	6	0	0	460	61	4	12	4 starch
✔Spinach Parmesan	1	320	3	8	1.5	5	560	60	3	15	4 starch
✔Trail Mix	1	380	6	14	3	0	560	71	3	11	4 1/2 starch, 1 fat
BAGUETTES											
✔Artisan French	1	120	0	0	0	0	340	25	1	5	1 1/2 starch
✔Fiesta Mini	1	130	2	14	1	5	310	24	1	6	1 1/2 starch
✔French	1	140	1	6	0	0	290	26	1	6	1 1/2 starch
✔Olive Mini	1	140	3	19	0	0	330	26	2	5	1 1/2 starch, 1/2 fat
✔Pesto Mini	1	130	1	7	0	0	250	26	1	5	1 1/2 starch
✔Sourdough	1	130	0	0	0	0	280	27	1	5	2 starch

(Continued)

✔ = Healthiest Bets; n/a = not available

BAGUETTES (Continued)	Amount	Cal.	Fat (g)	% Cal. Fat	Sat. Fat (g)	Chol. (mg)	Sod. (mg)	Carb. (g)	Fiber (g)	Pro. (g)	Servings/Exchanges
✓Sourdough Mini	1	130	0	0	0	0	280	27	1	5	2 starch
✓Sun-Dried Tomato Mini	1	130	0	0	0	0	270	27	1	5	2 starch
✓Three Seed	1	150	3	18	0	0	260	25	2	6	1 1/2 starch, 1/2 fat
BEVERAGES											
I.C. Java	20 oz	340	16	42	10	50	75	44	0	4	3 carb, 3 fat
I.C. Java	16 oz	270	13	43	8	40	55	35	0	3	2 carb, 2 fat
I.C. Java	12 oz	200	10	45	6	30	45	27	0	3	2 carb, 2 fat
I.C. Mocha	12 oz	240	10	38	6	30	50	35	0	3	2 carb, 2 fat
I.C. Mocha	16 oz	320	13	37	8	40	65	48	0	4	2 carb, 2 fat
I.C. Spice	12 oz	270	10	33	6	30	40	43	0	3	3 carb, 1 fat
I.C. Spice	16 oz	350	13	33	8	40	55	58	0	3	4 carb, 2 fat
I.C. Spice	20 oz	420	16	34	10	50	70	67	0	4	4 carb, 3 fat

Mocha Blast	12 oz	240	9	34	5	30	160	31	0	9	2 carb, 2 fat
Mocha Blast	16 oz	270	10	33	6	35	190	37	0	11	2 1/2 carb, 2 fat
Mocha Blast	20 oz	310	11	32	7	40	210	42	1	12	3 carb, 2 fat
BISCOTTI											
✔Caffe Crunch	1	170	9	48	3	35	30	21	2	4	1 1/2 starch, 1 fat
✔Honey Sesame	1	160	5	28	2.5	30	40	25	2	4	1 1/2 starch, 1 fat
BREAD BOWLS											
✔Sourdough	1	540	2	3	0	0	1160	110	5	21	7 starch
BREADS											
✔Artisan Cheese Demi Loaf	1 slice	130	2	14	1	5	270	23	1	6	1 1/2 starch
✔Artisan Cheese Loaf	1 slice	130	2	14	1	5	270	23	1	6	1 1/2 starch
✔Artisan Country Demi Loaf	1 slice	120	0	0	0	0	290	25	1	5	1 1/2 starch
✔Artisan Country Loaf	1 slice	120	0	0	0	0	290	25	1	5	1 1/2 starch

(Continued)

✔ = Healthiest Bets; n/a = not available

BREADS (*Continued*)	Amount	Cal.	Fat (g)	% Cal. Fat	Sat. Fat (g)	Chol. (mg)	Sod. (mg)	Carb. (g)	Fiber (g)	Pro. (g)	Servings/Exchanges
✔ Artisan Olive Demi Loaf	1 slice	140	2	13	0	0	270	26	1	5	1 1/2 starch
✔ Artisan Raisin Pecan Loaf	1 slice	140	3	19	0	0	280	26	1	4	1 1/2 starch, 1/2 fat
✔ Artisan Semolina Demi Loaf	1 slice	140	2	13	0	0	300	26	3	5	1 1/2 starch
✔ Artisan Three Seed	1 slice	140	3	19	0	0	270	24	2	5	1 1/2 starch, 1/2 fat
✔ Artisan Walnut Demi Loaf	1 slice	150	4	24	0	0	260	24	1	5	1 1/2 starch, 1 fat
✔ Artisan Walnut Loaf	1 slice	150	4	24	0	0	260	24	1	5	1 1/2 starch, 1 fat
✔ Asiago Loaf	1 piece	150	4	24	2	10	360	21	0	7	1 1/2 starch, 1 fat
✔ Asiago Mini	1 piece	150	4	24	2	10	360	21	0	7	1 1/2 starch, 1 fat
✔ Braided Challah	1 piece	160	3	17	0.5	40	280	28	1	6	2 starch, 1/2 fat
✔ Cinnamon Raisin	1 slice	160	2	11	0	5	220	33	1	5	2 starch
✔ French Loaf	1 slice	130	1	7	0	0	290	26	1	6	1 1/2 starch
✔ French Strip	1 slice	130	1	7	0	0	290	26	1	6	1 1/2 starch

✔ Hearty Grain	1 slice	150	3	18	0	0	200	28	3	6	2 starch
✔ Honey Wheat	1 slice	130	2	14	0	0	370	25	2	5	1 1/2 starch
✔ Large Pumpernickel Loaf	1 slice	150	2	12	0	0	160	28	2	6	2 starch
✔ Nine Grain	1 slice	140	2	13	0	0	300	27	2	6	2 starch
✔ Pumpernickel Loaf	1 slice	140	2	13	0.5	0	150	25	2	6	1 1/2 starch
✔ Rye Loaf	1 slice	130	2	14	0	0	330	25	2	5	1 1/2 starch
✔ Sourdough Loaf	1 slice	130	0	0	0	0	280	27	1	5	2 starch
✔ Sourdough Round	1 slice	130	0	0	0	0	280	27	1	5	2 starch
✔ Swirl Rye	1 slice	140	2	13	0	0	250	26	2	6	1 1/2 starch
✔ Tomato Basil	1 slice	130	1	7	0	0	360	27	1	5	2 starch
✔ XL French Loaf	1 slice	130	1	7	0	0	290	26	1	6	1 1/2 starch
✔ XL Rye Loaf	1 slice	150	2	12	0.5	0	370	28	3	6	2 starch
✔ XL Sourdough	1 slice	130	0	0	0	0	280	27	1	5	2 starch

(Continued)

✔ = Healthiest Bets; n/a = not available

	Amount	Cal.	Fat (g)	% Cal. Fat	Sat. Fat (g)	Chol. (mg)	Sod. (mg)	Carb. (g)	Fiber (g)	Pro. (g)	Servings/Exchanges
BREAKFAST SWEETS											
Bear Claw	1	460	22	43	7	45	380	58	4	12	4 starch, 3 fat
Cinnamon Roll	1	630	25	36	11	90	560	90	3	13	4 starch, 2 carb, 3 1/2 fat
✔ Coffee Cake	1	190	7	33	3	20	180	28	0	4	2 starch, 1 fat
Pecan Roll	1	540	26	43	4	30	270	68	3	8	4 1/2 starch, 4 fat
COOKIES											
Chocolate Chipper	1	410	22	48	14	60	320	53	1	4	3 1/2 carb, 3 fat
Chocolate Duet with Walnuts	1	380	21	50	11	50	270	47	2	5	3 carb, 3 fat
Nutty Chocolate Chipper	1	440	25	51	13	55	290	49	2	5	3 carb, 4 fat
Nutty Oatmeal Raisin	1	370	15	36	8	45	280	55	3	5	3 1/2 carb, 2 fat
Shortbread	1	390	25	58	17	65	200	39	0	4	2 1/2 carb, 4 fat

CROISSANTS

	Amount	Cal	Fat (g)	% Cal Fat	Sat Fat (g)	Chol (mg)	Sod (mg)	Carb (g)	Fiber (g)	Prot (g)	Exchanges/Choices
Apple	1	340	13	34	9	35	250	53	1	5	3 1/2 starch, 1 1/2 fat
Butter	1	310	17	49	12	45	260	33	1	6	2 starch, 3 fat
Cheese	1	360	19	48	13	50	300	42	1	6	3 starch, 3 fat
Chocolate	1	450	25	50	16	35	220	57	4	7	2 starch, 2 carb, 3 fat
Raspberry Cheese	1	320	15	42	10	40	250	43	1	6	2 starch, 1 carb, 2 fat

DANISHES

	Amount	Cal	Fat (g)	% Cal Fat	Sat Fat (g)	Chol (mg)	Sod (mg)	Carb (g)	Fiber (g)	Prot (g)	Exchanges/Choices
Apple	1	480	14	26	5	40	410	83	2	9	3 1/2 starch, 2 carb, 2 fat
Cheese	1	520	17	29	7	45	360	89	2	8	3 starch, 2 carb, 3 fat
Cherry	1	440	13	27	5	40	380	73	2	9	3 starch, 2 carb, 1 fat
German Chocolate	1	580	24	37	10	35	480	85	4	9	3 1/2 starch, 2 carb, 3 fat
Gooey Butter	1	600	22	33	9	45	430	92	2	10	3 starch, 3 carb, 3 fat

✔ = Healthiest Bets; n/a = not available

(Continued)

DANISHES (*Continued*)	Amount	Cal.	Fat (g)	% Cal. Fat	Sat. Fat (g)	Chol. (mg)	Sod. (mg)	Carb. (g)	Fiber (g)	Pro. (g)	Servings/Exchanges
Peach	1	450	13	26	5	40	360	78	2	8	3 starch, 2 carb, 1 fat
FOCACCIA											
✔Asiago	1 piece	160	6	34	2	5	340	20	1	6	1 1/2 starch, 1 fat
✔Rosemary & Onion	1 piece	140	5	32	1.5	5	290	20	1	5	1 starch, 1 fat
MUFFIES											
Banana Nut	1	290	14	43	2	20	290	36	2	6	2 1/2 starch, 2 fat
Chocolate Chip	1	270	11	37	3.5	20	280	40	1	4	2 1/2 starch, 2 fat
✔Pumpkin	1	270	9	30	1	20	260	41	1	3	2 1/2 starch, 2 fat
MUFFINS											
Blueberry	1	450	16	32	2.5	45	600	70	3	8	4 1/2 starch, 2 fat
Chocolate Chip	1	560	23	37	7	45	580	83	3	9	5 1/2 starch, 3 fat
✔Cobblestone	1	530	7	12	1.5	15	650	106	4	13	4 starch, 3 carb

✔Low Fat Tripleberry	1	320	4	11	0.5	30	310	67	3	7	4 starch
Pumpkin	1	550	19	31	2	50	550	85	2	6	5 1/2 starh, 2 fat
PANINI										
Cuban Pork & Ham	1	820	48	53	8	115	2590	71	4	37	4 1/2 starch, 3 lean meat, 6 fat
Frontega Chicken	1	860	47	49	10	95	1800	82	5	50	5 1/2 starch, 5 lean meat, 3 fat
Portobello & Mozzarella	1	620	35	51	10	40	1120	73	8	25	4 starch, 2 veg, 1 high-fat meat, 3 fat
ROLLS										
✔Combo	1	340	2	5	0	0	730	65	3	14	4 starch
✔French	1	160	1	6	0	0	340	30	1	7	2 starch

✔ = Healthiest Bets; n/a = not available

(Continued)

	Amount	Cal.	Fat (g)	% Cal. Fat	Sat. Fat (g)	Chol. (mg)	Sod. (mg)	Carb. (g)	Fiber (g)	Pro. (g)	Servings/Exchanges
✓Sourdough	1	170	1	5	0	0	360	34	1	6	2 starch
SALAD DRESSINGS											
✓Caesar	2 oz/4 T	160	15	84	1.5	90	380	0	0	0	3 1/2 fat
✓Fat Free Poppyseed	1 oz/2 T	40	0	0	0	0	95	11	0	0	1/2 carb
✓Fat Free Raspberry Vinaigrette	2 oz/4 T	45	0	0	0	0	85	10	1	0	1/2 carb
Greek	1 oz/2 T	140	16	103	2	0	280	0	0	0	3 fat
SALADS											
✓Asian Sesame Chicken	1	400	15	34	1.5	60	1070	43	4	26	2 starch, 3 veg, 2 very lean meat, 2 fat
Caesar	1	380	25	59	7	110	850	22	3	14	1 starch, 2 veg, 1 high-fat meat, 3 fat

Classic Café	1	400	36	81	5	0	340	12	4	5	2 veg, 8 fats
Fandango	1	400	28	63	7	25	410	23	7	13	3 veg, 1/2 carb, 1 high-fat meat, 4 fat
Greek	1	480	45	84	8	10	1850	15	5	9	3 veg, 9 fat
✓Strawberry Poppyseed	1	240	7	26	0.5	0	200	46	8	4	3 veg, 2 fruit, 1 fat
Tomato & Fresh Mozzarella	1	880	59	60	20	90	980	69	5	33	4 starch, 2 veg, 2 high-fat meat, 7 fat
SANDWICHES											
Asiago Roast Beef	1	730	35	43	14	110	1480	54	2	52	3 starch, 1 veg, 6 lean meat, 3 fat
Bacon Turkey Bravo	1	860	34	36	13	100	3320	84	5	56	5 starch, 1 veg, 5 lean meat, 3 fat

(Continued)

✓ = Healthiest Bets; n/a = not available

SANDWICHES (*Continued*)	Amount	Cal.	Fat (g)	% Cal. Fat	Sat. Fat (g)	Chol. (mg)	Sod. (mg)	Carb. (g)	Fiber (g)	Pro. (g)	Servings/Exchanges
Chicken Salad	1	480	24	45	2.5	75	1060	37	4	32	2 starch, 1 veg, 3 lean meat, 3 fat
Festiago Chicken	1	700	24	31	7	130	950	53	2	68	3 starch, 1 veg, 8 lean meat
Ham & Cheese	1	640	33	46	11	105	1130	46	6	44	3 starch, 1 veg, 5 lean meat, 2 fat
Italian Combo	1	760	44	52	6	25	1850	63	5	31	4 starch, 1 veg, 3 medium-fat meat, 4 fat
✔Peanut Butter & Jelly	1	440	16	33	3	0	580	64	3	16	4 starch, 1 high-fat meat
Sierra Turkey	1	760	44	52	3.5	75	2060	68	4	43	4 starch, 1 veg, 4 very lean meat, 6 fat
✔Smoked Turkey	1	460	15	29	0.5	40	1870	46	4	35	3 starch, 4 very lean meat, 2 fat

Tuna Salad	1	760	44	52	6	25	1850	63	5	31	4 starch, 1 veg, 3 lean meat, 6 fat
Tuscan Chicken	1	950	57	54	8	100	1560	82	5	45	5 starch, 1 veg, 4 lean meat, 7 fat
✔Veggie	1	440	16	33	8	35	1140	56	5	17	3 1/2 starch, 1 high-fat meat, 1 fat
SCONES										
Buttermilk with Orange Glaze	1	430	12	25	7	70	190	75	0	7	3 starch, 2 carb, 1 fat
Cinnamon Walnut	1	470	22	42	9	65	170	62	2	8	3 starch, 1 carb, 3 fat
Cranberry Hazelnut	1	440	17	35	8	65	170	63	3	8	3 starch, 1 carb, 3 fat
Lemon Poppyseed	1	410	14	31	8	70	180	64	1	8	3 starch, 1 carb, 2 fat
SOUPS										
Baked Potato	8 oz	240	15	56	6	25	910	20	1	6	1 starch, 4 fat

(Continued)

✔ = Healthiest Bets; n/a = not available

SOUPS *(Continued)*	Amount	Cal.	Fat (g)	% Cal. Fat	Sat. Fat (g)	Chol. (mg)	Sod. (mg)	Carb. (g)	Fiber (g)	Pro. (g)	Servings/Exchanges
Boston Clam Chowder	8 oz	210	12	51	7	45	980	19	1	7	1 starch, 1 very lean meat, 2 fat
Broccoli Cheddar	8 oz	220	17	70	10	55	980	13	1	8	1/2 starch, 1 veg, 3 1/2 fat
✓ Chicken Chili	8 oz	180	6	30	3	20	980	24	9	9	1 1/2 starch, 1 lean meat
✓ Chicken Noodle	8 oz	110	3	25	0.5	20	970	15	1	7	1 starch, 1 lean meat
✓ Corn & Green Chile Chowder	8 oz	190	8	38	3	15	720	25	3	6	1 1/2 starch, 2 fat
Cream of Chicken and Wild Rice	8 oz	210	13	56	7	50	880	18	0	7	1 starch, 1 very lean meat, 2 fat
Creamy Country Asparagus	8 oz	180	13	65	8	40	1100	13	2	3	1/2 starch, 1 veg, 3 fat
Fire Roasted Vegetable Bisque	8 oz	180	11	55	6	30	990	16	2	4	1 starch, 2 fat
✓ Forest Mushroom	8 oz	140	8	51	3.5	15	660	14	2	4	1 starch, 1 fat

French Onion	9 oz	180	11	55	7	35	1530	10	1	9	2 veg, 1 high-fat meat, 1/2 fat
✔Garden Vegetable	8 oz	100	1	9	0	0	740	20	3	4	1 starch, 1 veg
✔Mesa Bean & Vegetable	8 oz	100	1	9	0	0	710	18	3	4	1 starch
✔Potato Cream Cheese	8 oz	190	10	47	1	5	910	21	1	5	1 1/2 starch, 2 fat
✔Santa Fe Roasted Corn	8 oz	140	4	26	0	0	670	22	3	3	1 1/2 starch, 1 fat
✔Savory Vegetable Bean	8 oz	120	2	15	0	0	760	21	4	5	1 1/2 starch
✔Sirloin Steak Vegetable	8 oz	100	2	18	0.5	5	1140	16	2	5	1 starch
✔Tomato Mushroom & Barley	8 oz	110	2	16	0	0	810	21	4	4	1 1/2 starch
✔Vegetarian Black Bean	8 oz	180	1	5	0	0	800	32	17	11	2 starch
✔Vegetarian Lentil	8 oz	120	1	8	0	0	850	20	7	7	1 starch, 1/2 very lean meat

SPREADS

✔Plain Cream Cheese	2 oz/4 T	190	18	85	12	55	210	2	0	3	4 fat

✔ = Healthiest Bets; n/a = not available

(Continued)

SPREADS *(Continued)*	Amount	Cal.	Fat (g)	% Cal. Fat	Sat. Fat (g)	Chol. (mg)	Sod. (mg)	Carb. (g)	Fiber (g)	Pro. (g)	Servings/Exchanges
✔Reduced Fat Hazelnut Cream Cheese	2 oz/4 T	150	11	66	7	35	210	5	1	5	1 high-fat meat
✔Reduced Fat Honey Walnut Cream Cheese	2 oz/4 T	150	11	66	7	30	190	9	0	4	1 high-fat meat
✔Reduced Fat Plain Cream Cheese	2 oz/4 T	130	12	83	8	35	230	2	0	5	1 high-fat meat
✔Reduced Fat Raspberry Cream Cheese	2 oz/4 T	130	10	69	7	30	200	7	0	4	1/2 carb, 1 high-fat meat
✔Reduced Fat Salmon Cream Cheese	2 oz/4 T	120	10	75	6	30	270	2	0	6	1 high-fat meat

✔Reduced Fat Sundried Tomato Cream Cheese	2 oz/4 T	130	11	76	8	35	230	2	0	5	1 high-fat meat
✔Reduced Fat Veggie Cream Cheese	2 oz/4 T	130	11	76	7	35	230	4	1	5	1 high-fat meat
✔Roasted Garlic Hummus	2 T	45	3	60	0	0	95	4	2	0	1 fat

✔ = Healthiest Bets; n/a = not available

Schlotsky's Deli

❖Schlotsky's Deli provides nutrition information for all of its menu items on their website at www.schlotskys.com or www.cooldeli.com.

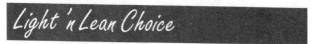
Light 'n Lean Choice

Santa Fe Chicken Sandwich (*small*)

Calories 431	Sodium (mg) 1,547
Fat (g) 13	Carbohydrate (g).........52
% calories from fat..27	Fiber (g) 3
Saturated fat (g)........6	Protein (g) 29
Cholesterol (mg) 72	

Exchanges: 3 starch, 1 veg, 3 lean meat

Healthy 'n Hearty Choice

Vegetable Club (*regular*)

Calories......................584	Sodium (mg) 1,435
Fat (g) 24	Carbohydrate (g).........76
% calories from fat..37	Fiber (g) 5
Saturated fat (g)........7	Protein (g) 19
Cholesterol (mg) 24	

Exchanges: 4 1/2 starch, 2 veg, 1 high fat meat, 2 fat

Schlotsky's Deli

	Amount	Cal.	Fat (g)	% Cal. Fat	Sat. Fat (g)	Chol. (mg)	Sod. (mg)	Carb. (g)	Fiber (g)	Pro. (g)	Servings/Exchanges
LIGHT & FLAVORFUL SANDWICHES											
Albacore Tuna on Wheat (small)	1	361	11	27	3	47	1122	50	3	21	3 starch, 2 lean meat, 1 fat
Albacore Tuna on Sourdough (large)	1	1000	26	23	6	122	3099	147	6	59	10 starch, 4 lean meat, 2 fat
Albacore Tuna on Wheat (regular)	1	533	15	25	4	69	1655	74	4	31	5 starch, 2 lean meat, 1 1/2 fat
Chicken Breast on Sourdough (large)	1	1008	15	13	4	155	4522	158	6	72	10 starch, 6 lean meat
Chicken Breast on Sourdough (regular)	1	535	10	17	3	85	2365	81	3	37	5 1/2 starch, 2 lean meat, 1 fat

(Continued)

✔ = Healthiest Bets; n/a = not available

LIGHT AND FLAVORFUL SANDWICHES (*Continued*)	Amount	Cal.	Fat (g)	% Cal. Fat	Sat. Fat (g)	Chol. (mg)	Sod. (mg)	Carb. (g)	Fiber (g)	Pro. (g)	Servings/Exchanges
Chicken Breast on Sourdough (small)	1	363	7	17	2	58	1596	55	2	25	4 1/2 starch, 2 lean meat
Dijon Chicken on Sourdough (large)	1	972	10	9	2	137	3981	150	8	74	10 starch, 6 very lean meat, 1 fat
Dijon Chicken on Wheat (regular)	1	497	6	11	1	68	2091	74	6	38	5 starch, 2 lean meat
Dijon Chicken on Wheat (small)	1	330	4	11	1	46	1373	50	4	25	3 starch, 2 lean meat
Pesto Chicken on Sourdough (large)	1	999	15	14	3	141	3799	145	7	73	10 starch, 6 very lean meat, 1 fat
Pesto Chicken on Sourdough (regular)	1	512	9	16	2	71	1927	73	4	37	5 starch, 2 lean meat, 1/2 fat
Pesto Chicken on Sourdough (small)	1	346	6	16	1	48	1297	49	2	25	3 starch, 2 lean meat

											Servings/Exchanges
Santa Fe Chicken on Jalapeno Cheese (regular)	1	642	19	27	9	106	2302	77	4	43	5 starch, 4 lean meat, 1 fat
Santa Fe Chicken on Jalapeno Cheese (small)	1	431	13	27	6	71	1547	52	3	29	3 1/2 starch, 3 lean meat, 1 fat
Santa Fe on Sourdough (large)	1	1182	29	22	14	185	4232	155	9	82	10 starch, 7 lean meat, 1 fat
Smoked Turkey Breast on Sourdough (large)	1	988	13	12	2	118	4229	150	6	68	10 starch, 5 lean meat
Smoked Turkey Breast on Sourdough (regular)	1	498	7	13	1	60	2123	75	3	34	5 starch, 2 lean meat
Smoked Turkey Breast on Sourdough (small)	1	335	5	13	1	40	1426	50	2	23	3 starch, 2 lean meat
The Vegetarian on Sourdough (large)	1	966	26	24	12	48	2398	150	8	34	10 starch, 5 fat

✔ = Healthiest Bets; n/a = not available

(Continued)

LIGHT AND FLAVORFUL SANDWICHES (*Continued*)	Amount	Cal.	Fat (g)	% Cal. Fat	Sat. Fat (g)	Chol. (mg)	Sod. (mg)	Carb. (g)	Fiber (g)	Pro. (g)	Servings/Exchanges
The Vegetarian on Wheat (regular)	1	519	17	29	7	32	1329	75	5	18	5 starch, 3 fat
✔The Vegetarian on Wheat (small)	1	351	11	28	5	22	889	51	4	12	3 1/2 starch, 2 fat
ORIGINAL SANDWICHES											
Cheese Original on Sourdough (large)	1	1857	98	47	56	180	4365	159	8	87	10 1/2 starch, 9 medium-fat meat, 10 fat
Cheese Original on Sourdough (regular)	1	854	44	46	23	72	2107	79	4	38	5 starch, 3 medium-fat meat, 6 fat
Cheese Original on Sourdough (small)	1	596	31	47	17	54	1432	53	3	27	3 1/2 starch, 3 medium-fat meat, 3 fat
Deluxe Original on Sourdough (regular)	1	970	47	44	18	128	1825	84	4	53	5 1/2 starch, 5 medium-fat meat, 4 fat

Item										Exchanges
Deluxe Original on Sourdough (small)	1	717	37	46	15	103	1280	57	3	39	4 starch, 4 medium-fat meat, 3 fat
Ham & Cheese Original on Sourdough (large)	1	1625	67	37	29	183	2974	163	6	93	11 starch, 9 medium-fat meat, 4 fat
Ham & Cheese Original on Sourdough (regular)	1	789	32	37	12	83	3428	82	4	44	5 1/2 starch, 3 medium-fat meat, 3 fat
Ham & Cheese Original on Sourdough (small)	1	537	22	37	9	58	2298	55	3	30	3 1/2 starch, 3 medium-fat meat, 1 fat
The Original on Sourdough (large)	1	1591	75	42	35	157	5019	157	8	74	10 starch, 6 medium-fat meat, 9 fat
The Original on Sourdough (regular)	1	778	36	42	16	75	2528	79	4	34	5 starch, 4 medium-fat meat, 7 fat

✔ = Healthiest Bets; n/a = not available

(Continued)

ORIGINAL SANDWICHES (*Continued*)	Amount	Cal.	Fat (g)	% Cal. Fat	Sat. Fat (g)	Chol. (mg)	Sod. (mg)	Carb. (g)	Fiber (g)	Pro. (g)	Servings/Exchanges
The Original on Sourdough (small)	1	550	27	44	12	55	1755	53	3	24	3 1/2 starch, 2 medium-fat meat, 9 fat
Turkey Original on Sourdough (large)	1	1772	77	39	34	241	6235	162	6	106	11 starch, 11 medium-fat meat, 4 fat
Turkey Original on Sourdough (regular)	1	862	37	39	15	112	1610	81	4	51	5 1/2 starch, 4 medium-fat meat, 3 fat
Turkey Original on Sourdough (small)	1	607	28	42	12	83	2136	54	3	36	3 1/2 starch, 4 medium-fat meat, 1 fat
SPECIALTY DELI SANDWICHES											
Albacore Tuna Melt on Sourdough (large)	1	1631	77	42	34	214	4474	158	7	93	10 1/2 starch, 9 medium-fat meat, 4 fat
Albacore Tuna Melt on Wheat (regular)	1	818	40	44	16	106	2293	79	5	45	5 starch, 4 medium-fat meat, 4 fat

Albacore Tuna Melt on Wheat (small)	1	562	28	45	12	74	1552	53	3	31	3 1/2 starch, 3 medium-fat meat, 3 fat
BLT on Sourdough (large)	1	1141	46	36	14	80	3066	140	6	41	9 starch, 4 medium-fat meat, 5 fat
BLT on Sourdough (regular)	1	578	24	37	7	41	1548	70	3	21	4 1/2 starch, 2 medium-fat meat, 3 fat
BLT on Sourdough (small)	1	379	15	36	5	26	1010	47	2	13	3 starch, 1 medium-fat meat, 2 fat
Chicken Club on Sourdough (large)	1	1351	45	30	17	209	4678	149	8	88	10 starch, 8 medium-fat meat, 1 fat
Chicken Club on Sourdough (regular)	1	686	23	30	9	106	2403	75	4	44	5 starch, 4 medium-fat meat, 1/2 fat

✔ = Healthiest Bets; n/a = not available

(Continued)

SPECIALTY DELI SANDWICHES (*Continued*)	Amount	Cal.	Fat (g)	% Cal. Fat	Sat. Fat (g)	Chol. (mg)	Sod. (mg)	Carb. (g)	Fiber (g)	Pro. (g)	Servings/Exchanges
Chicken Club on Sourdough (small)	1	458	15	29	6	71	1591	50	3	29	3 1/2 starch, 3 medium-fat meat
Corned Beef on Dark Rye (regular)	1	587	15	23	3	84	2488	70	4	40	4 1/2 starch, 4 lean meat, 1/2 fat
Corned Beef on Dark Rye (small)	1	388	10	23	2	56	1625	47	3	27	3 starch, 3 medium-fat meat, 1 fat
Corned Beef on Sourdough (large)	1	1134	25	20	5	167	4751	139	6	81	9 starch, 7 lean meat, 1 fat
Corned Beef Reuben on Dark Rye (regular)	1	833	35	38	13	132	3514	74	4	51	5 starch, 4 medium-fat meat, 3 fat
Corned Beef Reuben on Dark Rye (small)	1	528	21	36	7	80	2269	50	3	32	3 1/2 starch, 3 medium-fat meat, 1 fat

	✓										Exchanges
Corned Beef Reuben on Sourdough (large)	1	1594	62	35	25	262	6944	147	7	102	10 starch, 10 medium-fat meat, 2 fat
Pastrami & Swiss on Dark Rye (regular)	1	861	37	39	17	152	3718	74	4	57	5 starch, 6 medium-fat meat, 1 fat
Pastrami & Swiss on Dark Rye (small)	1	570	24	38	11	101	2445	49	3	38	3 starch, 3 medium-fat meat, 2 fat
Pastrami Reuben on Dark Rye (regular)	1	924	43	42	18	155	3924	77	4	56	5 starch, 6 medium-fat meat, 3 fat
Pastrami Reuben on Dark Rye (small)	1	619	29	42	12	103	2679	51	3	38	3 1/2 starch, 3 medium-fat meat, 3 fat
Pastrami Reuben on Sourdough (large)	1	1777	77	39	34	308	7765	152	7	113	10 starch, 10 medium-fat meat, 5 fat

(Continued)

✓ = Healthiest Bets; n/a = not available

SPECIALTY DELI SANDWICHES (*Continued*)	Amount	Cal.	Fat (g)	% Cal. Fat	Sat. Fat (g)	Chol. (mg)	Sod. (mg)	Carb. (g)	Fiber (g)	Pro. (g)	Servings/Exchanges
Roast Beef & Cheese on Sourdough (large)	1	1749	70	36	33	255	4987	163	8	120	11 starch, 12 medium-fat meat, 2 fat
Roast Beef & Cheese on Sourdough (regular)	1	848	34	36	14	119	2451	82	4	57	5 1/2 starch, 6 medium-fat meat, 1 fat
Roast Beef & Cheese on Sourdough (small)	1	580	24	37	10	83	1666	55	3	39	3 1/2 starch, 4 medium-fat meat, 1 fat
Roast Beef on Sourdough (large)	1	1185	28	21	6	164	3362	145	6	87	10 starch, 8 lean meat, 1 fat
Roast Beef on Sourdough (regular)	1	617	17	25	3	83	1733	73	3	43	5 starch, 4 lean meat, 1 fat
Roast Beef on Sourdough (small)	1	413	11	24	2	55	1162	49	2	29	3 starch, 3 lean meat
Texas Schlotsky's on Jalapeno Cheddar (regular)	1	816	37	41	16	98	3357	76	3	43	5 starch, 4 medium-fat meat, 3 fat

Texas Schlotsky's on Jalapeno Cheddar (small)	1	561	26	42	12	69	2263	51	2	31	3 1/2 starch, 3 medium-fat meat, 3 fat
Texas Schlotsky's on Sourdough (large)	1	1544	65	38	27	184	6446	155	6	84	10 starch, 8 medium-fat meat, 5 fat
The Philly on Sourdough (large)	1	1709	66	35	32	244	4477	157	7	121	10 starch, 12 medium-fat meat, 1 fat
The Philly on Sourdough (regular)	1	824	32	35	14	113	2189	78	4	57	5 starch, 3 medium-fat meat, 3 fat
The Philly on Sourdough (small)	1	559	22	35	10	78	1467	52	2	39	3 1/2 starch, 3 medium-fat meat, 1 fat
Turkey & Bacon Club on Sourdough (large)	1	1790	80	40	35	240	6086	161	7	108	11 starch, 10 medium-fat meat, 6 fat

(Continued)

✔ = Healthiest Bets; n/a = not available

SPECIALTY DELI SANDWICHES *(Continued)*	Amount	Cal.	Fat (g)	% Cal. Fat	Sat. Fat (g)	Chol. (mg)	Sod. (mg)	Carb. (g)	Fiber (g)	Pro. (g)	Servings/Exchanges
Turkey & Bacon Club on Wheat (regular)	1	874	40	41	15	113	3009	79	5	52	5 starch, 5 medium-fat meat, 3 fat
Turkey & Bacon Club on Wheat (small)	1	596	27	41	11	78	2012	53	3	35	3 1/2 starch, 3 medium-fat meat, 3 fat
Turkey Guacamole on Sourdough (large)	1	1317	42	29	6	118	5255	166	6	73	11 starch, 6 medium-fat meat, 2 fat
Turkey Guacamole on Sourdough (regular)	1	683	24	32	3	60	2680	84	3	36	5 1/2 starch, 3 medium-fat meat, 2 fat
Turkey Guacamole on Sourdough (small)	1	448	15	30	2	40	1764	56	2	24	3 1/2 starch, 2 medium-fat meat, 1 fat
Turkey Reuben on Dark Rye (regular)	1	863	39	41	16	124	3893	80	4	50	5 starch, 5 medium-fat meat, 3 fat

Turkey Reuben on Dark Rye (small)	1	579	26	40	11	83	2659	54	3	33	3 1/2 starch, 3 medium-fat meat, 2 fat
Turkey Reuben on Sourdough (large)	1	1656	69	38	31	247	7704	259	7	101	17 starch, 7 medium-fat meat, 7 fat
Vegetable Club on Sourdough (large)	1	1112	41	33	13	46	2716	151	9	39	10 starch, 1 medium-fat meat, 7 fat
Vegetable Club on Sourdough (regular)	1	581	24	37	7	24	1453	76	5	19	5 starch, 1 medium-fat meat, 3 fat
✔ Vegetable Club on Sourdough (small)	1	393	16	37	5	17	962	50	3	13	3 1/2 starch, 3 medium-fat meat, 3 fat
Western Vegetarian on Sourdough (large)	1	1261	61	44	28	125	2235	150	8	35	10 starch, 1 medium-fat meat, 11 fat

✔ = Healthiest Bets; n/a = not available

(Continued)

SPECIALTY DELI SANDWICHES (*Continued*)	Amount	Cal.	Fat (g)	% Cal. Fat	Sat. Fat (g)	Chol. (mg)	Sod. (mg)	Carb. (g)	Fiber (g)	Pro. (g)	Servings/Exchanges
Western Vegetarian on Sourdough (regular)	1	651	33	46	14	62	1161	75	4	18	5 starch, 6 1/2 fat
✓Western Vegetarian on Sourdough (small)	1	449	23	46	10	47	790	51	3	12	3 1/2 starch, 1 medium-fat meat, 3 1/2 fat
SPECIALTY SANDWICHES											
Pastrami & Swiss on Sourdough (large)	1	1681	69	37	32	304	7211	148	6	114	10 starch, 10 medium-fat meat, 7 fat

✓ = Healthiest Bets; n/a = not available

Subway

❖Subway provides nutrition information for most of its menu items on their website at www.subway.com.

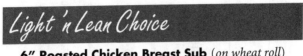

6" Roasted Chicken Breast Sub *(on wheat roll)*
Veggie Delite Salad
Fat Free Ranch Salad Dressing *(2 T, 1/2 packet)*

Calories......................391	Sodium (mg) 1,455
Fat (g) 7	Carbohydrate (g).........56
% calories from fat..16	Fiber (g) 6
Saturated fat (g)........2	Protein (g) 27
Cholesterol (mg) 48	

Exchanges: 3 starch, 2 veg, 2 lean meat

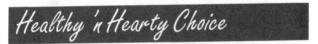

Asiago Caesar Chicken Wrap
Veggie Delite Salad
Fat Free French Salad Dressing *(2 T, 1/2 packet)*
Oatmeal Raisin Cookie

Calories......................695	Sodium (mg) 2,005
Fat (g) 24	Carbohydrate (g).........94
% calories from fat..31	Fiber (g) 6
Saturated fat (g)........5	Protein (g) 27
Cholesterol (mg) 61	

Exchanges: 3 starch, 2 veg, 2 carb, 2 lean meat, 3 fat

(Continued)

Subway

BREADS

	Amount	Cal.	Fat (g)	% Cal. Fat	Sat. Fat (g)	Chol. (mg)	Sod. (mg)	Carb. (g)	Fiber (g)	Pro. (g)	Servings/Exchanges
✔Asiago, 6"	1	220	5	20	3	8	490	34	2	9	2 starch, 1 fat
✔Country Wheat, 6"	1	206	3	13	0.5	0	360	39	3	8	2 1/2 starch, 1/2 fat
✔Deli Style Roll	1	150	3	18	0.5	0	260	27	1	5	2 starch, 1/2 fat
✔Hearty Italian, 6"	1	191	2	9	0.5	0	350	36	2	7	2 1/2 starch
✔Italian (white), 6"	1	178	2	10	0.5	0	350	33	2	7	2 starch
✔Parmesan Oregano, 6"	1	195	3	14	0.5	4	400	34	2	8	2 starch, 1/2 fat
✔Sesame Italian, 6"	1	210	5	21	0.5	0	360	34	2	8	2 starch, 1 fat
✔Sourdough, 6"	1	265	3	10	1.5	0	460	49	2	10	3 1/2 starch, 1/2 fat
✔Wheat, 6"	1	186	2	10	0.5	0	360	36	3	7	2 1/2 starch

✔ Wrap	1	200	2	9	0.5	0	670	39	1	6	2 1/2 starch

BREAKFAST SANDWICHES

✔ Bacon & Egg	1	305	15	44	4	184	500	29	1	13	2 starch, 1 medium-fat meat, 2 fat
✔ Cheese & Egg	1	302	15	45	4.5	187	520	29	1	13	2 starch, 1 medium-fat meat, 2 fat
✔ Ham & Egg	1	291	12	37	3	189	700	30	1	15	2 starch, 1 medium-fat meat, 1 fat
✔ Western Egg	1	285	12	38	2.5	182	510	31	2	13	2 starch, 1 medium-fat meat, 1 fat

6" COLD SUBS

Classic Italian B.M.T.	1	453	24	48	8	56	1740	40	3	21	2 1/2 starch, 2 lean meat, 3 fat

(Continued)

✔ = Healthiest Bets; n/a = not available

6" COLD SUBS (*Continued*)	Amount	Cal.	Fat (g)	% Cal. Fat	Sat. Fat (g)	Chol. (mg)	Sod. (mg)	Carb. (g)	Fiber (g)	Pro. (g)	Servings/Exchanges
Cold Cut Trio	1	415	20	43	7	57	1670	40	3	19	2 starch, 2 medium-fat meat, 2 fat
Ham	1	261	5	17	1.5	25	1260	39	3	17	2 1/2 starch, 2 lean meat
✔Roast Beef	1	264	5	17	1	20	840	39	3	18	2 1/2 starch, 2 lean meat
Subway Club (wheat bread)	1	294	5	15	1.5	33	1250	40	3	22	2 1/2 starch, 2 lean meat
Subway Seafood & Crab	1	378	16	38	4.5	24	1270	46	3	14	3 starch, 1 lean meat, 2 1/2 fat
Tuna	1	419	21	45	5	42	1180	39	3	18	2 1/2 starch, 2 lean meat, 3 fat
✔Turkey Breast	1	254	4	14	1	20	1000	39	3	16	2 1/2 starch, 1 lean meat
Turkey Breast & Ham	1	267	5	17	1	26	1210	40	3	18	2 1/2 starch, 2 lean meat
✔Veggie Delite	1	200	3	14	0.5	0	500	37	3	7	2 starch, 1 veg, 1/2 fat

CONDIMENTS & EXTRAS

	Amount	Calories	Fat (g)	% Cal. from Fat	Sat. Fat (g)	Chol. (mg)	Sodium (mg)	Carb. (g)	Fiber (g)	Protein (g)	Servings/Exchanges
✔Bacon	2 strips	45	4	80	1.5	8	180	0	0	2	1 fat
Cheddar Cheese	2 triangles	60	5	75	3	15	95	0	0	4	1 fat
✔Light Mayonnaise	1 T	46	5	98	1	6	100	1	0	0	1 fat
Mayonnaise	1 T	111	12	97	3	9	80	0	0	0	2 fat
Processed American Cheese	2 triangles	41	4	88	2	10	200	0	0	2	1 fat
Processed Pepperjack Cheese	2 triangles	40	4	90	2	11	210	0	0	2	1 fat
Provolone Cheese	2 half circles	51	4	71	2	11	125	0	0	4	1/2 high-fat meat
Swiss Cheese	2 triangles	53	4	68	3	13	30	0	0	4	1/2 high-fat meat

COOKIES

	Amount	Calories	Fat (g)	% Cal. from Fat	Sat. Fat (g)	Chol. (mg)	Sodium (mg)	Carb. (g)	Fiber (g)	Protein (g)	Servings/Exchanges
✔Chocolate Chip	1	209	10	43	3.5	12	135	29	1	3	2 carb, 2 fat

✔ = Healthiest Bets; n/a = not available

(Continued)

COOKIES (*Continued*)	Amount	Cal.	Fat (g)	% Cal. Fat	Sat. Fat (g)	Chol. (mg)	Sod. (mg)	Carb. (g)	Fiber (g)	Pro. (g)	Servings/Exchanges
✔Chocolate Chunk	1	210	10	43	3	12	150	30	1	2	2 carb, 2 fat
✔M&M	1	210	10	43	3	13	135	29	1	2	2 carb, 2 fat
✔Oatmeal Raisin	1	197	8	37	2	14	180	29	1	3	2 carb, 1 1/2 fat
Peanut Butter	1	220	12	49	3	0	200	26	1	3	2 carb, 2 fat
Sugar	1	222	12	49	3	18	170	28	1	2	2 carb, 2 fat
White Chocolate Macadamia Nut	1	221	12	49	3	13	140	27	1	2	2 carb, 2 fat
DELI SANDWICHES											
✔Bologna	1	292	12	37	2	20	744	38	2	10	2 1/2 starch, 1 medium-fat meat, 1 fat
✔Ham	1	194	4	19	1	12	750	30	2	10	2 starch, 1 lean meat
✔Roast Beef	1	206	4	17	1	13	600	31	2	12	2 starch, 1 lean meat
✔Tuna (light mayonnaise)	1	309	15	44	4	26	810	31	2	12	2 starch, 1 lean meat, 2 fat

✔Turkey Breast	1	200	4	18	1	13	700	31	2	12	2 starch, 1 lean meat

FRUIZLE EXPRESS

✔Berry Lishus (small)	13 oz	113	0	0	0	0	20	29	1	1	2 carb
✔Peach Pizzazz (small)	13 oz	103	0	0	0	0	25	29	1	1	2 carb
Pineapple Delight (small)	13 oz	133	0	0	0	0	25	33	1	1	2 carb
✔Sunrise Refresher	13 oz	119	0	0	0	0	20	29	1	1	2 carb

6" HOT SUBS

Meatball	1	501	25	45	10	56	1350	46	4	23	3 starch, 2 medium-fat meat, 3 fat
✔Roasted Chicken Breast	1	311	6	17	1.5	48	880	40	3	25	2 1/2 starch, 3 very lean meat, 1/2 fat
Steak & Cheese	1	362	13	32	4.5	37	1200	41	3	23	2 1/2 starch, 2 medium-fat meat

✔ = Healthiest Bets; n/a = not available

(Continued)

6" HOT SUBS *(Continued)*	Amount	Cal.	Fat (g)	% Cal. Fat	Sat. Fat (g)	Chol. (mg)	Sod. (mg)	Carb. (g)	Fiber (g)	Pro. (g)	Servings/Exchanges
Subway Melt (includes cheese)	1	384	15	35	5	44	1720	40	3	22	2 1/2 starch, 2 medium-fat meat, 1 fat
SALAD DRESSINGS											
✔Fat Free French	2 oz/4 T	70	0	0	0	0	390	17	0	0	1 carb
✔Fat Free Italian	2 oz/4 T	20	0	0	0	0	610	4	0	0	free
✔Fat Free Ranch	2 oz/4 T	60	0	0	0	0	530	14	0	0	1 carb
SALADS											
Classic B.M.T.	1	272	19	63	7	56	1440	11	3	16	2 veg, 2 high-fat meat
Cold Cut Trio	1	234	15	58	6	57	1370	11	3	14	2 veg, 1 medium-fat meat, 2 fat
✔Ham	1	112	3	24	1	25	1070	11	3	11	2 veg, 1 lean meat
Meatball	1	320	20	56	9	56	1050	17	4	17	1/2 starch, 2 veg, 1 medium-fat meat, 3 fat

✔Roast Beef	1	114	3	24	0.5	20	660	11	1	12	2 veg, 1 lean meat
✔Roasted Chicken Breast	1	137	3	20	0.5	36	730	12	3	16	2 veg, 2 very lean meat
✔Steak & Cheese (includes cheese)	1	181	8	40	3.5	37	890	12	4	17	2 veg, 2 lean meat
✔Subway Club	1	145	4	25	1	33	1070	12	3	17	2 veg, 1 lean meat
Subway Melt (includes cheese)	1	203	10	44	4.5	44	1410	11	3	17	2 veg, 2 medium-fat meat
✔Subway Seafood & Crab (light mayonnaise)	1	197	11	50	3.5	24	970	17	4	9	2 veg, 1 medium-fat meat, 1 fat
✔Tuna (light mayonnaise)	1	238	16	61	4	42	880	10	3	13	2 veg, 1 lean meat, 2 fat
✔Turkey Breast & Ham	1	117	3	23	0.5	26	1030	11	3	13	2 veg, 2 very lean meat
✔Turkey Breast	1	105	2	17	0	20	820	11	3	11	2 veg, 1 very lean meat
✔Veggie Delite	1	50	1	18	0	0	310	9	3	2	2 veg

✔ = Healthiest Bets; n/a = not available

(Continued)

	Amount	Cal.	Fat (g)	% Cal. Fat	Sat. Fat (g)	Chol. (mg)	Sod. (mg)	Carb. (g)	Fiber (g)	Pro. (g)	Servings/Exchanges
SELECT SANDWICHES											
✔Asiago Caesar Chicken	1	391	15	35	3	47	1000	41	3	22	2 1/2 starch, 2 medium-fat meat, 1 fat
SELECT SAUCES											
✔Asiago Caesar	2 oz/1 T	77	8	94	1.5	7	160	1	0	1	1 1/2 fat
✔Honey Mustard	2 oz/1 T	20	0	0	0	0	100	5	0	0	free
✔Horseradish	2 oz/1 T	100	9	81	1.5	5	130	2	0	0	2 fat
✔Southwest	2 oz/1 T	61	6	89		5	130	1	0	0	1 fat
SPECIALTY DELI SANDWICHES											
✔Horseradish Roast Beef	1	401	17	38	3	27	880	42	3	18	3 starch, 2 medium-fat meat, 1 fat

SPECIALTY SANDWICHES

Item											Exchanges
Caesar Italian BMT	1	530	31	53	10	66	1840	41	3	22	2 1/2 starch, 2 medium-fat meat, 4 fat
Honey Mustard Melt	1	376	11	26	5	44	1590	47	3	22	3 starch, 2 medium-fat meat
✔Honey Mustard Turkey w/Cucumber	1	275	4	13	1	20	990	46	2	16	3 starch, 1 medium-fat meat
Horseradish Steak & Cheese	1	468	22	42	6	44	1110	43	4	22	3 starch, 2 medium-fat meat, 2 fat
Southwest Steak & Cheese	1	412	18	39	6	44	1120	42		22	3 starch, 2 medium-fat meat, 1 1/2 fat
✔Southwest Turkey	1	362	13	32	2.5	43	960	40	2	21	2 1/2 starch, 2 medium-fat meat, 1/2 fat

✔ = Healthiest Bets; n/a = not available

(Continued)

WRAPS

	Amount	Cal.	Fat (g)	% Cal. Fat	Sat. Fat (g)	Chol. (mg)	Sod. (mg)	Carb. (g)	Fiber (g)	Pro. (g)	Servings/Exchanges
Asiago Caesar Chicken	1	413	15	33	3	47	1320	47	2	22	3 starch, 2 medium-fat meat, 1 fat
Steak & Cheese	1	353	9	23	4	37	1400	46	3	22	3 starch, 2 medium-fat meat
Turkey Breast & Bacon	1	321	7	20	2.5	28	1510	45	2	18	3 starch, 2 lean meat

✔ = Healthiest Bets; n/a = not available

Togo's Eatery

❖Togo's Eatery provided nutrition information for all of its menu items for use in this book.

Light 'n Lean Choice

Oriental Salad with Dressing

Calories 499	Sodium (mg)..........1,062
Fat (g) 21	Carbohydrate (g).........49
% calories from fat..38	Fiber (g) 3
Saturated fat (g) ....n/a	Protein (g) 25
Cholesterol (mg) 41	

Exchanges: 2 1/2 starch, 2 veg, 2 lean meat, 3 fat

Healthy 'n Hearty Choice

Tortellini Vegetable Soup (8 oz)
Spicy Chicken with
Jamaican Seasoning Sandwich

Calories......................624	Sodium (mg)..........1,760
Fat (g) 16	Carbohydrate (g).........86
% calories from fat..23	Fiber (g) 5
Saturated fat (g) ....n/a	Protein (g) 35
Cholesterol (mg) 100	

Exchanges: 5 starch, 1 veg, 3 lean meat

(Continued)

Togo's Eatery

	Amount	Cal.	Fat (g)	% Cal. Fat	Sat. Fat (g)	Chol. (mg)	Sod. (mg)	Carb. (g)	Fiber (g)	Pro. (g)	Servings/Exchanges
SALAD DRESSINGS											
✓1000 Island	1 pkt/4 T	231	22	86	n/a	30	532	9	0	1	1/2 carb, 4 fat
✓Blue Cheese	1 pkt/4 T	291	30	93	n/a	20	663	3	0	2	6 fat
✓Caesar	1 pkt/4 T	241	23	86	n/a	20	636	8	0	2	1/2 carb, 4 fat
✓Oriental	1 pkt/4 T	221	14	57	n/a	5	512	24	0	0	1 1/2 carb, 3 fat
Ranch	1 pkt/4 T	321	33	93	n/a	15	643	5	0	2	7 fat
✓Reduced Calorie Italian	1 pkt/4 T	60	5	75	n/a	0	693	4	0	0	1 fat
✓Reduced Calorie Ranch	1 pkt/4 T	191	16	75	n/a	25	603	10	0	1	1/2 carb, 3 fat
✓Sweet & Spicy	1 pkt/4 T	70	0	0	n/a	0	703	19	1	0	1 carb

SALADS

Item	Amount									Exchanges/Choices
Caesar	1	471	30	57	n/a	72	1189	23	2	30	2 veg, 1 carb, 3 medium-fat meat, 3 fat
Chef	1	387	19	44	n/a	65	1586	26	2	26	2 veg, 1 carb, 3 medium-fat meat, 3 fat
Cobb	1	487	24	44	n/a	293	984	29	2	40	2 veg, 1 carb, 5 medium-fat meat
✔Garden Salad	1 small	256	10	35	n/a	214	579	31	2	12	3 veg, 1 carb, 2 fat
✔Garden Salad with Avocado Scoop	1	357	19	48	n/a	214	586	35	n/a	13	3 veg, 1 1/2 carb, 4 fat
✔Garden Salad with Chicken Salad Scoop	1	369	18	44	n/a	232	796	34	n/a	26	3 veg, 1 1/2 carb, 2 medium-fat meat, 1 fat

(Continued)

✔ = Healthiest Bets; n/a = not available

SANDWICHES (*Continued*)	Amount	Cal.	Fat (g)	% Cal. Fat	Sat. Fat (g)	Chol. (mg)	Sod. (mg)	Carb. (g)	Fiber (g)	Pro. (g)	Servings/Exchanges
✓Garden Salad with Egg Salad Scoop	1	363	18	45	n/a	428	696	33	n/a	18	3 veg, 1 1/2 carb, 1 medium-fat meat, 2 fat
✓Garden Salad with Tuna Scoop	1	385	18	42	n/a	243	793	34	n/a	22	3 veg, 1 1/2 carb, 1 medium-fat meat, 2 fat
✓Oriental	1	499	21	38	n/a	41	1062	49	3	25	3 veg, 2 carb, 2 medium-fat meat, 2 fat
SANDWICHES											
Albacore Tuna	1 small	701	30	39	n/a	67	1653	78	3	32	5 starch, 2 lean meat, 4 fat
Avocado & Turkey	1 small	675	28	37	n/a	35	1606	80	6	27	5 starch, 2 lean meat, 3 fat
Avocado, Cucumber & Alfalfa Sprouts	1 small	637	28	40	n/a	6	1150	85	7	16	5 starch, 1 veg, 5 fat
Bar-B-Q Beef	1 small	724	22	27	n/a	88	2120	94	3	39	6 starch, 3 medium-fat meat, 1 fat

Item	Serving										Exchanges/Choices
California Roasted Chicken	1 small	510	15	26	n/a	65	1768	73	3	36	5 starch, 3 very lean meat
Cheese Sandwich—Swiss, American & Provolone	1 small	859	46	48	n/a	107	2195	77	3	42	5 starch, 4 high-fat meat, 1 fat
Egg Salad with Cheese	1 small	728	35	43	n/a	456	1765	76	3	29	5 starch, 2 medium-fat meat, 4 fat
Ham & Cheese	1 small	661	26	35	n/a	68	2899	76	3	33	5 starch, 3 medium-fat meat, 1 fat
Hot or Cold Roast Beef	1 small	552	11	18	n/a	84	1537	73	3	42	5 starch, 4 lean meat
Hot Pastrami	1 small	705	26	33	n/a	72	2260	85	3	34	5 1/2 starch, 3 medium-fat meat, 1 fat
Hummus	1 small	668	21	28	n/a	9	1510	102	4	20	7 starch, 4 fat
Italian Dry Salami & Cheese	1 small	770	33	39	n/a	118	3288	78	3	42	5 starch, 4 medium-fat meat, 2 fat

✔ = Healthiest Bets; n/a = not available

(Continued)

SIDE SALADS (*Continued*)	Amount	Cal.	Fat (g)	% Cal. Fat	Sat. Fat (g)	Chol. (mg)	Sod. (mg)	Carb. (g)	Fiber (g)	Pro. (g)	Servings/Exchanges
Italian Dry Salami, Capicolla, Mortadella, Cotto & Provolone	1 small	736	32	39	n/a	85	2191	74	3	31	5 starch, 2 medium-fat meat, 4 fat
Meatballs with Pizza Sauce, Veggies and Parmesan	1 small	707	28	36	n/a	97	1602	78	4	36	5 starch, 3 medium-fat meat, 3 fat
Pastrami Reuben	1 small	875	45	46	n/a	111	2460	85	2	44	5 1/2 starch, 4 medium-fat meat, 3 fat
Spicy Chicken with Jamaican Seasoning	1 small	562	14	22	n/a	85	1190	78	4	32	5 starch, 3 lean meat, 1 fat
Turkey & Cheese	1 small	638	23	32	n/a	71	2277	75	3	34	5 starch, 2 medium-fat meat, 2 fat
Turkey & Cranberry	1 small	623	13	19	n/a	49	1904	96	4	30	6 1/2 starch, 2 lean meat, 1 fat

Turkey & Ham with Cheese	1 small	670	25	34	n/a	76	2772	76	3	37	5 starch, 3 medium-fat meat, 2 fat

SIDE SALADS

Macaroni	4 oz	114	23	182	n/a	23	222	25	0	3	1 1/2 starch, 4 fat
Potato	4 oz	215	13	54	n/a	11	435	25	0	2	1 1/2 starch, 2 fat

SOUPS

✔Broccoli Cheese	8 oz	165	8	44	n/a	21	601	13	1	9	1 starch, 1 medium-fat meat
Broccoli Cheese	12 oz	247	12	44	n/a	31	902	20	1	14	1 starch, 2 medium-fat meat
✔Chicken Rice	8 oz	91	2	20	n/a	6	635	14	1	4	1 starch
✔Chicken Rice	12 oz	137	2	13	n/a	9	953	21	1	6	1 1/2 starch, 1 very lean meat
✔Chicken Vegetable	8 oz	71	2	25	n/a	13	613	7	1	5	1/2 starch, 1 lean meat
✔Chicken Vegetable	12 oz	106	3	25	n/a	19	920	11	1	7	1/2 starch, 1 lean meat

✔ = Healthiest Bets; n/a = not available

(Continued)

	Amount	Cal.	Fat (g)	% Cal. Fat	Sat. Fat (g)	Chol. (mg)	Sod. (mg)	Carb. (g)	Fiber (g)	Pro. (g)	Servings/Exchanges
✔Chili (no cheese)	8 oz	151	4	24	n/a	13	640	19	6	9	1 starch, 1 medium-fat meat
✔Chili (no cheese)	12 oz	226	6	24	n/a	20	960	29	9	13	2 starch, 1 medium-fat meat
✔Chili with cheese	8 oz	207	9	39	n/a	29	732	20	6	12	1 starch, 1 medium-fat meat, 1 fat
✔Chili with cheese	12 oz	282	6	19	n/a	35	1000	30	9	14	2 starch, 1 medium-fat meat
✔Clam Chowder	8 oz	162	6	33	n/a	23	601	16	1	10	1 starch, 1 lean meat, 1 fat
✔Clam Chowder	12 oz	243	10	37	n/a	34	902	24	1	14	1 1/2 starch, 1 lean meat, 1 fat
✔Corn Chicken	8 oz	151	4	24	n/a	16	482	19	1	9	1 starch, 1 lean meat
✔Corn Chicken	12 oz	226	6	24	n/a	24	723	29	2	13	2 starch, 1 lean meat
Lentil Rice	8 oz	165	2	11	n/a	0	1879	36	5	9	2 1/2 starch
Lentil Rice	12 oz	247	3	11	n/a	0	2818	54	7	13	3 1/2 starch

✓Minestrone	8 oz	66	2	27	n/a	3	670	9	1	3	1/2 starch
✓Minestrone	12 oz	99	3	27	n/a	5	1005	13	2	5	1 starch
✓Tortellini Vegetable	8 oz	62	2	29	n/a	15	571	8	1	3	1/2 starch
✓Tortellini Vegetable	12 oz	93	2	19	n/a	23	857	12	1	4	1 starch

✓ = Healthiest Bets; n/a = not available

Sweets, Desserts, and Frozen Treats

RESTAURANTS

Baskin Robbins

Freshëns Premium Yogurt

Häagen-Dazs Ice Cream Café

I Can't Believe It's Yogurt

Mrs. Fields Cookies

TCBY

The Scoop: Nutrition information is for 4-fluid-ounce servings. Yes, that's small, but it is the industry standard. In many cases the nutrition information is only for vanilla or several other flavors. Flavors that have nuts, fudge, or chocolate pieces will most likely have more calories. Several companies base their nutrition information on an average of all flavors.

No meals are provided for this chapter because these foods are usually eaten as a snack or in addition to a meal.

NUTRITION PROS

- Small portions are an option.
- Some restaurants offer a kiddie size. That's sometimes enough to satisfy your sweet tooth.
- Healthier toppings are easy to spot: fresh fruit, granola, nuts, or raisins.
- Low-fat, fat-free, and/or sugar-free frozen treats abound.

- Desserts are easy to split. Just ask for two forks or spoons.
- You can watch the server's every move. Make sure they do what you want.

NUTRITION CONS

- Overindulgence is easy.
- Unhealthy toppers are plentiful: candy bar pieces, cookies, hot fudge, or butterscotch.
- Sometimes the low-fat, fat-free, and/or sugar-free desserts are not that much lower in calories than the regular varieties. Check it out.
- Often the low-fat or fat-free products are higher in carbohydrate. The fat gets swapped for the carbohydrate.
- Fruit smoothies or shakes are often light on the "real fruit" and heavy on the sugar.

Healthy Tips

- ★ Don't think kiddie size is just for kids. It's a great small size for calorie counters too.
- ★ Order one dessert and two spoons. Just a few bites often quiets your sweet tooth.

Get It Your Way

★ Low-fat or fat-free; frozen yogurt, light ice cream, or sorbet; and kiddie and small— options are aplenty for healthful eating.

(*Continued*)

Baskin Robbins

❖Baskin Robbins provided nutrition information for all its menu items for use in this book. Their website is www.baskinrobbins.com.

Light 'n Lean Choice

These foods are usually eaten as snacks or in addition to meals.

Healthy 'n Hearty Choice

These foods are usually eaten as snacks or in addition to meals.

Baskin Robbins

BEVERAGES

	Amount	Cal.	Fat (g)	% Cal. Fat	Sat. Fat (g)	Chol. (mg)	Sod. (mg)	Carb. (g)	Fiber (g)	Pro. (g)	Servings/Exchanges
✔Cappuccino Blast w/ Whipped Cream (regular)	8 oz	160	7	39	4	30	60	22	0	2	1 1/2 carb, 1 fat
✔Cappuccino Nonfat Blast (large)	8 oz	90	0	0	0	0	60	20	0	2	1 carb
Chocolate Blast w/ Whipped Cream (regular)	8 oz	250	7	25	4.5	25	120	46	0	2	3 carb, 1 fat
Chocolate Nonfat Blast (regular)	8 oz	170	0	0	0	0	105	40	0	2	2 1/2 carb

✔ = Healthiest Bets; n/a = not available

(Continued)

BEVERAGES (*Continued*)	Amount	Cal.	Fat (g)	% Cal. Fat	Sat. Fat (g)	Chol. (mg)	Sod. (mg)	Carb. (g)	Fiber (g)	Pro. (g)	Servings/Exchanges
✔Mocha Cappuccino Blast w/ Whipped Cream (regular)	8 oz	180	6	30	4	25	70	28	0	2	2 carb, 1 fat
✔Mocha Cappuccino Nonfat Blast (regular)	8 oz	120	0	0	0	0	75	26	0	2	1 1/2 carb
FROZEN YOGURT SMOOTHIES											
Aloha Berry Banana, hardscoop (regular)	8 oz	210	0	0	0	0	85	46	2	2	3 carb
Aloha Berry Banana, soft serve (regular)	8 oz	180	0	0	0	5	80	40	2	2	2 1/2 carb
Bora Berry Bora, hardscoop (regular)	8 oz	190	0	0	0	0	75	40	2	2	2 1/2 carb
Bora Berry Bora, soft serve (regular)	8 oz	170	0	0	0	5	75	38	2	2	2 1/2 carb

Calypso Berry, hardscoop (regular)	8 oz	160	0	0	0	75	35	2	2	2 carb
Calypso Berry, soft serve (regular)	8 oz	160	0	0	0	75	35	2	2	2 carb
Copa Banana, hardscoop (regular)	8 oz	170	0	0	0	70	38	2	2	2 1/2 carb
✔ Copa Banana, soft serve (regular)	8 oz	140	0	0	5	65	30	1	2	2 carb
Sunset Orange, hardscoop (regular)	8 oz	170	0	0	0	75	38	2	2	2 1/2 carb
Sunset Orange, soft serve (regular)	8 oz	150	0	0	5	70	32	2	2	2 carb

✔ = Healthiest Bets; n/a = not available

(Continued)

	Amount	Cal.	Fat (g)	% Cal. Fat	Sat. Fat (g)	Chol. (mg)	Sod. (mg)	Carb. (g)	Fiber (g)	Pro. (g)	Servings/Exchanges
FROZEN YOGURT SMOOTHIES *(Continued)*											
Tropical Tango, hardscoop (regular)	8 oz	190	0	0	0	0	70	43	1	2	3 carb
Tropical Tango, soft serve (regular)	8 oz	160	1	6	0	5	65	36	1	2	2 carb
FROZONE											
✔ Cotton Candy	1/2 cup	150	8	48	4.5	25	45	18	0	1	1 carb, 1 fat
✔ Dirt 'N Worms	1/2 cup	160	8	45	4.5	25	80	22	0	1	1 1/2 carb, 1 fat
✔ Eerrie I Scream	1/2 cup	150	8	48	5	25	45	18	0	1	1 carb, 1 1/2 fat
✔ Neon Sour Apple Ice	1/2 cup	110	0	0	0	0	10	27	0	0	2 carb
✔ Pink Bubblegum	1/2 cup	150	8	48	5	30	40	19	0	2	1 carb, 1 1/2 fat
✔ Polar Paws	1/2 cup	160	10	56	6	30	45	17	0	1	1 carb, 2 fat
✔ Skullicious	1/2 cup	170	10	53	7	30	55	18	0	1	1 carb, 2 fat

	Serving	Cal	Fat (g)	% Fat	Sat Fat (g)	Chol (mg)	Sodium (mg)	Carb (g)	Fiber (g)		Exchanges
✔Strawberry Cone-Fetti	1/2 cup	150	8	48	6	25	50	19	0	1	1 carb, 1 fat
✔Volcanic Lava	1/2 cup	190	12	57	5	25	95	19	1	1	1 carb, 2 fat
✔Watermelon Ice	1/2 cup	110	0	0	0	0	10	28	0	0	2 carb

ICES

	Serving	Cal	Fat (g)	% Fat	Sat Fat (g)	Chol (mg)	Sodium (mg)	Carb (g)	Fiber (g)		Exchanges
✔Daiquiri	1/2 cup	110	0	0	0	0	10	28	0	0	2 carb
✔Neon Sour Apple	1/2 cup	110	0	0	0	0	10	27	0	0	1 1/2 carb
✔The Mask	1/2 cup	120	0	0	0	0	10	29	0	0	2 carb
✔Watermelon	1/2 cup	110	0	0	0	0	10	28	0	0	2 carb

LOW-FAT ICE CREAMS

	Serving	Cal	Fat (g)	% Fat	Sat Fat (g)	Chol (mg)	Sodium (mg)	Carb (g)	Fiber (g)		Exchanges
✔Espresso 'N Cream	1/2 cup	100	3	27	1	5	60	18	1	3	1 carb, 1/2 fat

ICE CREAMS—NO ADDED SUGAR

	Serving	Cal	Fat (g)	% Fat	Sat Fat (g)	Chol (mg)	Sodium (mg)	Carb (g)	Fiber (g)		Exchanges
✔Call Me Nuts	1/2 cup	110	2	16	1	5	55	21	1	2	1 1/2 carb
✔Cherry Cordial	1/2 cup	100	2	18	2	5	55	18	0	3	1 carb

✔ = Healthiest Bets; n/a = not available

(Continued)

NO ADDED SUGAR ICE CREAMS (*Continued*)	Amount	Cal.	Fat (g)	% Cal. Fat	Sat. Fat (g)	Chol. (mg)	Sod. (mg)	Carb. (g)	Fiber (g)	Pro. (g)	Servings/Exchanges
✔ Mad About Chocolate	1/2 cup	100	2	18	1	5	40	19	0	3	1 carb
✔ Pineapple Coconut	1/2 cup	90	2	20	1	5	60	16	0	3	1 carb
✔ Thin Mint	1/2 cup	100	3	27	2	5	65	16	0	3	1 carb, 1/2 fat
NONFAT ICE CREAMS											
✔ Berry Innocent Cheese	1/2 cup	110	0	0	0	0	100	24	0	3	1 1/2 carb
✔ Check-It-Out-Cherry	1/2 cup	100	0	0	0	0	90	22	0	3	1 1/2 carb
✔ Chocolate Vanilla Twist	1/2 cup	100	0	0	0	0	100	21	0	0	1 1/2 carb
✔ Jamoca Swirl	1/2 cup	110	0	0	5	5	105	23	0	3	1 1/2 carb
REGULAR DELUXE ICE CREAMS											
✔ Banana Strawberry	1/2 cup	130	7	48	4.5	25	40	17	0	2	1 carb, 1 fat
✔ Baseball Nut	1/2 cup	160	9	51	5	30	55	18	0	2	1 carb, 2 fat
✔ Black Walnut	1/2 cup	160	11	62	5	30	45	13	1	3	1 carb, 2 fat

	Amount	Calories	Fat (g)	% Fat Cal.	Sat. Fat (g)	Chol. (mg)	Sodium (mg)	Carb. (g)	Fiber (g)	Pro. (g)	Exchanges/Choices
✔ Blueberry Cheesecake	1/2 cup	150	8	48	5	35	70	18	0	1	1 carb, 1 1/2 fat
✔ Butter Brickle Cream	1/2 cup	170	9	48	6	35	65	19	0	1	1 carb, 2 fat
✔ Cappuccino & Espresso	1/2 cup	170	10	53	7	30	55	18	0	1	1 carb, 2 fat
✔ Cherries Jubilee	1/2 cup	140	7	45	4.5	30	40	16	0	2	1 carb, 1 fat
✔ Chocolate	1/2 cup	150	9	54	6	30	60	18	0	2	1 carb, 2 fat
✔ Chocolate Almond	1/2 cup	180	11	55	5	30	55	17	1	3	1 carb, 2 fat
✔ Chocolate Chip	1/2 cup	150	10	60	6	35	45	15	0	2	1 carb, 2 fat
✔ Chocolate Chip Cookie Dough	1/2 cup	170	9	48	6	35	70	20	0	2	1 carb, 2 fat
✔ Chocolate Fudge	1/2 cup	160	9	51	6	30	80	21	0	2	1 carb, 2 fat
✔ Chocolate Mousse Royale	1/2 cup	170	10	53	5	25	60	20	1	2	1 carb, 2 fat
✔ Chocolate Raspberry Truffle	1/2 cup	180	9	45	6	30	60	23	0	3	1 1/2 carb, 2 fat
✔ Choconutty Macaroon	1/2 cup	170	10	53	6	25	50	18	1	1	1 carb, 2 fat

(Continued)

✔ = Healthiest Bets; n/a = not available

REGULAR DELUXE ICE CREAMS (*Continued*)	Amount	Cal.	Fat (g)	% Cal. Fat	Sat. Fat (g)	Chol. (mg)	Sod. (mg)	Carb. (g)	Fiber (g)	Pro. (g)	Servings/Exchanges
✔ Chunky Heath Bar	1/2 cup	170	10	53	6	30	70	19	0	2	1 carb, 2 fat
✔ Coffee Biscotti Chocolati	1/2 cup	160	10	56	7	35	50	17	0	1	1 carb, 2 fat
✔ Cookies N Cream	1/2 cup	170	11	58	7	30	80	16	0	2	1 carb, 2 fat
✔ Egg Nog	1/2 cup	150	8	48	5	40	45	16	0	2	1 carb, 1 1/2 fat
✔ English Toffee	1/2 cup	160	9	51	6	30	70	19	0	1	1 carb, 2 fat
✔ Everybody's Favorite Candy Bar	1/2 cup	170	9	48	5	30	90	20	0	2	1 carb, 2 fat
✔ French Vanilla	1/2 cup	160	10	56	6	70	45	14	0	2	1 carb, 2 fat
✔ Fudge Brownie	1/2 cup	170	11	58	6	25	75	19	1	3	1 carb, 2 fat
✔ German Chocolate Cake	1/2 cup	180	10	50	6	25	75	20	0	3	1 carb, 2 fat
✔ Gold Medal Ribbon	1/2 cup	150	8	48	5	30	95	20	0	2	1 carb, 1 1/2 fat
✔ Jamoca	1/2 cup	140	9	58	5	35	45	14	0	2	1 carb, 1 1/2 fat

✔ Jamoca Almond Fudge	1/2 cup	160	9	51	4.5	25	40	17	0	3	1 carb, 2 fat
✔ Kahluaccino Chip	1/2 cup	150	8	48	5	25	45	18	0	1	1 carb, 1 fat
✔ Lemon Custard	1/2 cup	150	8	48	5	45	55	16	0	2	1 carb, 1 1/2 fat
✔ Mint Chocolate Chip	1/2 cup	150	10	60	6	35	45	15	0	3	1 carb, 2 fat
✔ Mississippi Mud	1/2 cup	160	8	45	4.5	25	85	22	0	1	1 carb, 2 fat
✔ Nutty Coconut	1/2 cup	170	12	64	6	30	45	15	1	1	1 carb, 2 fat
✔ Old Fashion Butter Pecan	1/2 cup	160	11	62	6	35	50	13	0	2	1 carb, 2 fat
✔ Peanut Butter N Chocolate	1/2 cup	180	12	60	6	30	95	16	1	3	1 carb, 2 fat
✔ Peppermint	1/2 cup	150	8	48	5	30	45	18	0	1	1 carb, 1 1/2 fat
✔ Pistachio Almond	1/2 cup	170	12	64	5	30	45	13	1	3	1 carb, 2 fat
✔ Pralines N Cream	1/2 cup	160	9	51	5	30	85	19	0	2	1 carb, 2 fat
✔ Pumpkin Pie	1/2 cup	130	7	48	4.5	30	50	16	0	2	1 carb, 1 fat
✔ Quarterback Crunch	1/2 cup	160	10	56	7	30	75	18	0	2	1 carb, 2 fat

✔ = Healthiest Bets; n/a = not available

(Continued)

REGULAR DELUXE ICE CREAMS (*Continued*)	Amount	Cal.	Fat (g)	% Cal. Fat	Sat. Fat (g)	Chol. (mg)	Sod. (mg)	Carb. (g)	Fiber (g)	Pro. (g)	Servings/Exchanges
✔Reeses Peanutbutter	1/2 cup	180	11	55	6	30	70	17	0	3	1 carb, 2 fat
✔Rocky Road	1/2 cup	170	10	53	5	30	60	19	0	3	1 carb, 2 fat
✔Rum Raisin	1/2 cup	140	7	45	4.5	30	40	18	0	2	1 carb, 1 fat
✔Strawberry Cheesecake	1/2 cup	150	9	54	5	35	65	17	0	2	1 carb, 2 fat
Tripple Chocolate Passion	1/2 cup	180	11	55	7	35	70	21	0	3	1 carb, 2 fat
✔Vanilla	1/2 cup	140	8	51	5	40	40	14	0	3	1 carb, 1 1/2 fat
✔Very Berry Strawberry	1/2 cup	130	7	48	4	25	40	16	0	1	1 carb, 1 fat
✔Winter White Chocolate	1/2 cup	150	9	54	6	25	50	18	0	2	1 carb, 2 fat
✔World Class Chocolate	1/2 cup	160	9	51	5	30	55	18	0	2	1 carb, 2 fat
SHERBETS											
✔Blue Raspberry	1/2 cup	120	2	15	1	5	30	25	0	1	1 1/2 carb
✔Orange	1/2 cup	120	2	15	1	5	25	26	0	1	1 1/2 carb

	Serving Size	Calories	Fat (g)	% Fat Cal	Sat Fat (g)	Chol (mg)	Sodium (mg)	Carb (g)	Fiber (g)	Protein (g)	Exchanges
✔Rainbow	1/2 cup	120	2	15	1	5	25	26	0	1	1 1/2 carb
✔Tangerine Pineapple	1/2 cup	120	1	8	0	5	25	22	0	1	1 1/2 carb
SORBETS											
✔Black Tie Bubbly	1/2 cup	120	0	0	0	0	15	31	0	1	2 carb
✔Mixed Berry Lemonade	1/2 cup	110	0	0	0	0	10	28	0	0	2 carb
✔Pink Raspberry Lemon	1/2 cup	120	0	0	0	0	10	29	0	0	2 carb
YOGURT GONE CRAZY											
✔Maui Brownie Madness	1/2 cup	140	3	19	1	5	80	26	1	2	1 1/2 carb, 1/2 fat
✔Perils of Praline	1/2 cup	140	3	19	1.5	5	105	25	0	4	1 1/2 carb, 1/2 fat
✔Raspberry Cheese Louise	1/2 cup	130	3	21	2	10	90	24	0	2	1 1/2 carb, 1/2 fat

✔ = Healthiest Bets; n/a = not available

Freshëns Premium Yogurt

❖Freshëns Premium Yogurt provides nutrition
information for some of its menu items on its
website at www.freshens.com.

Light 'n Lean Choice

These foods are usually eaten as snacks or in addition
to meals.

Healthy 'n Hearty Choice

These foods are usually eaten as snacks or in addition
to meals.

Freshëns Premium Yogurt

	Amount	Cal.	Fat (g)	% Cal. Fat	Sat. Fat (g)	Chol. (mg)	Sod. (mg)	Carb. (g)	Fiber (g)	Pro. (g)	Servings/Exchanges
CITRUS SMOOTHIES											
Orange Shooter	1	369	3	7	n/a	11	39	81	3	3	5 1/2 carb
Orange Sunrise	1	399	3	7	n/a	11	39	90	3	3	6 carb
Pineapple Passion	1	442	4	8	n/a	0	11	100	3	3	6 1/2 carb
Raspberry Rumba	1	407	1	2	n/a	0	12	95	4	5	6 carb
DECADENT SMOOTHIES											
Coffee Fudge Ripple	1	733	12	15	n/a	17	319	138	2	16	9 carb, 1 fat
Fudge Oreo Supreme	1	663	11	15	n/a	12	413	126	2	15	8 1/2 carb
Peanut Butter	1	978	34	31	n/a	17	514	141	3	27	9 carb, 6 fat
Peanut Butter Banana Supreme	1	763	23	27	n/a	7	401	114	4	25	7 1/2 carb, 3 fat

✔ = Healthiest Bets; n/a = not available

(Continued)

	Amount	Cal.	Fat (g)	% Cal. Fat	Sat. Fat (g)	Chol. (mg)	Sod. (mg)	Carb. (g)	Fiber (g)	Pro. (g)	Servings/Exchanges
FROZEN YOGURT											
✔ All Flavors (average)	4 oz	100	0	0	n/a	10	75	19	n/a	4	1 carb
ICE CREAMS											
✔ Outrageous	4 oz	150	9	54	n/a	n/a	35	16	n/a	3	1 carb, 1 fat
(average of all flavors)											
PRETZELS											
Pretzel	1	510	6	11	0.5	0	780	98	4	14	6 1/2 starch, 1 fat
YOGURT SMOOTHIES											
Caribbean Craze	1	349	1	3	n/a	0	11	84	4	2	5 1/2 carb
Jamaican Jammer	1	495	1	2	n/a	5	156	110	4	12	7 carb
Pina Colider	1	584	4	6	n/a	5	156	126	4	11	8 1/2 carb
Raspberry Rapture	1	541	1	2	n/a	5	157	121	4	12	8 carb

Raspberry Rhapsody	1	379	1	2	n/a	0	12	88	4	5	6 carb
Raspberry Rocker	1	509	1	2	n/a	5	157	113	4	25	7 1/2 carb
Strawberry Shooter	1	256	0	0	n/a	0	11	63	2	1	4 carb
Strawberry Squeeze	1	405	1	2	n/a	5	156	88	2	11	6 carb

✔ = Healthiest Bets; n/a = not available

Häagen-Dazs Ice Cream Café

❖Häagen-Dazs Ice Cream Café provided nutrition
  information for most of its menu items for use in
  this book. Their website is www.haagendazs.com.

Light 'n Lean Choice

These foods are usually eaten as snacks or in addition
to meals.

Healthy 'n Hearty Choice

These foods are usually eaten as snacks or in addition
to meals.

Häagen-Dazs Ice Cream Café

	Amount	Cal.	Fat (g)	% Cal. Fat	Sat. Fat (g)	Chol. (mg)	Sod. (mg)	Carb. (g)	Fiber (g)	Pro. (g)	Servings/Exchanges
FROZEN YOGURTS											
Vanilla Fudge	1/2 cup	160	0	0	0	5	100	34	0	6	2 carb
✔ Vanilla Raspberry Swirl	1/2 cup	130	0	0	0	5	30	29	0	4	2 carb
ICE CREAM											
Baileys Irish Cream	1/2 cup	270	17	57	10	115	70	23	0	5	1 1/2 carb, 3 fat
Belgian Chocolate Chocolate	1/2 cup	330	21	57	12	85	50	29	3	5	2 carb, 4 fat
Brownies a la mode	1/2 cup	280	16	51	10	30	135	28	0	5	2 carb, 3 fat
Butter Pecan	1/2 cup	300	22	66	10	105	110	20	0	5	1 1/2 carb, 4 fat
Cappuccino Commotion	1/2 cup	310	21	61	12	100	90	25	1	5	1 1/2 carb, 4 fat
Chocolate	1/2 cup	260	17	59	10	110	60	21	1	5	1 1/2 carb, 3 fat

✔ = Healthiest Bets; n/a = not available

(Continued)

ICE CREAM (*Continued*)	Amount	Cal.	Fat (g)	% Cal. Fat	Sat. Fat (g)	Chol. (mg)	Sod. (mg)	Carb. (g)	Fiber (g)	Pro. (g)	Servings/Exchanges
Chocolate Chocolate Chip	1/2 cup	300	19	57	11	100	55	26	2	5	1 1/2 carb, 4 fat
Chocolate Chocolate Mint	1/2 cup	300	20	60	11	95	50	25	1	5	1 1/2 carb, 4 fat
Chocolate Swiss Almond	1/2 cup	300	20	60	11	100	55	24	2	5	1 1/2 carb, 4 fat
Coffee	1/2 cup	250	17	61	10	115	65	20	0	5	1 1/2 carb, 3 fat
Coffee Mocha Chip	1/2 cup	270	18	60	12	105	75	24	0	4	1 1/2 carb, 3 fat
Cookie Dough Dynamo	1/2 cup	310	20	58	12	95	125	29	0	4	2 carb, 3 1/2 fat
Cookies & Cream	1/2 cup	270	17	57	10	105	95	23	0	5	1 1/2 carb, 3 fat
Deep Chocolate Peanut Butter	1/2 cup	350	24	62	11	80	85	26	4	8	1 1/2 carb, 5 fat
Dulce De Leche Caramel	1/2 cup	270	16	53	10	95	90	27	0	5	2 carb, 2 1/2 fat
Macadamia Brittle	1/2 cup	280	19	61	11	105	105	24	0	4	1 1/2 carb, 4 fat
Macadamia Nut	1/2 cup	320	24	68	12	110	100	20	0	5	1 carb, 5 fat
Mint Chip	1/2 cup	280	18	58	12	105	85	25	0	4	1 1/2 carb, 4 fat

Pineapple Coconut	1/2 cup	230	13	51	8	90	55	25	0	4	1 1/2 carb, 2 1/2 fat
Pistachio	1/2 cup	280	19	61	10	110	80	21	0	5	1 1/2 carb, 3 1/2 fat
Pralines & Cream	1/2 cup	280	17	55	9	95	160	28	0	4	2 carb, 3 fat
Rum Raisin	1/2 cup	260	17	59	10	105	55	21	0	4	1 1/2 carb, 3 fat
Strawberry	1/2 cup	250	16	58	9	90	60	22	0	4	1 1/2 carb, 3 fat
Vanilla	1/2 cup	250	17	61	10	115	65	20	0	4	1 1/2 carb, 3 fat
Vanilla Chocolate Chip	1/2 cup	290	19	59	12	100	70	25	0	5	1 1/2 carb, 4 fat
Vanilla Swiss Almond	1/2 cup	290	20	62	11	100	70	23	0	5	1 1/2 carb, 4 fat
ICE CREAM BARS											
Chocolate & Dark Chocolate	1	350	24	62	15	85	45	28	2	5	2 carb, 4 fat
Coffee & Almond Crunch	1	370	27	66	15	90	80	27	0	5	2 carb, 4 1/2 fat
Vanilla & Almonds	1	380	28	66	14	90	70	26	1	6	1 1/2 carb, 5 fat
Vanilla & Milk Chocolate	1	340	24	64	14	90	65	25	0	5	1 1/2 carb, 5 fat

(Continued)

✓ = Healthiest Bets; n/a = not available

	Amount	Cal.	Fat (g)	% Cal. Fat	Sat. Fat (g)	Chol. (mg)	Sod. (mg)	Carb. (g)	Fiber (g)	Pro. (g)	Servings/Exchanges
LOW-FAT ICE CREAM											
Coffee Fudge	1/2 cup	170	3	16	1.5	25	95	32	0	5	2 carb
Cookies & Fudge	1/2 cup	180	3	15	1.5	15	115	33	0	7	2 carb
SOFT-SERVE FROZEN YOGURTS											
✔Chocolate	1/2 cup	110	0	0	0	0	65	23	0	4	1 1/2 carb
✔Chocolate Mousse	1/2 cup	80	0	0	0	0	65	24	1	5	1 1/2 carb
✔Coffee	1/2 cup	110	0	0	0	5	70	22	0	5	1 1/2 carb
✔Strawberry	1/2 cup	110	0	0	0	0	60	24	0	4	1 1/2 carb
✔Vanilla	1/2 cup	110	0	0	0	5	75	22	0	5	1 1/2 carb
✔Vanilla Mousse	1/2 cup	70	0	0	0	5	65	23	0	4	1 1/2 carb
✔White Chocolate	1/2 cup	110	0	0	0	5	75	22	0	5	1 1/2 carb
SORBET											
✔Mango	1/2 cup	120	0	0	0	0	0	31	0	0	2 carb

	Amount	Cal	Fat (g)	% Cal Fat	Sat Fat (g)	Chol (mg)	Sod (mg)	Carb (g)	Fiber (g)	Pro (g)	Choices/Exchanges
✓Orange	1/2 cup	120	0		0	0	0	30	0	0	2 carb
✓Raspberry	1/2 cup	120	0		0	0	0	30	0	0	2 carb
✓Strawberry	1/2 cup	120	0		0	0	0	30	0	0	2 carb
✓Zesty Lemon	1/2 cup	120	0		0	0	0	31	0	0	2 carb
SORBET BARS											
✓Raspberry	1	90	0		0	0	15	21	0	2	1 1/2 carb
✓Vanilla	1	90	0		0	0	15	21	0	2	1 1/2 carb
SORBET SOFT SERVE											
✓Raspberry	1/2 cup	110	0		0	0	0	28	2	0	2 carb
UNCOATED ICE CREAM BARS											
✓Chocolate	1	200	13	59	8	85	55	16	0	4	1 carb, 2 1/2 fat
✓Coffee	1	190	13	62	8	85	65	15	0	3	1 carb, 2 1/2 fat
✓Vanilla	1	190	13	62	8	85	50	15	0	3	1 carb, 2 1/2 fat

✓ = Healthiest Bets; n/a = not available

I Can't Believe It's Yogurt

❖I Can't Believe It's Yogurt provides nutrition
information for some of its menu items in a
brochure.

Light 'n Lean Choice

These foods are usually eaten as snacks or in addition
to meals.

Healthy 'n Hearty Choice

These foods are usually eaten as snacks or in addition
to meals.

I Can't Believe It's Yogurt

	Amount	Cal.	Fat (g)	% Cal. Fat	Sat. Fat (g)	Chol. (mg)	Sod. (mg)	Carb. (g)	Fiber (g)	Pro. (g)	Servings/Exchanges
HAND-SCOOPED FROZEN YOGURT											
✔ Amaretto Cherry Crunch	1/2 cup	170	5	26	2	25	95	27	1	5	2 carb, 1 fat
✔ Chocolate	1/2 cup	150	4	24	3	10	135	25	1	5	1 1/2 carb, 1 fat
Chocolate Cherry Cheesecake	1/2 cup	180	5	25	3	25	110	32	0	5	2 carb, 1 fat
✔ Chocolate Chip Cookie Dough	1/2 cup	180	5	25	3	40	120	30	0	5	2 carb, 1 fat
✔ Chocolate Mint Chip	1/2 cup	180	7	35	5	25	95	27	0	5	2 carb, 1 fat
✔ Chunky Chocolate Brownie	1/2 cup	180	6	30	3	10	135	28	1	5	2 carb, 1 fat

✔ = Healthiest Bets; n/a = not available

(Continued)

HAND-SCOOPED FROZEN YOGURT (*Continued*)	Amount	Cal.	Fat (g)	% Cal. Fat	Sat. Fat (g)	Chol. (mg)	Sod. (mg)	Carb. (g)	Fiber (g)	Pro. (g)	Servings/Exchanges
✔Classic Vanilla	1/2 cup	160	4	23	2	40	115	26	0	6	1 1/2 carb, 1 fat
✔Cookies 'N Cream	1/2 cup	170	5	26	3	25	120	28	0	5	2 carb, 1 fat
✔Macadamia Mania	1/2 cup	180	6	30	4	25	150	30	0	5	2 carb, 1 fat
✔Peanut Butter Cup	1/2 cup	200	8	36	4	25	135	27	0	6	2 carb, 1 1/2 fat
✔Pralines 'N Cream	1/2 cup	180	5	25	3	25	130	31	0	5	2 carb, 1 fat
✔Rocky Road	1/2 cup	180	6	30	3	10	125	27	2	5	2 carb, 1 fat
✔Rum Raisin	1/2 cup	170	4	21	2	25	95	31	0	5	2 carb, 1 fat
✔Tin Roof Fudge	1/2 cup	180	6	30	3	25	110	28	0	6	2 carb, 1 fat
NONFAT FROZEN YOGURT											
✔Chocolicious	1/2 cup	100	0	0	0	5	70	21	1	3	1 1/2 carb
✔Coffee Break	1/2 cup	90	0	0	0	0	70	20	0	3	1 carb
✔Eggnog Extravaganza	1/2 cup	110	0	0	0	5	65	24	0	3	1 1/2 carb

✓German Chocolate Cakes	1/2 cup	100	0	0	0	80	23	1	3	1 1/2 carb
✓Go Bananas	1/2 cup	100	0	0	0	60	21	0	3	1 1/2 carb
✓Key Lime Pie	1/2 cup	100	0	0	0	65	22	0	3	1 1/2 carb
✓N.Y. Cheesecake	1/2 cup	100	0	0	0	70	22	0	3	1 1/2 carb
✓New Orleans Praline	1/2 cup	100	0	0	0	90	23	0	3	1 1/2 carb
✓Not Just Plain Vanilla	1/2 cup	90	0	0	0	70	20	0	3	1 carb
✓Peppermint Stick	1/2 cup	100	0	0	0	65	23	0	3	1 1/2 carb
✓Strictly Strawberry	1/2 cup	110	0	0	0	70	24	0	2	1 1/2 carb
✓The Great Pumpkin	1/2 cup	100	0	0	0	70	23	0	3	1 1/2 carb
NONFAT FROZEN YOGURT W/ NUTRASWEET										
✓After Dinner Mint	1/2 cup	90	0	0	0	75	19	1	3	1 carb
✓All American Cherry	1/2 cup	90	0	0	0	75	18	0	3	1 carb

(Continued)

✓ = Healthiest Bets; n/a = not available

NONFAT FROZEN YOGURT W/ NUTRASWEET *(Continued)*	Amount	Cal.	Fat (g)	% Cal. Fat	Sat. Fat (g)	Chol. (mg)	Sod. (mg)	Carb. (g)	Fiber (g)	Pro. (g)	Servings/Exchanges
✔Butterscotch Burst	1/2 cup	90	0	0	0	0	75	18	0	3	1 carb
✔Chocolicious	1/2 cup	100	0	0	0	0	70	21	1	3	1 1/2 carb
✔Decaf Coffee Break	1/2 cup	90	0	0	0	0	75	18	0	3	1 carb
✔Just Peachy	1/2 cup	90	0	0	0	0	75	18	0	3	1 carb
✔Orange Appeal	1/2 cup	90	0	0	0	0	75	18	0	3	1 carb
ORIGINAL FROZEN YOGURT											
✔Awesome Amaretto	1/2 cup	130	3	21	2	10	105	23	0	3	1 1/2 carb, 1/2 fat
✔Cookies 'N Cream	1/2 cup	120	2	15	1	5	90	25	0	3	1 1/2 carb
✔French Vanilla	1/2 cup	120	3	23	2	20	90	21	0	3	1 1/2 carb, 1/2 fat
✔Peanut Butter Bliss	1/2 cup	140	6	39	2	5	95	21	0	3	1 1/2 carb, 1 fat
YOGLACE FROZEN DAIRY DESSERT											
✔Belgian Chocolate	1/2 cup	60	0	0	0	0	45	14	1	3	1 carb

✔Lemon Spritzer	1/2 cup	45	0	0	0	5	30	12	0	2	1 carb
✔Margarita	1/2 cup	50	0	0	0	5	30	13	0	2	1 carb
✔Swiss Vanilla	1/2 cup	45	0	0	0	5	30	12	0	2	1 carb

✔ = Healthiest Bets; n/a = not available

Mrs. Fields Cookies

❖Mrs. Fields Cookies provides nutrition information for most of its products on their website at www.mrsfields.com.

Light 'n Lean Choice

These foods are usually eaten as snacks or in addition to meals.

Healthy 'n Hearty Choice

These foods are usually eaten as snacks or in addition to meals.

Mrs. Fields Cookies

	Amount	Cal.	Fat (g)	% Cal. Fat	Sat. Fat (g)	Chol. (mg)	Sod. (mg)	Carb. (g)	Fiber (g)	Pro. (g)	Servings/Exchanges
BAGELS											
✔Cinnamon Raisin	1	300	2	6	0.5	0	230	61	4	11	4 starch
✔Cinnamon Sugar	1	310	2	6	0.5	0	330	64	3	12	4 starch
✔Everything	1	290	2	6	0.5	0	330	59	3	12	4 starch
✔Onion	1	290	2	6	0.5	0	330	59	3	12	4 starch
✔Plain	1	290	2	6	0.5	0	330	59	3	12	4 starch
✔Poppyseed	1	290	2	6	0.5	0	330	59	3	12	4 starch
✔Sesame	1	290	2	6	0.5	0	330	59	3	12	4 starch
BREAKFAST COOKIES											
Banana Nut	1	340	20	53	4	40	290	34	2	7	2 starch, 4 fat

✔ = Healthiest Bets; n/a = not available

(Continued)

BREAKFAST COOKIES (*Continued*)	Amount	Cal.	Fat (g)	% Cal. Fat	Sat. Fat (g)	Chol. (mg)	Sod. (mg)	Carb. (g)	Fiber (g)	Pro. (g)	Servings/Exchanges
Blueberry	1	330	16	44	7	50	340	43	2	5	3 starch, 2 fat
Chocolate Chip	1	320	14	39	7	60	410	42	2	5	3 starch, 2 fat
Mandarin Orange	1	290	13	40	6	50	340	37	0	5	2 1/2 starch, 2 fat
Raspberry	1	280	12	39	6	50	350	38	0	4	2 1/2 starch, 2 fat
BROWNIES											
Double Fudge	1	360	19	48	11	80	240	49	2	4	3 carb, 3 fat
Frosted Fudge	1	440	21	43	12	80	265	62	2	4	4 carb, 2 1/2 fat
German Chocolate	1	570	35	55	16	45	290	69	4	6	4 1/2 carb, 4 fat
Peanut Butter Dreamba	1	670	42	56	21	85	460	70	3	10	4 1/2 carb, 7 1/2 fat
Pecan Fudge	1	340	21	56	9	70	220	40	2	4	2 1/2 carb, 3 fat
✓Pecan Pie	1	140	7	45	4	15	110	20	0	1	1 carb, 1 fat
Rocky Mountain Mogul	1	610	35	52	18	60	280	76	4	6	5 carb, 4 1/2 fat

	Amount	Cal	Fat (g)	% Cal Fat	Sat Fat (g)	Chol (mg)	Sod (mg)	Carb (g)	Fiber (g)	Pro (g)	Exchanges
Walnut Fudge	1	340	20	53	9	70	220	40	2	5	2 1/2 carb, 3 fat
CINNAMON ROLLS											
Cinnamon Roll	1	440	17	35	3	0	500	64	0	6	4 starch, 2 1/2 fat
Cinnamon Roll w/ Icing	1	470	18	34	3.5	5	500	69	0	6	4 1/2 starch, 2 fat
Sticky Bun	1	440	17	35	3	0	500	64	0	6	4 starch, 2 1/2 fat
COOKIE CUPS											
✔ Butter	1	220	9	37	6	30	190	29	0	2	2 carb, 1 fat
Butter Toffee	1	420	18	39	11	70	400	60	0	4	4 carb, 2 fat
Chewy Fudge	1	410	20	44	12	45	180	61	3	4	4 carb, 2 fat
Coconut Macadamia	1	440	24	49	12	55	380	55	2	4	4 carb, 2 1/2 fat
Debra's Special	1	410	17	37	8	50	370	60	3	5	4 carb, 2 fat
Milk Chocolate	1	430	20	42	12	55	340	60	1	4	4 carb, 3 fat
Milk Chocolate Macadamia	1	450	24	48	12	50	310	56	2	4	4 carb, 3 fat

(Continued)

✔ = Healthiest Bets; n/a = not available

COOKIE CUPS (*Continued*)	Amount	Cal.	Fat (g)	% Cal. Fat	Sat. Fat (g)	Chol. (mg)	Sod. (mg)	Carb. (g)	Fiber (g)	Pro. (g)	Servings/Exchanges
Milk Chocolate w/ Walnuts	1	440	23	47	12	55	330	58	2	5	4 carb, 3 fat
Oatmeal Raisin	1	410	17	37	8	50	380	60	2	5	4 carb, 2 fat
Peanut Butter	1	430	22	46	10	65	450	54	1	7	4 carb, 2 1/2 fat
Pumpkin Harvest	1	370	19	46	10	50	200	47	1	4	3 carb, 3 fat
Semi-Sweet Chocolate	1	420	20	43	12	20	320	62	2	4	4 carb, 2 fat
Semi-Sweet Chocolate w/ Walnuts	1	440	23	47	12	50	310	58	2	4	4 carb, 3 fat
Triple Chocolate	1	430	21	44	12	55	340	60	2	4	4 carb, 2 fat
White Chunk Macadamia	1	460	24	47	12	20	310	58	1	4	4 carb, 3 fat
COOKIE NIBBLERS											
✔ Butter	2	110	5	41	3	15	90	15	0	1	1 carb, 1/2 fat
✔ Chewy Chocolate Fudge	2	110	5	41	3.4	10	30	15	0	1	1 carb, 1/2 fat
✔ Cinnamon Sugar	2	120	5	38	3	15	90	17	0	1	1 carb, 1/2 fat

Item											Exchanges
✔Debra's Special—Oatmeal Raisin Walnut	2	100	5	45	2	10	80	13	0	1	1 carb, 1/2 fat
✔Milk Chocolate	2	110	5	41	3	15	70	15	0	1	1 carb, 1/2 fat
✔Milk Chocolate w/Walnuts	2	120	6	45	3	10	65	14	0	1	1 carb, 1 fat
✔Peanut Butter	2	110	6	49	2.5	15	95	13	0	2	1 carb, 1 fat
✔Semi-Sweet Chocolate	2	110	5	41	3	10	60	15	0	1	1 carb, 1/2 fat
✔Triple Chocolate	2	110	6	49	3	15	65	15	0	1	1 carb, 1/2 fat
✔White Chunk Macadamia	2	120	7	53	3.5	10	60	13	0	1	1 carb, 1 fat
COOKIES											
Butter	1	290	12	37	8	50	250	39	0	3	2 1/2 carb, 2 fat
Butter Toffee	1	290	13	40	8	55	190	40	0	3	2 1/2 carb, 2 fat
Chewy Fudge	1	300	14	42	9	35	80	40	3	3	2 1/2 carb, 2 fat
Cinnamon Sugar	1	300	12	36	8	50	250	41	0	3	2 1/2 carb, 2 fat

✔ = Healthiest Bets; n/a = not available

(Continued)

COOKIES (Continued)	Amount	Cal.	Fat (g)	% Cal. Fat	Sat. Fat (g)	Chol. (mg)	Sod. (mg)	Carb. (g)	Fiber (g)	Pro. (g)	Servings/Exchanges
Coconut Macadamia	1	280	13	42	5	20	220	39	0	3	2 1/2 carb, 2 fat
Debra's Special	1	280	12	39	6	40	180	39	2	4	2 1/2 carb, 2 fat
M & M	1	330	14	38	9	50	255	45	0	2	3 carb, 2 fat
Milk Chocolate	1	280	13	42	8	40	180	38	0	3	2 1/2 carb, 2 fat
Milk Chocolate Macadamia	1	320	18	51	9	40	180	36	0	4	2 1/2 carb, 3 fat
Milk Chocolate with Walnuts	1	320	17	48	9	40	180	37	1	4	2 1/2 carb, 3 fat
Oatmeal Chocolate Chip	1	280	13	42	8	35	140	40	1	3	2 1/2 carb, 2 fat
Peanut Butter	1	310	16	46	8	45	260	34	0	5	2 carb, 3 fat
Peanut Butter Milk Chocolate	1	300	17	51	8	40	160	35	0	5	2 carb, 3 fat
Pumpkin Harvest	1	260	14	48	7	40	270	31	0	4	2 carb, 2 fat
Semi-Sweet Chocolate	1	280	14	45	8	30	160	40	1	2	2 1/2 carb, 2 fat
Semi-Sweet Chocolate w/ Pecans	1	320	18	51	9	40	180	36	0	4	2 1/2 carb, 3 fat

Semi-Sweet Chocolate w/ Walnuts	1	310	16	46	8	35	170	38	2	3	2 1/2 carb, 2 fat
White Chunk Macadamia	1	310	17	49	9	35	170	37	0	4	2 1/2 carb, 2 fat

CROISSANTS

Almond	1	430	26	54	15	50	265	43	2	8	3 starch, 4 fat
✔Apple Filled	1	250	8	29	4	20	260	39	2	5	2 1/2 starch, 1 fat
Butter	1	320	20	56	15	48	257	30	1	6	2 starch, 3 1/2 fat
Chocolate Filled	1	339	15	40	8	22	250	44	2	6	3 starch, 2 fat
Cream Cheese	1	284	13	41	7	27	277	37	1	6	2 1/2 starch, 2 fat

FAT-FREE MUFFINS

✔Apple Cinnamon	1	360	1	3	0	0	620	79	2	8	5 starch

LOW-FAT MUFFINS

✔Apple Bran	1	340	3	8	1	5	680	74	5	6	5 starch

(Continued)

✔ = Healthiest Bets; n/a = not available

LOW FAT MUFFINS (Continued)	Amount	Cal.	Fat (g)	% Cal. Fat	Sat. Fat (g)	Chol. (mg)	Sod. (mg)	Carb. (g)	Fiber (g)	Pro. (g)	Servings/Exchanges
✔Fruit	1	250	2	7	1	0	320	55	1	4	3 1/2 starch
✔Poppyseed	1	290	3	9	1	0	370	60	1	6	4 starch
MINI COOKIE CUPS											
✔Butter	1	110	5	41	3	15	90	15	0	1	1 carb, 1/2 fat
✔Chewy Chocolate Fudge	1	140	7	45	4	15	60	20	0	1	1 carb, 1 fat
✔Debra's Special	1	140	6	39	2.5	20	130	20	0	2	1 carb, 1 fat
✔Milk Chocolate	1	140	7	45	4	20	115	20	0	1	1 carb, 1 fat
✔Milk Chocolate w/ Walnuts	1	150	8	48	4	20	110	19	0	2	1 carb, 1 1/2 fat
✔Peanut Butter	1	140	7	45	3.5	20	150	18	0	2	1 carb, 1 fat
✔Semi-Sweet Chocolate	1	140	7	45	4	15	110	20	0	1	1 carb, 1 1/2 fat
✔Semi-Sweet Chocolate w/ Walnuts	1	150	8	48	4	15	100	20	0	1	1 carb, 1 1/2 fat

✔Triple Chocolate	1	140	7	45	4	20	115	20	0	1	1 carb, 1 fat
✔White Chunk Macadamia	1	150	8	48	4	15	105	19	0	1	1 carb, 1 1/2 fat

MINI MUFFINS

✔Banana Nut	1	80	5	56	1	10	70	8	0	2	1/2 starch, 1 fat
✔Blueberry	1	80	4	45	2	10	85	11	0	1	1/2 starch, 1/2 fat
✔Chocolate Chip	1	80	4	45	1.5	15	100	10	0	1	1/2 starch, 1 fat
✔Coco White	1	90	5	50	2.5	10	80	10	0	1	1/2 starch, 1 fat
✔Mandarin Orange	1	70	3	39	1.5	15	85	9	0	1	1/2 starch, 1/2 fat
✔Mandarin Orange Chocolate Chip	1	80	4	45	2	10	70	10	0	1	1/2 starch, 1 fat
✔Pumpkin	1	70	4	51	1	10	85	9	0	1	1/2 starch, 1/2 fat
✔Raspberry	1	70	3	39	1.5	15	90	8	0	1	1/2 starch, 1/2 fat
✔White Chunk Macadamia	1	70	3	39	1.5	10	85	10	0	1	1/2 starch, 1/2 fat

(Continued)

✔ = Healthiest Bets; n/a = not available

	Amount	Cal.	Fat (g)	% Cal. Fat	Sat. Fat (g)	Chol. (mg)	Sod. (mg)	Carb. (g)	Fiber (g)	Pro. (g)	Servings/Exchanges
MUFFINS											
Banana Nut	1	420	25	54	5	50	360	42	3	8	3 starch, 4 fat
Blueberry	1	400	20	45	9	60	420	53	2	6	3 1/2 starch, 3 fat
Bran	1	400	16	36	4	15	470	59	4	7	4 starch, 1 1/2 fat
Chocolate Chip	1	390	17	39	8	70	500	51	0	6	3 1/2 starch, 2 fat
Mandarin Orange	1	360	16	40	7	65	420	46	1	6	3 starch, 2 1/2 fat
Raspberry	1	340	15	40	7	60	430	46	1	5	3 starch, 2 fat
SUGAR-FREE COOKIES											
✔Chocolatey Chunk	1	130	5	35	2.5	15	55	19	0	2	1 carb, 1 fat
✔Old Fashioned Oatmeal Spice	1	120	4	30	1.5	15	70	19	0	2	1 carb, 1 fat
✔White Chunk Fudge	1	120	5	38	2.5	20	75	18	0	2	1 carb, 1 fat

✔ = Healthiest Bets; n/a = not available

TCBY

❖TCBY provides nutrition information for some of
its items in a brochure.

Light 'n Lean Choice

These foods are usually eaten as snacks or in addition
to meals.

Healthy 'n Hearty Choice

These foods are usually eaten as snacks or in addition
to meals.

(*Continued*)

TCBY

	Amount	Cal.	Fat (g)	% Cal. Fat	Sat. Fat (g)	Chol. (mg)	Sod. (mg)	Carb. (g)	Fiber (g)	Pro. (g)	Servings/Exchanges
FROZEN SOFT-SERVE YOGURT											
✔ 96% Fat Free Frozen Yogurt	1/2 cup	130	3	21	2	15	60	23	0	4	1 1/2 carb, 1/2 fat
✔ No Sugar Added Nonfat Frozen Yogurt	1/2 cup	80	0	0	0	0	35	20	0	4	1 carb
✔ Nonfat & Nondairy Sorbet	1/2 cup	100	0	0	0	0	30	24	0	0	1 1/2 carb
✔ Nonfat Frozen Yogurt	1/2 cup	110	0	0	0	0	60	23	0	4	1 1/2 carb
HAND-DIPPED											
✔ Low Fat Ice Cream	1/2 cup	120	3	23	1	5	75	22	0	3	1 1/2 carb, 1/2 fat
✔ No Sugar Added Lowfat Ice Cream	1/2 cup	100	3	27	1.5	10	55	20	0	3	1 carb, 1/2 fat

✔ = Healthiest Bets; n/a = not available

Tacos, Burritos, and All Else Mexican

RESTAURANTS

Del Taco

Taco Bell

Taco John's

Taco Time

NUTRITION PROS

- Beans used in Mexican cooking, such as pinto beans and black beans, add soluble fiber. This is the kind of fiber that allows your blood glucose to rise slowly and not as high.
- In most of the fast-food Mexican restaurants, ordering is à la carte—an enchilada, a burrito, a Mexican salad. This helps you order and eat less.
- High-fat items, such as guacamole, cheese, and sour cream, are added onto and not mixed into some dishes. That's a plus because you can ask the kitchen to hold or serve them on the side.
- Do opt for guacamole over sour cream, as it contains healthier monounsaturated fat rather than saturated fat and cholesterol.
- Hot and spicy sauces—red sauce, green sauce, or salsa—add zest without the fat and calories of sour cream, cheese, and guacamole.
- Garlic, cilantro, chilies, and onions add flavor with few calories.

- Mexican cuisine is naturally low in protein. You don't get 8-oz hunks of meat. You find a small amount of protein mixed into dishes.
- Mexican cuisine is naturally high in carbohydrate. Beans, flour or corn tortillas, and rice are staples.
- Most fast-food Mexican restaurants now fry in 100% vegetable oil. That's better than lard because it contains no cholesterol and less saturated fat. But remember, teaspoon for teaspoon, the calories are the same.
- In the fast-food Mexican restaurants, the tortilla chips don't greet you at the table.

NUTRITION CONS

- Fried items seem almost unavoidable—tortilla chips, taco shells, tortilla shells (which salad might be served in), and chimichangas.
- Cheese—shredded, melted, or sauced—is a mainstay ingredient.
- Vegetables are few and far between—a few shreds of lettuce or pieces of tomato.
- Fruit is unavailable.
- High-fiber beans are often served refried. Some restaurants still use lard to make them.
- The bet-you-can't-eat-just-one tortilla chips are waiting at your table in most sit-down Mexican or Tex-Mex restaurants.

Healthy Tips

★ If the fried tortilla chips greet you when you sit down, hands off. Send them back or at least to the opposite side of the table.

★ Use extra salsa and other hot sauces to add flavor with very few calories.

★ Use salsa or another hot sauce as a salad dressing.

★ Don't feel you have to order an entree. Choose from appetizers and side dishes to control your portions.

★ Take advantage of ordering à la carte. Mix and match a healthy meal.

★ As a starter, try a cup of black bean soup or chili to fill you up and not out.

★ Make a bowl of black bean soup or chili the main course with a salad on the side.

★ Look for menu items that use soft tortillas rather than crispy fried ones. For example, choose a burrito or an enchilada rather than a taco or a chimichanga.

★ Fajitas are great to split. There's always enough for two.

★ Split a side dish—Mexican rice, refried beans, or black beans—to get more carbohydrates and fiber.

★ Take advantage of lite or nonfat sour cream if it's served.

Get It Your Way

★ Hold the guacamole, cheese, and sour cream, or ask for them on the side.
★ If a menu item is served with melted cheese, request a light helping.
★ Substitute black beans for refried beans (if available).
★ Ask for extra tomatoes and lettuce.
★ Request extra salsa or other zesty, low-calorie topper.

Del Taco

❖Del Taco provided nutrition information for all its menu items for use in this book. Their website is www.deltaco.com.

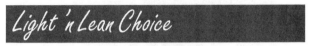

Light 'n Lean Choice

**Chicken Soft Taco
1/2 Beans 'n Cheese Cup**

Calories......................470	Sodium (mg).............630
Fat (g) 15	Carbohydrate (g).........60
% calories from fat..29	Fiber (g) 17
Saturated fat (g)........6	Protein (g) 27
Cholesterol (mg) 35	

Exchanges: 4 starch, 2 lean meat, 1 fat

Healthy 'n Hearty Choice

**Soft Taco
Bean & Cheese Green Burrito
Rice Cup**

Calories......................580	Sodium (mg)..........2,270
Fat (g) 18	Carbohydrate (g).........81
% calories from fat..29	Fiber (g) 8
Saturated fat (g)......10	Protein (g) 22
Cholesterol (mg) 37	

Exchanges: 5 1/2 starch, 1 medium-fat meat, 1 1/2 fat

(Continued)

Del Taco

	Amount	Cal.	Fat (g)	% Cal. Fat	Sat. Fat (g)	Chol. (mg)	Sod. (mg)	Carb. (g)	Fiber (g)	Pro. (g)	Servings/Exchanges
BREAKFAST											
✓Bacon	2 slices	50	4	72	1.5	10	170	0	0	3	1 fat
Bacon & Egg Quesadilla	1	450	23	46	12	260	920	40	2	21	2 1/2 starch, 2 medium-fat meat, 2 fat
✓Breakfast Burrito	1	250	11	40	6	160	520	24	1	10	1 1/2 starch, 1 medium-fat meat, 1 fat
Egg & Cheese Burrito	1	450	24	48	13	530	740	39	3	23	2 1/2 starch, 2 lean meat, 3 fat
Macho Bacon & Egg Burrito	1	1030	60	52	20	790	1760	82	6	40	6 starch, 3 medium-fat meat, 7 fat

Steak & Egg Burrito	1	580	34	53	16	560	1270	41	3	33	2 1/2 starch, 4 medium-fat meat, 2 fat

BURGERS

Bacon Double Cheeseburger	1	610	39	58	14	95	1130	35	4	29	2 starch, 3 medium-fat meat, 5 fat
✔ Bun Taco	1	440	21	43	12	65	830	37	4	24	2 1/2 starch, 3 medium-fat meat, 1/2 fat
✔ Cheeseburger	1	330	13	35	6	35	870	37	3	16	2 1/2 starch, 1 medium-fat meat, 1 1/2 fat
✔ Del Burger	1	380	21	50	5	35	490	35	4	13	2 starch, 1 medium-fat meat, 3 fat
Del Cheeseburger	1	430	25	52	7	45	710	35	4	16	2 starch, 2 medium-fat meat, 3 fat

✔ = Healthiest Bets; n/a = not available

(Continued)

BURGERS *(Continued)*	Amount	Cal.	Fat (g)	% Cal. Fat	Sat. Fat (g)	Chol. (mg)	Sod. (mg)	Carb. (g)	Fiber (g)	Pro. (g)	Servings/Exchanges
Double Del Cheeseburger	1	560	35	56	12	85	960	35	4	26	2 starch, 3 medium-fat meat, 4 fat
✔Hamburger	1	280	9	29	3	25	640	37	3	13	2 1/2 starch, 1 medium-fat meat, 1 fat
BURRITOS											
✔Bean & Cheese Green Burrito	1	280	8	26	5	15	1030	38	6	11	2 1/2 starch, 1 medium-fat meat, 1/2 fat
✔Bean & Cheese Red Burrito	1	270	8	27	5	15	1020	38	6	11	2 1/2 starch, 1 medium-fat meat, 1/2 fat
Chicken Works Burrito	1	520	23	40	12	65	1620	57	4	26	4 starch, 2 lean meat, 2 fat
Del Beef Burrito	1	550	30	49	17	90	1090	42	3	31	3 starch, 3 medium-fat meat, 3 fat

											Exchanges
Del Classic Chicken Burrito	1	560	36	58	13	70	1100	41	3	24	2 1/2 starch, 2 lean meat, 6 fat
Del Combo Burrito	1	530	22	37	13	55	1680	61	11	28	4 starch, 2 medium-fat meat, 2 fat
Deluxe Combo Burrito	1	530	25	42	15	60	1390	56	9	27	3 1/2 starch, 2 medium-fat meat, 3 fat
Deluxe Del Beef Burrito	1	590	33	50	19	95	1110	45	4	32	3 starch, 3 medium-fat meat, 3 1/2 fat
Half Pound Green Burrito	1	430	12	25	9	20	1690	59	13	20	4 starch, 1 medium-fat meat, 1 fat
Half Pound Red Burrito	1	430	12	25	9	20	1670	65	13	20	4 starch, 1 medium-fat meat, 1 fat

(Continued)

✔ = Healthiest Bets; n/a = not available

BURRITOS (*Continued*)	Amount	Cal.	Fat (g)	% Cal. Fat	Sat. Fat (g)	Chol. (mg)	Sod. (mg)	Carb. (g)	Fiber (g)	Pro. (g)	Servings/Exchanges
Macho Beef Burrito	1	1170	62	48	29	190	2190	89	7	60	6 starch, 7 medium-fat meat, 5 fat
Macho Combo Burrito	1	1050	44	38	21	115	2760	113	17	49	7 1/2 starch, 4 medium-fat meat, 3 fat
Spicy Chicken Burrito	1	480	16	30	10	40	1850	66	8	23	4 1/2 starch, 2 lean meat
Steak Works Burrito	1	590	31	47	16	70	1820	58	5	27	4 starch, 2 medium-fat meat, 3 fat
Veggie Works Burrito	1	490	18	33	11	25	1660	69	9	18	4 1/2 starch, 1 medium-fat meat, 1 fat
FRENCH FRIES											
Large Fries	1 order	490	32	59	5	0	380	47	5	5	3 starch, 6 fat
Chili Cheese Fries	1 order	670	46	62	15	45	880	51	5	17	3 1/2 starch, 1 high-fat meat, 7 fat

	Amount	Cal.	Fat (g)	% Fat Cal.	Sat. Fat (g)	Chol. (mg)	Sod. (mg)	Carb. (g)	Fiber (g)	Prot. (g)	Exchanges
Deluxe Chili Cheese Fries	1 order	710	49	62	16	50	880	53	6	17	3 1/2 starch, 10 fat
Macho Fries	1 order	690	46	60	7	0	550	68	6	7	4 1/2 starch, 9 fat
Regular Fries	1 order	350	23	59	4	0	270	34	3	3	2 starch, 4 1/2 fat
Small Fries	1 order	210	14	60	2	0	160	20	2	2	1 starch, 3 fat
NACHOS											
Macho Nachos	1 order	1100	63	52	42	55	2640	113	15	31	8 starch, 1 high-fat meat, 11 fat
Nachos	1 order	380	24	57	8	5	630	40	2	5	2 1/2 starch, 5 fat
QUESADILLAS											
Chicken Quesadilla	1	580	31	48	21	104	1240	41	2	33	2 1/2 starch, 4 lean meat, 3 fat
Regular Quesadilla	1	500	27	49	20	75	860	39	2	23	2 1/2 starch, 2 medium-fat meat, 3 fat

(Continued)

✔ = Healthiest Bets; n/a = not available

QUESADILLAS (Continued)	Amount	Cal.	Fat (g)	% Cal. Fat	Sat. Fat (g)	Chol. (mg)	Sod. (mg)	Carb. (g)	Fiber (g)	Pro. (g)	Servings/Exchanges
Spicy Jack Chicken Quesadilla	1	570	30	47	16	105	1300	40	2	32	2 1/2 starch, 4 lean meat, 4 fat
Spicy Jack Regular Quesadilla	1	490	26	48	17	75	920	38	2	23	2 1/2 starch, 2 medium-fat meat, 3 fat
SALADS											
Chicken Fiesta Bowl w/ Ancho Chile Sauce	1	550	27	44	5	80	2210	50	6	27	2 starch, 2 veg, 2 lean meat, 5 fat
Chicken Fiesta Bowl w/o Ancho Chile Sauce	1	420	13	28	3	60	2010	49	6	26	2 starch, 2 veg, 2 lean meat, 2 fat
Deluxe Chicken Salad	1	740	34	41	15	70	2610	77	16	33	4 starch, 3 veg, 2 lean meat, 5 fat

Deluxe Taco Salad	1	780	40	46	18	80	2250	76	14	33	4 starch, 3 veg, 2 medium-fat meat, 5 fat
Taco Salad	1	350	30	77	10	45	390	10	2	10	2 veg, 1 medium-fat meat, 5 fat
Veggie Fiesta Bowl w/ Ancho Chile Sauce	1	490	22	40	4	20	1830	64	9	10	3 starch, 2 veg, 4 fat

SHAKES

Chocolate (large)	1	680	16	21	12	45	350	117	1	16	1 low-fat milk, 7 carb
Chocolate (small)	1	520	12	21	9	35	270	89	1	12	1 low-fat milk, 5 carb
Strawberry (large)	1	540	8	13	6	40	280	100	1	14	1 low-fat milk, 5 carb
Strawberry (small)	1	410	6	13	4	30	220	76	1	11	1 low-fat milk, 4 carb
Vanilla (large)	1	550	10	16	6	50	320	97	0	16	1 low-fat milk, 5 carb, 1 fat
Vanilla (small)	1	420	7	15	5	35	250	75	0	12	1 low-fat milk, 4 carb

✔ = Healthiest Bets; n/a = not available

(Continued)

	Amount	Cal.	Fat (g)	% Cal. Fat	Sat. Fat (g)	Chol. (mg)	Sod. (mg)	Carb. (g)	Fiber (g)	Pro. (g)	Servings/Exchanges
SIDES											
Beans 'n Cheese Cup	1	260	3	10	2	5	1810	44	16	16	3 starch, 1 lean meat
✔Rice Cup	1	140	2	13	1	2	910	27	1	3	2 starch
TACOS											
✔Big Fat Chicken Taco	1	340	13	34	4	45	840	38	3	18	2 1/2 starch, 1 lean meat, 2 fat
Big Fat Crispy Chicken Taco	1	620	38	55	9	60	1070	52	3	21	3 1/2 starch, 2 lean meat, 5 fat
✔Big Fat Steak Taco	1	390	19	44	6	45	960	38	3	18	2 1/2 starch, 2 medium-fat meat, 2 fat
✔Big Fat Taco	1	320	11	31	5	35	650	39	3	16	2 1/2 starch, 1 medium-fat meat, 1 fat

											Exchanges
✔Chicken Soft Taco	1	210	12	51	4	30	520	16	1	11	1 starch, 1 lean meat, 1 fat
✔Soft Taco	1	160	8	45	4	20	330	16	1	8	1 starch, 1 lean meat, 1 fat
✔Taco	1	160	10	56	4	20	150	11	1	7	1 starch, 1 medium-fat meat, 1 fat
✔Ultimate Taco	1	260	17	59	8	50	470	13	2	14	1 starch, 1 medium-fat meat, 2 fat

✔ = Healthiest Bets; n/a = not available

Taco Bell

❖Taco Bell provides nutrition information for all of its menu items on their website at www.tacobell.com.

Light 'n Lean Choice

Gordita Nacho Cheese—Chicken
Soft Taco Beef
Pico de Gallo (*2 orders*)
1/2 Mexican Rice

Calories......................600	Sodium (mg)..........1,585
Fat (g) 27	Carbohydrate (g).........61
% calories from fat..40	Fiber (g) 6
Saturated fat (g)........9	Protein (g) 29
Cholesterol (mg).........63	

Exchanges: 4 starch, 2 medium-fat meat, 3 fat

Healthy 'n Hearty Choice

Tostada
Beef Soft Taco
Salsa (*1 order*)
Pintos 'n Cheese
1/2 Mexican Rice

Calories......................740	Sodium (mg)..........2,175
Fat (g) 35	Carbohydrate (g).........77
% calories from fat..40	Fiber (g) 24
Saturated fat (g)......14	Protein (g) 33
Cholesterol (mg).........74	

Exchanges: 5 starch, 3 medium-fat meat, 2 1/2 fat

Taco Bell

	Amount	Cal.	Fat (g)	% Cal. Fat	Sat. Fat (g)	Chol. (mg)	Sod. (mg)	Carb. (g)	Fiber (g)	Pro. (g)	Servings/Exchanges
BURRITOS											
7-Layer Burrito	1	520	22	38	7	25	1270	65	13	16	4 starch, 1 high-fat meat, 2 fat
Bean Burrito	1	370	12	29	3.5	10	1080	54	12	13	3 1/2 starch, 2 fat
Burrito Supreme—Beef	1	430	18	38	7	40	1210	50	9	17	3 starch, 1 medium-fat meat, 2 1/2 fat
Burrito Supreme—Steak	1	420	16	34	6	45	1140	48	8	21	3 starch, 2 medium-fat meat, 1 fat
Burrito Supreme—Chicken	1	410	16	35	6	45	1120	45	8	20	3 starch, 2 lean meat, 1 1/2 fat

(Continued)

✔ = Healthiest Bets; n/a = not available

BURRITOS *(Continued)*	Amount	Cal.	Fat (g)	% Cal. Fat	Sat. Fat (g)	Chol. (mg)	Sod. (mg)	Carb. (g)	Fiber (g)	Pro. (g)	Servings/Exchanges
✔Chili Cheese Burrito	1	330	13	35	5	25	900	40	4	13	2 1/2 starch, 1 medium-fat meat, 1 fat
Double Burrito Supreme—Beef	1	510	23	41	9	60	1500	52	11	23	3 1/2 starch, 2 medium-fat meat, 2 meat
Double Burrito Supreme—Chicken	1	460	17	33	6	70	1200	50	3	27	3 starch, 3 lean meat, 1 fat
Double Burrito Supreme—Steak	1	470	18	34	7	55	1230	48	3	28	3 starch, 3 lean meat, 1 fat
Fiesta Burrito—Beef	1	380	15	36	5	30	1100	49	4	14	3 starch, 1 medium-fat meat, 2 fat
✔Fiesta Burrito—Chicken	1	370	12	29	3.5	35	1000	48	3	17	3 starch, 2 lean meat, 1 fat
Grilled Stuft Chicken Burrito	1	690	29	38	8	70	1900	73	8	33	5 starch, 2 lean fat meat, 4 fat

CHALUPAS

	Amount	Cal.	Fat (g)	% Cal. Fat	Sat. Fat (g)	Chol. (mg)	Sod. (mg)	Carb. (g)	Fiber (g)	Pro. (g)	Exchanges/Choices
Chalupa Baja—Beef	1	420	27	58	7	35	760	30	3	14	2 starch, 1 medium-fat meat, 4 fat
Chalupa Baja—Chicken	1	400	24	54	5	40	660	28	2	17	2 starch, 2 lean meat, 3 fat
Chalupa Baja—Steak	1	400	24	54	6	30	680	27	2	17	2 starch, 2 lean meat, 3 fat
Chalupa Nacho Cheese—Beef	1	370	22	54	6	25	740	30	3	13	2 starch, 1 lean meat, 3 1/2 fat
✔Chalupa Nacho Cheese—Chicken	1	350	19	49	4.5	25	640	29	6	16	2 starch, 1 lean meat, 3 fat
✔Chalupa Nacho Cheese—Steak	1	350	19	49	4.5	20	660	28	1	16	2 starch, 1 lean meat, 3 fat
Chalupa Santa Fe—Beef	1	440	29	59	7	35	660	31	4	14	2 starch, 1 medium-fat meat, 4 1/2 fat
Chalupa Santa Fe—Chicken	1	420	26	56	6	40	560	30	2	17	2 starch, 2 lean meat, 5 1/2 fat

(Continued)

✔ = Healthiest Bets; n/a = not available

CHALUPAS (Continued)	Amount	Cal.	Fat (g)	% Cal. Fat	Sat. Fat (g)	Chol. (mg)	Sod. (mg)	Carb. (g)	Fiber (g)	Pro. (g)	Servings/Exchanges
Chalupa Santa Fe—Steak	1	430	27	57	6	35	580	29	2	18	2 starch, 2 lean meat, 5 fat
Chalupa Supreme—Beef	1	380	23	54	8	40	580	29	3	14	2 starch, 1 lean meat, 3 fat
Chalupa Supreme—Chicken	1	360	20	50	7	45	490	28	2	17	2 starch, 2 lean meat, 2 fat
Chalupa Supreme—Steak	1	360	20	50	7	35	500	27	2	17	2 starch, 2 lean meat, 2 fat
CONDIMENTS											
✔Border Sauce—Fire	1/3 oz/1 T	0	0	0	0	0	110	1	0	0	free
✔Border Sauce—Hot	1/3 oz/1 T	0	0	0	0	0	85	0	0	0	free
✔Border Sauce—Mild	1/3 oz/1 T	0	0	0	0	0	75	0	0	0	free
Burger Sauce	1/2 oz/1 T	60	5	75	1	5	110	2	0	0	1 fat
✔Cheddar Cheese	1/4 oz/1/2 T	30	2	60	1.5	5	45	0	0	2	free
Club Sauce	1/2 oz/1 T	80	8	90	1	10	105	1	0	0	1 1/2 fat
✔Green Sauce	1 oz/1 T	5	0	0	0	0	150	1	0	0	free

✔ Guacamole	3/4 oz/1 1/2 T	35	3	77	0	0	80	1	1	0	1/2 fat
✔ Nacho Cheese Sauce	2 oz/4 T	120	10	75	2.5	5	470	5	0	2	2 fat
✔ Picante Sauce	1/3 oz/1 T	0	0	0	0	0	110	1	0	0	free
✔ Pico de Gallo	3/4 oz/1 1/2 T	5	0	0	0	0	65	1	0	1	free
✔ Red Sauce	1 oz/2 T	10	0	0	0	0	260	2	0	0	free
✔ Salsa	3 oz/6 T	25	0	0	0	0	220	5	0	3	free
✔ Sour Cream	3/4 oz/1 1/2 T	40	4	90	2.5	10	10	1	0	1	1 fat

DESSERTS

Choco Taco Ice Cream	1	310	17	49	10	50	100	37	1	3	2 1/2 carb, 3 fat

ENCHIRITOS

Beef	1	370	19	46	9	50	1300	33	9	18	2 starch, 2 medium-fat meat, 1 1/2 fat

(Continued)

✔ = Healthiest Bets; n/a = not available

ENCHIRITOS (*Continued*)	Amount	Cal.	Fat (g)	% Cal. Fat	Sat. Fat (g)	Chol. (mg)	Sod. (mg)	Carb. (g)	Fiber (g)	Pro. (g)	Servings/Exchanges
Chicken	1	350	16	41	8	55	1210	32	7	21	2 starch, 2 medium-fat meat, 1 fat
Steak	1	350	16	41	8	45	1220	31	7	22	2 starch, 2 medium-fat meat, 1 fat
GORDITAS											
Gordita Baja Beef	1	360	21	53	5	35	810	29	4	13	2 starch, 1 medium-fat meat, 3 fat
Gordita Baja Chicken	1	340	18	48	4	40	710	28	3	16	2 starch, 1 lean meat, 3 fat
Gordita Baja Steak	1	340	18	48	4	35	760	28	3	15	2 starch, 1 medium-fat meat, 2 fat
✔Gordita Nacho Cheese—Beef	1	310	15	44	4	25	780	30	4	13	2 starch, 1 medium-fat meat, 2 fat

										Exchanges
✔ Gordita Nacho Cheese—Chicken	1	290	13	40	2.5	25	690	29	3	15	2 starch, 1 medium-fat meat, 1 fat
✔ Gordita Nacho Cheese—Steak	1	290	13	40	3	20	700	28	2	16	2 starch, 1 medium-fat meat, 1 fat
Gordita Santa Fe—Beef	1	380	23	54	5	35	700	31	5	14	2 starch, 1 lean meat, 3 fat
✔ Gordita Santa Fe—Chicken	1	370	20	49	4	40	610	33	4	14	2 starch, 1 medium-fat meat, 3 fat
✔ Gordita Supreme Beef	1	300	14	42	5	35	550	27	3	17	2 starch, 2 lean meat, 1 fat
✔ Gordita Supreme Chicken	1	300	13	39	5	45	530	28	3	16	2 starch, 1 lean meat, 2 fat
✔ Gordita Supreme Steak	1	300	13	39	5	45	530	28	3	16	2 starch, 2 lean meat, 1 fat

NACHOS

										Exchanges
Mucho Grande Nachos	1	1320	82	56	25	75	2670	116	18	31	7 1/2 starch, 1 medium-fat meat, 14 fat

✔ = Healthiest Bets; n/a = not available

(Continued)

OTHER ENTREES

	Amount	Cal.	Fat (g)	% Cal. Fat	Sat. Fat (g)	Chol. (mg)	Sod. (mg)	Carb. (g)	Fiber (g)	Pro. (g)	Servings/Exchanges
Cheese Quesadilla	1	350	18	46	9	50	860	31	3	16	2 starch, 1 medium-fat meat, 2 1/2 fat
Chicken Quesadilla	1	540	30	50	12	80	1270	40	4	28	2 1/2 starch, 3 lean meat, 2 fat
Mexican Pizza	1	390	25	58	8	45	930	28	8	18	2 starch, 2 medium-fat meat, 2 fat
✓MexiMelt	1	290	15	47	7	45	830	22	4	15	1 1/2 starch, 1 high-fat meat, 1 1/2 fat
Nachos BellGrande	1	760	39	46	11	35	1300	83	17	20	5 1/2 starch, 1 medium-fat meat, 5 1/2 fat

	Amount										
Nachos Supreme	1	440	24	49	7	37	800	44	9	14	3 starch, 1 medium-fat meat, 3 fat
✓Tostada	1	250	12	43	4.5	15	640	27	11	10	2 starch, 1 medium-fat meat, 1/2 fat

SALADS

Taco Salad w/ Salsa	1	850	52	55	14	70	2250	69	16	30	4 1/2 starch, 3 medium-fat meat, 6 fat
Taco Salad w/ Salsa w/o Shell	1	400	22	50	10	70	1510	31	15	24	2 starch, 3 medium-fat meat, 1/2 fat

SIDES

✓Cinnamon Twists	1 order	150	5	30	1	0	190	27	1	1	1 starch, 1 fat
✓Mexican Rice	1	190	9	43	3.5	15	750	23	1	5	1 1/2 starch, 2 fat
Nachos	1	320	18	51	4	5	560	34	3	5	2 starch, 3 1/2 fat

(Continued)

✓ = Healthiest Bets; n/a = not available

SIDES (*Continued*)	Amount	Cal.	Fat (g)	% Cal. Fat	Sat. Fat (g)	Chol. (mg)	Sod. (mg)	Carb. (g)	Fiber (g)	Pro. (g)	Servings/Exchanges
✔Pintos 'n Cheese	1	180	8	40	4	15	640	18	10	9	1 starch, 1 medium-fat meat, 1/2 fat
TACOS											
BLT Soft Taco	1	340	23	61	8	40	610	22	2	11	1 1/2 starch, 1 medium-fat meat, 3 1/2 fat
DOUBLE DECKER Taco	1	380	17	40	5	30	740	43	9	15	3 starch, 1 medium-fat meat, 2 fat
DOUBLE DECKER Taco Supreme	1	420	21	45	8	38	760	45	10	15	3 starch, 1 medium-fat meat, 3 fat
✔Grilled Chicken Soft Taco	1	190	7	33	2.5	35	480	19	2	13	1 starch, 1 lean meat, 1 fat
✔Grilled Steak Soft Taco	1	280	17	55	4	35	630	20	2	12	1 starch, 1 medium-fat meat, 3 fat

✔ Soft Taco—Beef	1	210	10	43	4	30	570	20	3	11	1 starch, 1 medium-fat meat, 1 fat
Taco	1	210	12	51	4	30	330	18	3	9	1 starch, 1 medium-fat meat, 1 fat
Taco Supreme	1	260	16	55	6	40	350	20	4	10	1 starch, 1 medium-fat meat, 2 fat

✔ = Healthiest Bets; n/a = not available

Taco John's

❖Taco John's provides nutrition information
  for all its menu items on their website at
  www.tacojohns.com.

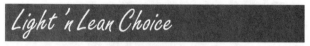

Chicken Fajita Burrito
Bean Burrito

Calories......................700	Sodium (mg)..........1,710
Fat (g) 21	Carbohydrate (g).........94
% calories from fat..27	Fiber (g) 19
Saturated fat (g)........9	Protein (g) 33
Cholesterol (mg).........50	

Exchanges: 6 starch, 2 lean meat, 2 1/2 fat

Healthy 'n Hearty Choice

Chicken Fajita Burrito
Soft Shell Tacos—Chicken
Refried Beans *(split)*
Mexican Rice *(split)*

Calories......................795	Sodium (mg)..........2,440
Fat (g) 23	Carbohydrate (g).......106
% calories from fat..26	Fiber (g) 19
Saturated fat (g)......11	Protein (g) 41
Cholesterol (mg).......133	

Exchanges: 6 starch, 2 veg, 3 lean meat, 2 fat

Taco John's

BURRITOS

	Amount	Cal.	(g)	% Fat	Sat. (g)	(mg)	(mg)	(g)	(g)	(g)	Servings/Exchanges
✓Bean Burrito	1	380	11	26	5	15	820	53	12	15	3 1/2 starch, 1 medium-fat meat, 1 fat
Beefy Burrito	1	440	20	41	9	55	860	44	6	22	3 starch, 2 medium-fat meat, 1 fat
Chicken & Potato Burrito	1	450	18	36	5	20	1310	56	9	15	3 1/2 starch, 1 lean meat, 2 1/2 fat
Chicken Festiva	1	550	28	46	7	40	1150	56	9	17	3 1/2 starch, 1 medium-fat meat, 4 fat

(Continued)

✓ = Healthiest Bets; n/a = not available

BURRITOS (*Continued*)	Amount	Cal.	Fat (g)	% Cal. Fat	Sat. Fat (g)	Chol. (mg)	Sod. (mg)	Carb. (g)	Fiber (g)	Pro. (g)	Servings/Exchanges
Combination Burrito	1	410	15	33	7	35	840	49	9	18	3 starch, 1 medium-fat meat, 2 fat
El Grande Burrito	1	730	36	44	15	85	1630	69	8	33	4 1/2 starch, 3 medium-fat meat, 3 fat
El Grande Chicken Burrito	1	630	26	37	11	75	1850	66	8	33	4 1/2 starch, 3 lean meat, 2 fat
Meat & Potato Burrito	1	500	23	41	7	25	1200	58	8	15	4 starch, 1 medium-fat meat, 2 1/2 fat
Ranch Burrito—Beef	1	440	22	45	8	45	830	43	7	16	3 starch, 1 medium-fat meat, 3 fat
✔Ranch Burrito—Chicken	1	380	17	40	6	40	940	41	7	16	2 1/2 starch, 1 medium-fat meat, 2 fat

	Amount										Exchanges/Choices
Smothered Burrito	1	540	24	40	9	50	1120	57	11	25	4 starch, 2 medium-fat meat, 2 fat
Super Burrito	1	450	19	38	7	35	910	51	10	19	3 1/2 starch, 1 medium-fat meat, 2 fat
DESSERTS											
✓Apple Grande	1	258	9	31	3	7	240	40	1	5	1 fruit, 1 1/2 carb, 2 fat
Choco Taco	1	311	17	49	10	20	100	37	1	3	2 1/2 carb, 3 fat
✓Churro	1	158	11	63	2	10	115	13	1	2	1 carb, 2 fat
✓Taco John's Cinnamon Mint Swirl	1	60	0	n/a	n/a	n/a	5	14	n/a	0	1 carb
✓Taco John's Cookies	1 bag	130	5	35	2	0	70	20	0	1	1 carb
FAJITAS											
✓Chicken Fajita Burrito	1	320	10	28	4	35	890	41	7	18	2 1/2 starch, 2 lean meat

(Continued)

✓ = Healthiest Bets; n/a = not available

OTHER ENTREES

	Amount	Cal.	Fat (g)	% Cal. Fat	Sat. Fat (g)	Chol. (mg)	Sod. (mg)	Carb. (g)	Fiber (g)	Pro. (g)	Servings/Exchanges
✔Bean Tostada	1	160	7	39	3	5	230	17	3	6	1 starch, 1 lean meat, 1 fat
✔Cheese Crisp	1	220	16	65	8	35	250	9	0	10	1/2 starch, 3 fat
Chicken Festiva Salad	1	690	50	65	12	75	1450	39	5	22	2 starch, 2 veg, 2 medium-fat meat, 7 fat
✔Chicken Festiva Salad w/o dressing	1	370	20	49	7	55	680	27	5	21	2 starch, 2 lean meat, 2 fat
Chicken Quesadilla	1 order	430	20	42	8	45	990	42	7	20	3 starch, 1 lean meat, 3 fat
Chicken Super Nacho	1	810	54	60	13	55	1530	57	7	26	4 starch, 2 lean meat, 8 fat
Chilito	1 order	440	22	45	12	60	1060	41	7	21	2 1/2 starch, 2 medium-fat meat, 2 fat

Double Enchilada	1	780	43	50	18	100	1950	58	8	38	4 starch, 4 medium-fat meat, 4 fat
Mexi Rolls	1 order	670	40	54	12	65	1470	53	2	28	4 1/2 starch, 2 medium-fat meat, 4 fat
Potato Oles Bravo	1 order	570	35	55	9	10	1750	55	6	9	3 1/2 starch, 7 fat
Quesadilla	1 order	460	24	47	10	45	860	41	7	18	3 1/2 starch, 1 medium-fat meat, 2 1/2 fat
Sierra Chicken Fillet Sandwich	1	480	27	51	6	65	880	37	2	25	2 1/2 starch, 3 lean meat, 2 1/2 fat
Super Nachos	1 order	900	60	60	15	45	1350	68	10	23	4 1/2 starch, 2 high-fat meat, 7 1/2 fat
Taco John's Mexican Pizza	1	560	31	50	8	50	720	47	4	23	3 starch, 2 medium-fat meat, 4 fat

(Continued)

✔ = Healthiest Bets; n/a = not available

OTHER ENTREES (Continued)	Amount	Cal.	Fat (g)	% Cal. Fat	Sat. Fat (g)	Chol. (mg)	Sod. (mg)	Carb. (g)	Fiber (g)	Pro. (g)	Servings/Exchanges
Taco Salad	1	770	50	58	15	55	1890	55	3	24	3 starch, 2 veg, 2 medium-fat meat, 7 fat
Taco Salad (includes bowl, no dressing)	1	600	33	50	12	55	970	50	3	24	2 starch, 3 veg, 2 medium-fat meat, 8 fat
✔Tostada	1	200	12	54	5	25	250	13	0	9	1 starch, 1 medium-fat meat, 2 fat
PLATTERS											
Beef & Chimi Platter	1	740	33	40	9	40	1780	82	10	26	5 1/2 starch, 2 medium-fat meat, 3 fat
Beef Enchilada Platter	1	830	41	44	15	70	2190	79	11	34	5 starch, 2 medium-fat meat, 6 fat

Chicken Enchilada Platter	1	690	32	42	11	50	2220	71	10	27	4 1/2 starch, 2 medium-fat meat, 4 fat
Smothered Burrito Platter	1	880	36	37	12	55	1930	101	17	35	7 starch, 2 medium-fat meat, 3 fat

SIDES

Mexican Rice	1 order	250	45	162	5	1	860	44	0	6	3 starch, 9 fat
Nacho Cheese	2 oz/4 T	300	10	30	0	0	600	0	n/a	5	1 high-fat meat
Nachos	1 order	440	30	61	7	10	740	35	4	7	2 starch, 6 fat
Potato Oles (small)	1 order	310	18	52	5	n/a	880	33	3	3	2 starch, 3 fat
Potato Oles	1 order	410	24	53	6	n/a	1190	45	4	4	3 starch, 5 fat
Potato Oles (large)	1 order	484	30	56	7	0	1285	50	n/a	4	3 starch, 6 fat
Potato Oles (super)	1 order	970	61	57	18	45	2920	82	10	22	5 1/2 starch, 10 fat

(Continued)

✔ = Healthiest Bets; n/a = not available

SIDES (*Continued*)	Amount	Cal.	Fat (g)	% Cal. Fat	Sat. Fat (g)	Chol. (mg)	Sod. (mg)	Carb. (g)	Fiber (g)	Pro. (g)	Servings/Exchanges
Potato Oles (with Nacho Cheese)	1 order	530	34	58	10	10	1930	50	4	7	3 starch, 7 fat
Refried Beans	9.5 oz	360	11	28	5	15	1020	45	15	18	3 starch, 1 lean meat, 1 fat
Side Salad	1	290	25	78	5	20	560	15	2	3	2 veg, 5 fat
✓Sour Cream	1 oz/2 T	60	6	90	0	0	15	1	n/a	1	1 fat
Texas Style Chili	9.5 oz	380	22	52	10	55	950	23	4	21	1 1/2 starch, 2 lean meat, 5 fat

TACOS

	Amount	Cal.	Fat (g)	% Cal. Fat	Sat. Fat (g)	Chol. (mg)	Sod. (mg)	Carb. (g)	Fiber (g)	Pro. (g)	Servings/Exchanges
Crispy Tacos	1 order	190	12	57	5	25	250	13	0	9	1 starch, 1 medium-fat meat, 1 fat
El Grande Chicken Taco	1	330	18	49	5	40	740	24	1	17	1 1/2 starch, 2 lean meat, 2 fat

El Grande Taco	1	480	29	54	10	65	760	30	1	24	2 starch, 3 lean meat, 3 1/2 fat
Sierra Taco—Beef	1	500	30	54	7	45	530	39	2	18	2 1/2 starch, 2 medium-fat meat, 3 fat
Sierra Taco—Chicken	1	430	24	50	5	40	670	37	3	18	2 1/2 starch, 1 lean meat, 4 fat
✔Softshell Chicken Taco	1	170	5	26	3	20	610	21	4	11	1 1/2 starch, 1 lean meat
✔Softshell Tacos	1 order	230	10	39	5	25	500	23	3	11	1 1/2 starch, 1 medium-fat meat, 1 fat
✔Taco Bravo	1	360	15	38	5	25	660	40	6	15	2 1/2 starch, 1 medium-fat meat, 2 fat
✔Taco Burger	1	280	11	35	5	35	580	29	1	14	2 starch, 1 medium-fat meat, 1 fat

✔ = Healthiest Bets; n/a = not available

Taco Time

❖Taco Time provides nutrition information for all of its menu items on their website at www.tacotime.com.

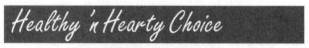

Light 'n Lean Choice

Super Shredded Beef Soft Taco
Mexican Rice

Calories......................527

Fat (g) 13

  % calories from fat..22

  Saturated fat (g)........7

Cholesterol (mg) 22

Sodium (mg) 1,086

Carbohydrate (g).........68

  Fiber (g) 8

Protein (g) 15

Exchanges: 4 starch, 1 medium-fat meat, 1 fat

Healthy 'n Hearty Choice

Value Soft Bean Burrito (*single*)
Chicken Soft Taco
1/2 Refritos (*refried beans*)

Calories......................864

Fat (g) 26

  % calories from fat..27

  Saturated fat (g)......10

Cholesterol (mg) 63

Sodium (mg) 1,749

Carbohydrate (g).......118

  Fiber (g) 20

Protein (g) 43

Exchanges: 8 1/2 starch, 4 lean meat, 2 fat

Taco Time

	Amount	Cal.	Fat (g)	% Cal. Fat	Sat. Fat (g)	Chol. (mg)	Sod. (mg)	Carb. (g)	Fiber (g)	Pro. (g)	Servings/Exchanges
BURRITOS											
Casita Burrito, Meat	1	647	31	43	15	89	1233	54	16	40	3 1/2 starch, 4 medium-fat meat, 2 fat
Crisp Burrito, Bean	1	427	18	38	5	12	453	53	9	15	3 1/2 starch, 1 lean meat, 3 fat
Crisp Burrito, Chicken	1	422	25	53	8	54	795	32	2	17	2 starch, 2 lean meat, 4 fat
Crisp Burrito, Meat	1	552	30	49	10	58	1000	39	7	34	2 1/2 starch, 4 medium-fat meat, 2 fat
Double Soft Bean Burrito	1	506	12	21	6	22	860	77	19	23	5 starch, 1 lean meat, 2 fat

✔ = Healthiest Bets; n/a = not available

(Continued)

BURRITOS *(Continued)*	Amount	Cal.	Fat (g)	% Cal. Fat	Sat. Fat (g)	Chol. (mg)	Sod. (mg)	Carb. (g)	Fiber (g)	Pro. (g)	Servings/Exchanges
Double Soft Combination Burrito	1	617	23	34	10	63	1343	66	18	39	4 starch, 4 medium-fat meat, 1/2 fat
Double Soft Meat Burrito	1	726	33	41	14	99	1809	55	17	57	3 1/2 starch, 7 lean meat, 2 1/2 fat
✓Value Soft Bean Burrito (single)	1	380	10	24	4	15	715	58	13	16	4 starch, 1 lean meat, 1 fat
Value Soft Meat Burrito (single)	1	491	21	38	8	56	1197	48	12	31	3 1/2 starch, 3 lean meat, 2 fat
Veggie Burrito	1	491	16	29	6	24	643	70	10	21	4 1/2 starch, 3 fat
CONDIMENTS											
✓Enchilada Sauce	1 oz/2 T	12	0	0	0	0	133	3	1	0	free
✓Guacamole	1 oz/2 T	29	2	62	0	0	94	2	1	0	free
✓Hot Sauce	1 oz/2 T	10	0	0	0	0	120	2	0	0	free

	Serving	Cal	Fat (g)	% Fat	Sat Fat (g)	Chol (mg)	Sodium (mg)	Carb (g)	Fiber (g)	Prot (g)	Exchanges
✓ Ranchero Salsa	2 oz/4 T	21	1	43	0	0	192	3	1	1	free
✓ Sour Cream	1 oz/2 T	55	5	82	3	19	11	1	0	1	1 fat
✓ Sour Cream Dressing	1.5 oz/3 T	137	14	92	5	8	207	2	0	1	3 fat
Thousand Island Dressing	1 oz/2 T	160	16	90	2	10	220	4	0	0	3 fat
DESSERTS											
✓ Cherry Empanada	1	250	9	32	n/a	0	46	37	n/a	5	2 1/2 carb, 2 fat
OTHER ENTREES											
✓ Cheese Quesadilla	1	205	11	48	6	30	255	17	1	11	1 starch, 1 high-fat meat
Nachos	1 order	680	38	50	19	78	1250	61	11	26	4 starch, 2 medium-fat meat, 4 fat
Nachos Deluxe	1 order	1048	57	49	23	109	2252	91	17	46	6 starch, 4 medium-fat meat, 7 fat

(Continued)

✓ = Healthiest Bets; n/a = not available

OTHER ENTREES (*Continued*)	Amount	Cal.	Fat (g)	% Cal. Fat	Sat. Fat (g)	Chol. (mg)	Sod. (mg)	Carb. (g)	Fiber (g)	Pro. (g)	Servings/Exchanges
Taco Cheeseburger	1	633	36	51	10	66	1291	48	7	31	3 starch, 3 medium-fat meat, 4 fat
SALADS											
✔ Chicken Taco Salad w/o Dressing (regular)	1	370	21	51	7	48	861	27	3	19	2 starch, 2 medium-fat meat, 2 fat
Taco Salad w/o Dressing (regular)	1	479	28	53	11	63	895	30	7	30	1 starch, 2 veg, 3 medium-fat meat, 2 1/2 fat
Tostada Delight Salad, Meat	1	628	32	46	14	82	1004	48	13	36	3 starch, 4 medium-fat meat, 2 fat
SIDES AND INGREDIENTS											
Cheddar Cheese	0.75 oz/1 1/2 T	86	7	73	4	22	132	0	0	5	1 high-fat meat
Chips	1 order	266	12	41	3	0	461	35	3	4	2 starch, 2 fat

Crustos	1 order	373	15	36	n/a	7	1250	47	n/a	9	3 carb, 3 fat
Mexi-Fries (large)	1 order	532	34	58	n/a	0	1598	54	n/a	6	3 1/2 starch, 7 fat
Mexi-Fries (regular)	1 order	266	17	58	n/a	0	799	27	n/a	3	2 starch, 3 fat
✔Mexican Rice	4 oz	159	2	11	1	0	530	30	1	3	2 starch
Refritos	7 oz	326	10	28	5	22	525	44	13	18	3 starch, l lean meat, 1 fat
TACOS											
✔Chicken Soft Taco	1	387	16	37	6	48	933	41	7	21	3 starch, 2 medium-fat meat, 1 fat
✔Crisp Taco	1	295	17	52	7	48	609	16	5	22	1 starch, 3 medium-fat meat
Natural Super Taco—Meat	1	627	27	39	13	82	915	60	14	41	4 starch, 4 medium-fat meat
Rolled Soft Flour Taco	1	512	23	40	10	63	1111	46	12	33	3 starch, 3 medium-fat meat, 1 1/2 fat

✔ = Healthiest Bets; n/a = not available

(Continued)

TACOS (*Continued*)	Amount	Cal.	Fat (g)	% Cal. Fat	Sat. Fat (g)	Chol. (mg)	Sod. (mg)	Carb. (g)	Fiber (g)	Pro. (g)	Servings/Exchanges
✔Super Shredded Beef Soft Taco	1	368	11	27	6	12	556	38	7	12	2 1/2 starch, 1 medium-fat meat, 2 fat
✔Value Soft Taco	1	316	15	43	7	48	599	23	5	24	1 1/2 starch, 3 medium-fat meat

✔ = Healthiest Bets; n/a = not available

Books from the American Diabetes Association

Keeping Your Heart Healthy Despite Diabetes
Marie McCarren

Heart healthy tips you can actually use right away. No lengthy diets. No cumbersome exercise programs. No exotic meal plans. Simple, easy, quick tips you can start to use now to pump up your heart health. Turn your daily newspaper pickup into a heart-healthy walk. Eat an apple to load up on heart-healthy fiber. Instead of giving up butter, try baking and cooking with oil. You'll find all kinds of one-minute miracle makers including how to increase your chances of surviving a heart attack if you do have one.

- Best fish for your heart.
- Top ways to work soy into your meals—without sacrificing taste.
- Ditch health robbers like trans fats—steer clear of these 7 foods.

64 pages, softcover.
#4854-01 One low price: $7.95

The Diabetes Food & Nutrition Bible
Hope S. Warshaw, MMSc, RD, CDE;
and Robyn Webb, MS

Get the nutrition advice you need and the flavor-rich recipes you crave. Learn about superfoods with the power to protect and heal, and get scrumptious recipes to work into your eating plan.

What you learn can have a dramatic impact on the way you eat, what you eat, and how long you live.

325 pages, softcover.
#4714-01 Nonmember: $18.95 Member: $16.95

Complete Guide to Carb Counting
Hope Warshaw, MMSc, RD, CDE;
and Karmeen Kulkarni, MS, RD, CDE

Unravel the mystery of knowing what blood sugar is going to do. Here are tips to help you know when your blood sugar will rise or fall before you eat and what it will do tomorrow and the next day. You can stop eating the same old foods and add variety to your meal planning—without worrying about upsetting the balance. Learn to count carbs, easy and effortlessly, and you can simplify your life, feel better, and avoid long-term diabetes complications.

192 pages, softcover.
#4715-01 One low price: $16.95

ADA Complete Guide to Convenience Food Counts
Lea Ann Holzmeister, RD, CDE

Quick eating, healthy eating—a reality for people on the go. Fast food no longer means greasy burgers and fries. Instead, an entirely new crop of convenience foods has been popping up all over our grocer's shelves, and these foods are making it easy for you to eat healthy without the fuss or the muss. ADA's all new guide details the convenience foods now available to you (many you never even thought of), where you can find them, and how to combine them to make super meals in minutes, along with lists of the nutrients in every serving. Guaranteed to cut your shopping, prep, and cooking time.

- Top convenience foods to always have on hand for meals in minutes
- Clues from takeout food that say "toss out now."
- Common sources of added sugar.
- One hidden danger in convenience foods.

Plus 7 days of super handy, super healthy convenience menus that include Teriyaki Chicken Salad with Mini Bagels…Chicken Parmesan Pocket with Fresh Pear … Breakfast Burrito with Melon … Chicken and Herb Rice with Steamed Broccoli, and many more.

256 pages, softcover.
#4710-01 Nonmember: $16.95 Member: $14.95

Diabetes Nutrition A to Z
American Diabetes Association

New to the popular best-selling A to Z series, this fact-packed book delivers complete nutrition and health information. Readers will appreciate the book's comprehensive coverage from adolescents to weight loss, and everything in between. Learn surprising facts about the safety of cow's milk. Protect yourself from heart disease and cancer with the super healing vitamins. Plus:

- Learn why herbals and supplements may not be the safest choice for you.
- Improve your diabetes control with beans—research proves it!

Read it cover to cover, or just flip to those sections of interest.

192 pages, softcover.
#4843-01 One low price: $14.95

The Diabetes Travel Guide
How to travel with diabetes—anywhere in the world
Davida F. Kruger, MSN, RN, CS, CDE

Travel stress-free, worry-free with this handy survival kit—the perfect prescription for being prepared. It covers all the essentials from planning and packing, to rules on insulin, directives for diabetes pills, and what to do if you get sick. Tips and tricks, checklists, and charts get you organized. 172 pages, softcover. All royalties from the sale of this book are donated to the American Diabetes Association Research Foundation.

#6060-04 Nonmember: $14.95 Member: $12.95

FREE with purchase

Order The Diabetes Travel Guide and we'll send you this handy foreign language translation guide absolutely FREE. It contains phrases you need to know to ask for medical help in Spanish, German, French, Italian, Russian, Japanese, and Chinese.

For super speedy service order online at
http://store.diabetes.org
or call toll free
1-800-232-6733

About the American Diabetes Association

The American Diabetes Association is the nation's leading voluntary health organization supporting diabetes research, information, and advocacy. Founded in 1940, the Association provides services to communities across the country. Its mission is to prevent and cure diabetes and to improve the lives of all people affected by diabetes.

For more than 50 years, the American Diabetes Association has been the leading publisher of comprehensive diabetes information for people with diabetes and the health care professionals who treat them. Its huge library of practical and authoritative books for people with diabetes covers every aspect of self care—cooking and nutrition, fitness, weight control, medications, complications, emotional issues, and general self care. The Association also publishes books and medical treatment guides for physicians and other health care professionals.

Membership in the Association is available to health care professionals and people with diabetes and includes subscriptions to one or more of the Association's periodicals. People with diabetes receive *Diabetes Forecast*, the nation's leading health and wellness magazine for people with diabetes. Health care professionals receive one or more of the Association's five scientific and medical journals.

For more information, please call toll-free:

Questions about diabetes:	1-800-DIABETES
Membership, people with diabetes:	1-800-806-7801
Membership, health professionals:	1-800-232-3472
Free catalog of ADA books:	1-800-232-6733
Visit us on the Web:	www.diabetes.org
Visit us at our Web bookstore:	merchant.diabetes.org